Pediatrics

Rehabilitation Medicine Quick Reference

Ralph M. Buschbacher, MD

Series Editor

Professor, Department of Physical Medicine and Rehabilitation
Indiana University School of Medicine
Indianapolis, Indiana

◼ Spine

Andre N. Panagos

◼ Spinal Cord Injury

Thomas N. Bryce

◼ Traumatic Brain Injury

David X. Cifu and Deborah Caruso

◼ Pediatrics

Maureen R. Nelson

◼ Musculoskeletal, Sports, and Occupational Medicine

William Micheo

Forthcoming Volumes in the Series

Neuromuscular/EMG

Prosthetics

Stroke

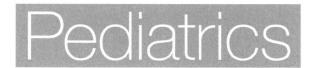

Pediatrics

Rehabilitation Medicine Quick Reference

Maureen R. Nelson, MD

Director
Pediatric Rehabilitation Services
Levine Children's Hospital
Charlotte, North Carolina

Adjunct Associate Professor
Department of Physical Medicine and Rehabilitation
University of North Carolina
Chapel Hill, North Carolina

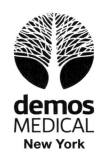

demos
MEDICAL
New York

Acquisitions Editor: Beth Barry
Cover Design: Steven Pisano
Compositor: Newgen Imaging Systems
Printer: Bang Printing

Visit our Web site at www.demosmedpub.com

Medicine is an ever-changing science. Research and clinical experience are continually expanding our knowledge, in particular our understanding of proper treatment and drug therapy. The authors, editors, and publisher have made every effort to ensure that all information in this book is in accordance with the state of knowledge at the time of production of the book. Nevertheless, the authors, editors, and publisher are not responsible for errors or omissions or for any consequences from application of the information in this book and make no warranty, express or implied, with respect to the contents of the publication. Every reader should examine carefully the package inserts accompanying each drug and should carefully check whether the dosage schedules mentioned therein or the contraindications stated by the manufacturer differ from the statements made in this book. Such examination is particularly important with drugs that are either rarely used or have been newly released on the market.

Library of Congress Cataloging-in-Publication Data
Nelson, Maureen R.
Pediatrics / Maureen R. Nelson.
      p. ; cm.—(Rehabilitation medicine quick reference)
 Includes bibliographical references and index.
 ISBN 978-1-933864-60-0
 1. Children with disabilities—Rehabilitation—Handbooks, manuals, etc.
2. Pediatrics—Handbooks, manuals, etc. I. Title. II. Series: Rehabilitation medicine quick reference.
 [DNLM: 1. Disabled Children—rehabilitation—Handbooks. 2. Pediatrics—methods—Handbooks. WS 368]
 RJ138.N42 2011
 618.92—dc22   2010038161

Special discounts on bulk quantities of Demos Medical Publishing books are available to corporations, professional associations, pharmaceutical companies, health care organizations, and other qualifying groups. For details, please contact:

Special Sales Department
Demos Medical Publishing
11 West 42nd Street, 15th Floor
New York, NY 10036
Phone: 800-532-8663 or 212-683-0072
Fax: 212-941-7842
Email: rsantana@demosmedpub.com

Made in the United States of America

10 11 12 13   5 4 3 2 1

I would like to thank the amazing babies, children, teenagers, and their families who I have had the privilege to work with over the years. They have taught me so much.

They are exemplified by Maddie, who is pictured below two weeks after she had a muscle tendon transfer surgery and would be wearing this splint constantly for 6 weeks. Her mother told me about the day after the operation, when they maneuvered through the crowded airport with Maddie wearing the bulky splint, boarded an airplane, sat on the runway for an hour, and then the plane was brought back to the terminal due to a mechanical problem. After collecting their bags, a hungry Maddie opened her snack box and counted the pieces, then beaming, yelled to her parents, "Look! I got two extra pieces...This must be my lucky day!"

Wow! What a role model this little girl is! Could there be a better example of a positive attitude, of making the most of what you have? It seems the very definition of rehabilitation to me. This is one of the best examples of the lessons I am reminded of every day by the children I am privileged to see. This is why pediatric rehabilitation is such a great profession and why I am grateful to be a part of it every day.

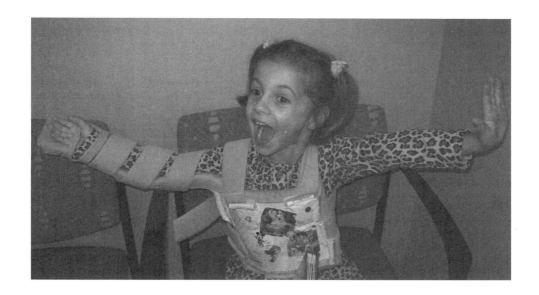

Contents

I Diagnostic Considerations

II Pediatric Diseases and Complications

Series Foreword

The Rehabilitation Medicine Quick Reference (RMQR) series is dedicated to the busy clinician. While we all strive to keep up with the latest medical knowledge, there are many times when things come up in our daily practices that we need to look up. Even more importantly…look up quickly.

Those aren't the times to do a complete literature search, or to read a detailed chapter, or review an article. We just need to get a quick grasp of a topic that we may not see routinely or just to refresh our memory. Sometimes a subject comes up that is outside our usual scope of practice, but that may still impact our care. It is for such moments that this series has been created.

Whether you need to quickly look up what a Tarlov cyst is, or you need to read about a neurorehabilitation complication or treatment, RMQR has you covered.

RMQR is designed to include the most common problems found in a busy practice and also a lot of the less common ones as well.

I was extremely lucky to have been able to assemble an absolutely fantastic group of editors. They in turn have harnessed an excellent set of authors. So what we have in this series is, I hope and believe, a tremendous reference set to be used often in daily clinical practice. As series editor, I have of course been privy to these books before actual publication. I can tell you that I have already started to rely on them in my clinic—often. They have helped me become more efficient in practice.

Each chapter is organized into succinct facts, presented in a bullet point style. The chapters are set up in the same way throughout all of the volumes in the series, so once you get used to the format, it is incredibly easy to look things up.

And while the focus of the RMQR series is, of course, rehabilitation medicine, the clinical applications are much broader.

I hope that each reader grows to appreciate the RMQR series as much as I have. I congratulate a fine group of editors and authors on creating readable and useful texts.

Ralph M. Buschbacher, MD

Preface

The field of pediatric physical medicine and rehabilitation is extremely broad. In this text our goal is to describe a logical, efficient, and orderly approach to diagnosis and excellent clinical care of children with the most common 100 diagnoses related to our field. We have also covered some additional related issues even though they weren't diagnoses, including aging with a pediatric-onset disability and an electrodiagnostic approach to children. The book is divided into three sections: General Diagnostic Considerations, Diagnoses, and Special Issues.

Our goal was to have a functional medical guide for daily physician care of children, and training residents and students regarding a broad spectrum of diagnoses.

We aimed to have the crucial information so that one would be able to see a child and start an effective care plan and have the guidance toward more detailed information, if necessary.

The main goals were efficiency and efficacy for both the practical care of children with disabilities and the access to gain knowledge related to doing so. We have assembled a great group of pediatric physiatrists who have contributed their knowledge and experience to this text and I believe we have accomplished our goals with this book.

Maureen R. Nelson, MD

Acknowledgments

Pediatric physical medicine and rehabilitation is a challenging, rewarding, and fun field. I would like to thank some of the people who have helped to guide me to it and through it. First, my parents, Bob and Mary, who made me believe I could do anything, and that I should be grateful for the opportunities given. I would like to thank the teachers who inspired me; Mr. Bunn and Sister Nancy at IHM, my University of Illinois professors and TAs, the University of Illinois College of Medicine faculty especially Dr. Olsson and the pediatrics group. I would also like to thank my residency teachers Drs. Kalantri, Dumitru, Currie, and Chris Johnson; and in fellowship Drs. Alexander and Steg. Additional thanks to Gloria, Carlos, Kate (Kathy), and Diane who helped guide and inspire me.

Contributors

Christine Aguilar, MD
Medical Director, Pediatric Rehabilitation
Department of Pediatric Rehabilitation
Children's Hospital Oakland Research Institute
Oakland, California

Joshua Jacob Alexander, MD, FAAP, FAAPMR
Clinical Associate Professor
Departments of Physical Medicine and Rehabilitation,
    and Pediatrics
University of North Carolina School of Medicine
Chapel Hill, North Carolina

Michael A. Alexander, MD
Professor
Departments of Pediatrics, and Physical Medicine and
    Rehabilitation
Thomas Jefferson University
Philadelphia, Pennsylvania
Chief of Pediatric Rehabilitation
Alfred I. duPont Hospital for Children
Wilmington, Delaware

Susan D. Apkon, MD
Associate Professor
Department of Rehabilitation Medicine
University of Washington School of Medicine
Director
Department of Rehabilitation Medicine
Seattle Children's Hospital
Seattle, Washington

Rita Ayyangar, MBBS
Associate Professor (Clinical)
Department of Physical Medicine and Rehabilitation
University of Michigan
Attending Physician
Department of Pediatric Physical Medicine and
    Rehabilitation
C.S. Mott Children's Hospital
Ann Arbor, Michigan

Susan Biffl, MPT, MD
Assistant Professor
Department of Pediatric Physical Medicine and
    Rehabilitation
The Children's Hospital
Denver Health and Hospital
Denver, Colorado

Deborah Bilder, MD
Assistant Professor (Clinical)
Department of Psychiatry, Division of Child and
    Adolescent Psychiatry
University of Utah School of Medicine
Salt Lake City, Utah

Glendaliz Bosques, MD
Instructor
Pediatric Rehabilitation Medicine
Department of Physical Medicine and Rehabilitation
Johns Hopkins University School of Medicine
International Center for Spinal Cord Injury
Kennedy Krieger Institute
Baltimore, Maryland

Paul S. Carbone, MD
Assistant Professor of Pediatrics
Department of Pediatrics
University of Utah
Salt Lake City, Utah

Gregory T. Carter, MD
Professor
Department of Rehabilitation Medicine
University of Washington School of Medicine
Seattle, Washington

James R. Christensen, MD
Research Scientist
Kennedy Krieger Institute
Associate Professor
Departments of Physical Medicine and Rehabilitation,
    and Pediatrics
Johns Hopkins University School of Medicine
Baltimore, Maryland

Supreet Deshpande, MD
Attending Physician
Department of Pediatric Rehabilitation
Gillette Children's Specialty Healthcare
St. Paul, Minnesota

Joshua Benjamin Ewen, MD
Assistant Professor
Department of Neurology
Johns Hopkins University School of Medicine
Director of Clinical Neurophysiology Laboratory
Department of Neurology and Developmental Medicine
The Kennedy Krieger Institute
Baltimore, Maryland

Deborah Gaebler-Spira, MD
Attending Physician
Professor of Physical Medicine and Rehabilitation and
    Pediatrics
Department of Physical Medicine and Rehabilitation
The Rehabilitation Institute of Chicago
Professor
Department of Physical Medicine and Rehabilitation
Feinberg School of Medicine
Northwestern University
Chicago, Illinois

Carl D. Gelfius, MD
Clinical Assistant Professor
Department of Physical Medicine and Rehabilitation
The Ohio State University College of Medicine
Pediatric Physiatrist
Department of Physical Medicine and Rehabilitation
Nationwide Children's Hospital
Columbus, Ohio

Judith L. Gooch, MD
Professor
Department of Physical Medicine and Rehabilitation
University of Utah
Salt Lake City, Utah

Liza Green, MD, MS
Lecturer
Medical Director, Pediatric Inpatient Service
Department of Physical Medicine and Rehabilitation
C.S. Mott Children's Hospital
University of Michigan
Ann Arbor, Michigan

Jay J. Han, MD
Associate Professor
Department of Physical Medicine and Rehabilitation
University of California Davis School of Medicine
Sacramento, California

Joseph E. Hornyak, MD, PhD
Associate Professor
Director, Down Syndrome Clinic
Department of Physical Medicine and Rehabilitation
C.S. Mott Children's Hospital
University of Michigan
Ann Arbor, Michigan

Edward A. Hurvitz, MD
Associate Professor and Chair
James W. Rae Collegiate Professor
Department of Physical Medicine and Rehabilitation
C.S. Mott Children's Hospital
University of Michigan
Ann Arbor, Michigan

Kenneth M. Jaffe, MD
Professor
Departments of Rehabilitation Medicine, Pediatrics, and
    Neurological Surgery
University of Washington School of Medicine
Seattle, Washington

Nanette C. Joyce, DO
Clinical Research Fellow
California Institute of Regenerative Medicine
Department of Physical Medicine and Rehabilitation
University of California Davis Medical School
Sacramento, California

Ellen S. Kaitz, MD
Assistant Professor
Department of Physical Medicine and Rehabilitation
Ohio State University
Physiatrist and Fellowship Director
Department of Pediatric Rehabilitation Medicine
Nationwide Children's Hospital
Columbus, Ohio

Benjamin Katholi, MD
Associate Staff
Department of Developmental and Rehabilitation
    Pediatrics
Cleveland Clinic Children's Hospital for Rehabilitation
Cleveland, Ohio

Brian M. Kelly, DO
Associate Professor
Medical Director, Rehabilitation Medical Service
Assistant Program Director, Resident Training Program
Department of Physical Medicine and Rehabilitation
University of Michigan Health System
Ann Arbor, Michigan

Heakyung Kim, MD
Associate Professor and Medical Director
Departments of Physical Medicine and
    Rehabilitation, and Pediatrics
Section of Pediatric Rehabilitation Medicine
The Children's Hospital of Philadelphia
University of Pennsylvania
Philadelphia, Pennsylvania

Douglas G. Kinnett, MD
Associate Professor of Pediatrics and Physical Medicine
    and Rehabilitation
Division of Pediatric Physical Medicine and
    Rehabilitation
Cincinnati Children's Hospital Medical Center
Cincinnati, Ohio

Stephen Kirkby, MD
Assistant Professor of Pediatrics
Section of Pediatric Pulmonary Medicine
Nationwide Children's Hospital
Assistant Professor of Internal Medicine
Division of Pulmonary Allergy, Critical Care, and
    Sleep Medicine
The Ohio State University Medical Center
Columbus, Ohio

Paul Bryan Kornberg, MD, FAAPMR, MSRT
Medical Director Rehabilitation Services
St. Joseph's Hospital
Head, Pediatric Rehabilitation Program
St. Joseph's Children's Hospital of Tampa
Medical Director, Pediatric Rehabilitation Services
Tampa General Hospital
Tampa, Florida

Linda E. Krach, MD
Director, Research Administration
Department of Pediatric Rehabilitation Medicine
Gillette Children's Specialty Healthcare
St. Paul, Minnesota

Brad G. Kurowski, MD, MS
Instructor
Department of Physical Medicine and Rehabilitation
University of Cincinnati College of Medicine
Instructor
Department of Pediatrics
Cincinnati Children's Hospital Medical Center
Cincinnati, Ohio

Aga Julia Lewelt, MD
Assistant Professor
Department of Physical Medicine and
    Rehabilitation
University of Utah
Assistant Professor
Department of Pediatric Rehabilitation
Primary Children's Medical Center
Salt Lake City, Utah

Benjamin Reyes Mandac, MD
Department Chief, Pediatric Rehabilitation
Department of Physical Medicine and Rehabilitation
Kaiser Permanente
Santa Clara, California

Teresa L. Massagli, MD
Professor
Department of Rehabilitation Medicine
University of Washington
Attending Physician
Department of Rehabilitation Medicine
Seattle Children's Hospital
Seattle, Washington

Dennis J. Matthews, MD
Professor and Chair
Department of Physical Medicine and Rehabilitation
University of Colorado School of Medicine
Medical Director
Department of Rehabilitation Medicine
The Children's Hospital
Aurora, Colorado

Anne May, MD
Assistant Professor of Clinical Medicine
Section of Pediatric Pulmonary Medicine
Assistant Professor of Clinical Pediatrics
Department of Pediatrics
Nationwide Children's Hospital
The Ohio State University
Columbus, Ohio

Mary McMahon, MD
Associate Professor
Departments of Physical Medicine and Rehabilitation,
    and Pediatrics
Division of Pediatric Rehabilitation
Cincinnati Children's Medical Center
University of Cincinnati
Cincinnati, Ohio

Thomas E. McNalley, MD
Acting Assistant Professor
Department of Rehabilitation Medicine
University of Washington
Seattle Children's Hospital
Seattle, Washington

Linda J. Michaud, MD
Director, Pediatric Physical Medicine and
    Rehabilitation
Associate Professor, Clinical Physical Medicine and
    Rehabilitation and Clinical Pediatrics
Departments of Physical Medicine and Rehabilitation,
    and Pediatrics
Cincinnati Children's Hospital Medical Center
University of Cincinnati College of Medicine
Cincinnati, Ohio

Michelle A. Miller, MD
Clinical Assistant Professor
Division Director, Pediatric Physical Medicine and
    Rehabilitation
Department of Physical Medicine and
    Rehabilitation
The Ohio State University
Section Chief, Pediatric Physical Medicine and
    Rehabilitation
Department of Physical Medicine and
    Rehabilitation
Nationwide Children's Hospital
Columbus, Ohio

Elizabeth Moberg-Wolff, MD
Associate Professor
Director of Tone Management
Department of Physical Medicine and
    Rehabilitation
Children's Hospital of Wisconsin
Milwaukee, Wisconsin

Olga Morozova, MD
Pediatric Physiatrist
Department of Physical Medicine and
    Rehabilitation
Children's National Medical Center
Assistant Professor
Department of Pediatrics
George Washington University
Washington, DC

Kevin P. Murphy, MD
Medical Director
Gillette Specialty Healthcare Northern Clinics
Department of Rehabilitation Medicine
Gillette Children's Specialty Healthcare
Duluth, Minnesota
Medical Director, Pediatric Rehabilitation Medicine
Department of Physical Medicine and Rehabilitation
Med Center One Health System
Bismarck, North Dakota

Nancy A. Murphy, MD, FAAP, FAAPMR
Associate Professor of Pediatrics
Department of Pediatrics
University of Utah School of Medicine
Salt Lake City, Utah

Maureen R. Nelson, MD
Director
Pediatric Rehabilitation Services
Levine Children's Hospital
Charlotte, North Carolina
Adjunct Associate Professor
Department of Physical Medicine and Rehabilitation
University of North Carolina
Chapel Hill, North Carolina

Virginia Simson Nelson, MD, MPH
Professor
Department of Physical Medicine and Rehabilitation
University of Michigan Medical School
Chief
Pediatric and Adolescent Physical Medicine and
    Rehabilitation
C.S. Mott Children's Hospital
University of Michigan
Ann Arbor, Michigan

Joyce Oleszek, MD
Assistant Professor
Department of Rehabilitation
The Children's Hospital
University of Colorado at Denver
Aurora, Colorado

Andre N. Panagos, MD
Medical Director
Spine and Sports Medicine of New York
New York, New York

Scott M. Paul, BES, MD
Senior Staff Clinician and Research Coordinator
Department of Rehabilitation Medicine
Clinical Center
National Institutes of Health
Adjunct Assistant Professor
Department of Biomedical Engineering
The Johns Hopkins University School of Medicine
Baltimore, Maryland

Frank S. Pidcock, MD
Associate Professor
Departments of Physical Medicine and Rehabilitation,
    and Pediatrics
The Johns Hopkins University School of Medicine
Vice President
Department of Rehabilitation
Kennedy Krieger Institute
Baltimore, Maryland

David W. Pruitt, MD
Assistant Professor
Department of Physical Medicine and Rehabilitation
University of Cincinnati College of Medicine
Department of Pediatrics
Cincinnati Children's Hospital Medical Center
Cincinnati, Ohio

Susan Quigley, MD
Medical Director of Inpatient Rehabilitation Services
Department of Pediatric Physical Medicine and
    Rehabilitation
Gillette Children's Specialty Healthcare
St. Paul, Minnesota

Melanie Rak, MD
Attending Physician
Departments of Physical Medicine and Rehabilitation,
    Pediatrics
The Rehabilitation Institute of Chicago
Northwestern Feinberg School of Medicine
Chicago, Illinois

Gadi Revivo, DO
Clinical Assistant Professor
Department of Physical Medicine and Rehabilitation
Assistant Medical Director
Department of Pediatric and Adolescent Rehabilitation
    Program
Rehabilitation Institute of Chicago
Chicago, Illinois

Maria R. Reyes, MD
Assistant Professor
Department of Rehabilitation Medicine
University of Washington
Seattle, Washington

Stephanie Ried, MD
Assistant Professor (Clinical)
Department of Physical Medicine and Rehabilitation
University of Pennsylvania School of Medicine
Medical Director for Rehabilitation
Shriners Hospital for Children, Philadelphia
Philadelphia, Pennsylvania

Robert J. Rinaldi, MD
Assistant Professor of Pediatrics
Section of Pediatric Rehabilitation Medicine
The Children's Mercy Hospitals and Clinics
Kansas City, Missouri

Desirée Rogé, MD
Assistant Professor
Department of Pediatric Physical Medicine and
    Rehabilitation
Children's Mercy Hospital and Clinics
Kansas City, Missouri
Clinical Instructor
Department of Physical Medicine and Rehabilitation
    Residency Program
University of Kansas Medical Center
Kansas City, Kansas

Aloysia Schwabe, MD
Assistant Professor
Department of Physical Medicine and Rehabilitation
Texas Children's Hospital
Baylor College of Medicine
Houston, Texas

Maurice Sholas, MD, PhD
Medical and Practice Director
Rehabilitation Services
Children's Healthcare of Atlanta
Clinical Assistant Professor
Department of Rehabilitation Medicine
Emory School of Medicine
Atlanta, Georgia

Charles E. Sisung, MD
Assistant Professor
Departments of Pediatrics, and Physical Medicine and
  Rehabilitation
Feinberg School of Medicine
Northwestern University
Director
Department of Pediatric Rehabiltation
The Rehabilitation Institute of Chicago
Chicago, Illinois

Andrew J. Skalsky, BS, MD
Assistant Professor
Department of Pediatrics
Rady Children's Hospital
University of California, San Diego
San Diego, California

Mark Splaingard, MD
Professor of Pediatrics
Ohio State University College of Medicine
Director
Sleep Disorders Center
Nationwide Children's Hospital
Columbus, Ohio

Rajashree Srinivasan, MD
Assistant Professor
Pediatric Physiatrist
Our Children's House
Baylor Health Care System
Dallas, Texas

Teresa Such-Neibar, DO
Assistant Professor (Clinical)
Department of Physical Medicine and Rehabilitation
Primary Children's Medical Center
University of Utah School of Medicine
Salt Lake City, Utah

Stacy J. Suskauer, MD
Research Scientist
Kennedy Krieger Institute
Assistant Professor
Department of Physical Medicine and Rehabilitation
Johns Hopkins University School of Medicine
Baltimore, Maryland

Adrienne G. Tilbor, DO
Program Director, National Childrens' Center for
  Rehabilitation
Department of Pediatric Physical Medicine and
  Rehabilitation
Childrens' National Medical Center
National Rehabilitation Hospital
Washington, DC

Melissa K. Trovato, MD
Assistant Professor
Department of Physical Medicine and Rehabilitation
Johns Hopkins School of Medicine
Baltimore, Maryland

Margaret Turk, MD
Professor
Departments of Physical Medicine and Rehabilitation,
  and Pediatrics
SUNY Upstate Medical University
Syracuse, New York

Marcie Ward, MD
Pediatric Rehabilitation Medicine
Department of Physical Medicine and Rehabilitation
Gillette Children's Specialty Healthcare
St. Paul, Minnesota
Adjunct Instructor, Physical Medicine and
  Rehabilitation
Department of Physical Medicine and Rehabilitation
University of Minnesota
Minneapolis, Minnesota

Joshua Wellington, MD, MS
Assistant Professor of Clinical Anesthesia and
  Physical Medicine and Rehabilitation
Medical Director
Indiana University Pain Medicine Center
Departments of Anesthesia, and Physical Medicine and
  Rehabilitation
Indiana University Medical Center
Indianapolis, Indiana

Pamela E. Wilson, MD
Associate Professor
Department of Pediatric Rehabilitation Medicine
The Children's Hospital
University of Colorado School of Medicine
Aurora, Colorado

Edward A. Wright, MD
Pediatric Physiatrist
The Children's Center
Bethany, Oklahoma

Colleen A. Wunderlich, MD
Associate Director
Pediatric Rehabilitation
Levine Children's Hospital and Carolinas Rehabilitation
Charlotte, North Carolina

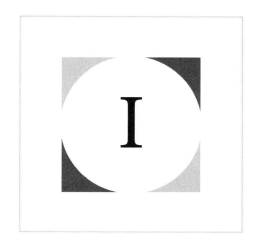

Diagnostic
Considerations

Normal Development

Maureen R. Nelson MD

Description

There are general developmental milestones that are considered normal although there is some variability. It is helpful to consider classic development when evaluating a child in whom there are concerns about abnormalities or deficits. There is cause for further evaluation, if there is a large deviation from the normal values in one area or if there are smaller differences in several areas.

Reflexes

A part of the normal development is the progression, then disappearance of primitive reflexes. These reflexes should be extinguishable, not obligate. It is important to keep head midline to assess the reflexes.

- Root—baby turns head toward anything that strokes lip or cheek near mouth
- Moro—baby abducts arms, extends and then flexes elbows, and may cry, after sudden neck extension, release of grasp, or loud noise
- Galant—baby curves body toward side when that side of the back is stroked
- Stepping—child "takes steps" if trunk is supported upright, tilted forward and to sides, and feet placed on surface
- Tonic labyrinthine—when supine and head extended the baby's tone will increase into extension, and tone will decrease when in the lap or prone, with neck flexed
- Asymmetrical tonic neck reflex—with passive rotation of the neck of a supine baby to the side, the baby will extend the arm on the side he or she is facing and flex the other elbow and fist
- Palmar grasp—flexes fingers and grips with stimulation/touch to palm
- Symmetric tonic neck—baby's arms flex and legs extend when neck is flexed; while arms extend and legs flex when neck is extended
- Placing—flexes leg with touch to dorsum of foot
- Plantar grasp—flexes toes and forefoot with stimulation/touch to distal sole of foot
- These protective reactions are important in prevention of injuries from falls

Reflex	Present	Disappears
Root	birth	3–4 months
Moro/startle	birth	4–6 months
Galant/truncal incurvature	birth	2–6 months
Stepping/walking	birth	3–5 months
Tonic labyrinthine	birth	4–6 months
Asymmetric tonic neck/fencer	birth	4–7 months
Palmar grasp	birth	5–6 months
Symmetric tonic neck	2 months	6–7 months
Placing	birth	12 months
Plantar grasp	birth	12–14 months

Protective Reactions	Appears at	
Forward/parachute	5–7 months	continues
Lateral	6–8 months	continues

Development

Speech and language development

Birth to 12 months	Appears at
• Smiles interactively	by birth to 4 months
• Phonation: pre-ooing	birth–2 months
• Primitive articulation: cooing	2–4 months
• Expansion: vowels, raspberries	4–6 months
• Canonical: syllables, sequences	6–10 months
• Gesture	by 9 months
• Listen selectively, including name and "no"	by 12 months

12–24 months
• Point to body parts and pictures
• Use two word phrases
• Understand 50 words, uses much less
• Express wants and needs
• Follow one-step commands

Speech and language development

24–42 months

- Know colors
- Use three-word phrases
- Ask questions
- Understand prepositions and conditionals
- Use pronouns
- Vocabulary boom to hundreds of words
- Know about past and future
- Follow two-step commands

Motor development

Gross motor

Lift up head from prone	3 months
Support chest up on two hands in prone	4 months
Balance on one arm and reach with other	5 months
Roll supine to prone	6 months
Sit unsupported	8 months
Crawl and pull to stand	10 months
Walk with support	12 months
Walk without support	14 months
Walk up stairs, both feet on one step	2 years
Run	2 years
Walk up stairs alternating feet	3 years
Pedal tricycle	3 years
Go down stairs alternating feet	4 years
Hop/jump	4 years
Skip	5 years

Motor development

Fine motor

Reach for objects	5 months
Grasp with first three fingers	8–10 months
Thumb-index pincer grasp	12 months
Scribble	13 months
Use a cup	13–15 months
Stack two to three cubes	15 months
Use spoon	15 months
Hand dominance	12–18 months
Remove shoes and socks	18 months
Put on socks	24 months
Turn single pages	24 months
Stack more than five cubes	24 months
Throw overhand	24 months
Potty trained	30 months
Draw circle, imitate cross	3 years
Dress self except buttons	3 years
Copy square	5 years
Tie shoe	5 years
Copy diamond	6 years

Suggested Readings

Matthews DJ. Examination of the pediatric patient. In: Braddom RL, ed. *Physical Medicine and Rehabilitation*. Philadelphia, PA: WB Saunders; 1996:43–48.

Schott JM, Rossor MN. The grasp and other primitive reflexes. *J Neurol Neurosurg Psychiatr*. 2003;75(5):558–560.

Section I: Diagnostic Considerations

History and Physical in Pediatric Rehabilitation

Christine Aguilar MD ■ Benjamin Reyes Mandac MD

History
- Prenatal, birth, family, and social history
- Developmental history
- Nutritional history
- Dysmorphology
- Bowel, bladder issues including continence, bowel and bladder program, constipation, and diarrhea
- Functional concerns in activities: play and school, including regular and/or special classes, grades, and any change in performance
- Preadolescent and older: sexual history, illicit drug, tobacco and alcohol use, behavioral changes, peer interactions, and family/caregiver concerns

Considerations Prior to Physiatric Evaluation
- Examination room with wall-mounted toys may be helpful
- The initial behavior noted at the time of entering the examination room can be significant and can guide how examination conduct may proceed
- Have a general idea of the general developmental considerations for the age of child to be examined
- Gather documented history prior to going into the examination
- Consider removal of white coat; hair, glasses, ties, badges; all that is brought into the room attached to the examiner may be pulled. Any of these can also be used for the examination
- Parents'/caregivers' reactions can be helpful in guiding the examination
- Do not examine an adolescent alone without the parent or chaperone
- Wash hands before and after the examination

Helpful Hints
- Interact with the children
- Play with them
- Engage them
- Watch them in play
  - Have toys available in the room for children to explore
- How to enter the room: Greet the family as well as the child
- Children's temperaments will be variable—affects ability to physically examine child. Utilize toys they bring in
- Look at clothes: check the images printed and see if they will identify or talk about it
- Look at the growth and development chart for height, weight, and body mass index (BMI)
  - Specific growth charts may be available for specific conditions, for example, Trisomy 21 growth charts
  - Age correction for premature children may be done for the first 12 to 18 months of age
- Cognitive development is key consideration in how patients are examined throughout the ages

Physical Examination with Different Age Groups

Infant
- Watch movement, alertness, and interest in the environment in caregiver's arms, on exam table, and as the provider handles the infant
- Consider exam on caregiver's lap if possible
- Head control, facial symmetry, and neck movements
- Visual and auditory tracking
- Listen for cry
- Check suck and swallow
- Cervical, thoracic, lumbar, and sacral spine
- Scapular position/thorax symmetry and respiratory effort
- Resting upper and lower extremity position at rest and with movement
- Muscle tone proximal and distal
- Reflexes: DTR's infantile reflexes, emerging reflexes
- Age-appropriate reflexes/maneuvers
- Hips, including joint maneuvers
- Genitalia
- Anus and anal wink
- Dysmorphologies: head circumference (FOC), height, weight, skin abnormalities, and body disproportions

Child

- Watch movement in way they come into examination room and manner during interactions with caregiver
- Engage child through play
- Eyes, ears, nose, and mouth functions
- Upper and lower extremity tone, function
- Gait pattern, movement patterns if not yet ambulating, including run, jump, skip, and balance
- Ability to arise from a squatting position; is there a Gower's sign (using the hands to "walk up" the body due to hip weakness and inability to directly arise)?
- Spine alignment
- Hip position and range of motion
- Leg length discrepancy
- Reflexes emerging, retained, postural, and deep tendon reflexes
- Strength testing by function

Preadolescent

- Engage via discussing age-appropriate topics
- As in child examination plus:
  - Tanner stage examination findings (see Ratings Scales chapter)
  - Isolated manual motor test is possible
- Check reading

Adolescent

- As in preadolescent plus:
- Take note of types of clothes worn
- Skin check for tattoos, piercings, and abnormal scars
- Engage via discussing age appropriate topics to build an environment of trust
- Evaluate affect and mood
- Examine and obtain history without family in examination room
  - Use a chaperone during examination
- Cognitive screen

Key Principles and Procedures

1 to 8 months

Key principles

- Rapid growth of the infant
- Consider use of Denver Developmental screen
  - Plot on growth chart
  - Anterior fontanelle and posterior fontanelle are open during this period but sutures are not widened or overlapped
  - Primitive reflexes must be age appropriate
  - Must undress infant

Key procedures

- Move extremities, symmetric
- Hips evaluation: Ortolani (baby supine with hips flexed to 90°, abduct and hear clunk if relocate a hip)/Barlow (baby supine, hips flexed to 90°, adduct with pressure down and lateral, hear a clunk if dislocates)/Galeazzi (baby supine, flex hips and knees, if asymmetrical, short side is dislocated)
- Sense should be intact: hearing, vision, and response to touch
- Gross grasp, no persistent cortical thumb position
- Social—social smile usually occurs by 1 month of age
- Speech—cry should not be high pitched
- Anticipated problems
  - Four months of age—infants began to laugh and social contacts are pleasurable. If infant is crying and inconsolable, look for a physical or environmental problem
  - The Moro reflex should never be asymmetrical
  - Six months of age—preference to be with their mother or caretaker over medical provider
  - Social—by 8 months of age
    Attentive to their name
    Babbling speech by 8 months
  - Stranger anxiety begins
    Avoid eye contact if stranger

9 to 12 months

Key principles

- Abnormal if not curious

Key procedures

- Gross motor—abnormal if not walking by 18 months of age
- Fine motor—a fine pincher grasp; gives objects on request such as a ball or small toy
- Social—by 9 months of age waves bye-bye; by 12 months they may play peek-a-boo with caretaker
- Speech—abnormal if not babbling with specific sounds
- Abnormal if doesn't respond to inhibitory words such as no-no
- Anticipated problems
  - May see initial stranger anxiety but should be able to overcome

12 to 18 months

Key principles

- Abnormal if not exploring and willing to separate from parent after initial anxiety

Key procedures

- Gross motor—abnormal if walking does not occur by 18 months of age
- Fine motor—abnormal if no finger isolation, that is, pointing with index finger
- Social—abnormal if not locating familiar objects or familiar persons, animals or toys on request
- By 18 months can point to at least one body part with good accuracy
- Speech—says at least 5 to 10 words (these are usually nouns)
- Anticipated problems
  - Noncooperative—may not perform for examiner
  - Utilize parents to encourage performance
  - Cling to parents
    Examine on parent's lap
  - Resists active examination
  - Poor attention
    Entice with toys, play
  - Interaction with parents and siblings in the same room

18 months to 2-year old

Key principles

- Very independent when comfortable with surroundings. Play is very important

Key procedures

- Gross motor—squats in play; walks up and down stairs with one hand held-step to step; kicks ball; throws ball; picks up toy from floor without falling
- Fine motor—good normal grasp of small objects; folds paper, strings beads; stacks cubes
- Social—usually initially fearful and then becomes curious
- Speech—clear but usually no more than two to three words in a sentence

2-year old to 4-year old—Preschool age group

Description

Abnormal if play is not a large part of their activity and engagement

Key principles

- The child is evolving from the sensorimotor stage to preoperational
- Egocentric thought and language is noted
- There is no concept of conservation, for example, a same amount liquid poured into a tall glass will be considered more than the same liquid poured into a short glass
- Stranger anxiety may remain for the 2-year old
- Approach child in play, nonthreatening manner

- Language is evolving rapidly, sings, says "No"
- Evolve with identifying colors and matching shapes
- Toileting considerations
- Functional activities of daily living dressing, undressing
- Handedness solidifying
- Attention span to a task can be limited—1 to 5 minutes to a task may be maximum limit

Procedural steps

- Get down to their level
- Give high 5's, engage
- Examine while on parent lap then consider move to examination table
- Watch play activity
- Watch level of attention—may be limited
- Assess separation anxiety
- Gross and fine motor
  - Movement quality with gait, manipulation of objects/toys
- Language/cognitive
  - Sentence structure and word use
  - Identification of toys/objects/colors/shapes
- Social
  - Follows multiple steps
  - Cooperative play

Helpful hints

- Engage with play
- Utilize family member/care giver
- Use toys to entice activity—stickers are useful
- Examine on parent lap
- Back off early if not cooperative and keep initial distance until child engages
- May need to rely on family report for certain skills such as dressing and undressing
- Subsequent clinic visits should improve cooperation

5 to 11 years old—School age group

Description

This age group represents an expanding skill set from vocabulary to social abilities. Motor skills continue to improve and independence in self-care as well as expanding confidence outside of the realm of the caregivers. Early experiences in the preschool age group shape this group's abilities. Gender roles are evolving.

Key principles

- Language comprehension and manipulation continue to evolve
- Academic and cognitive development include key skills of attention and memory

- Cognitive development is in the preoperational stage evolving to concrete operational stage
  - Conservation concept is completed. Operations are concrete and can be reversible; for example, both: 3 apples + 2 apples = 5 apples; and 3 apples = 5 apples – 2 apples
- No problems noted with separation from parent/caregiver

Procedural steps
- Engagement with language is easier; deficiencies can easily be determined with direct interaction
- Concrete directions may be followed
- More isolated testing can be done with simple explanations
- Play activities may be more complex thereby increasing ability to check specific skills
- Climbing onto the examination table will be without difficulty
- Writing skills may be assessed—pen/crayon paper can be handy
- Note sexual characteristic maturation—early maturation may be abnormal

Anticipated problems
- May dominate examination—need to have ability to distract and redirect
- Short attention and hyperactivity can easily be distinguished—have a plan to redirect or elicit the help of the family/caregiver
- May play with instruments on the wall—be prepared to redirect. Can use toys appropriate for age
- More resistance if unable to separate from parent/caregiver

Helpful hints
- Books may be enough to keep attention; if not, age-specific toys may be useful
- Individual play may assist with redirection as well as assessment of function—gross motor, fine motor, language, and social

Preteen—Early adolescence
Description
Differences between male and female start to emerge aside from toy and clothes preference. Gender roles are more definitive. This is the start of rapid changes in development akin to that seen in the first year of life.

Key principles
- Formal operational cognitive abilities are evolving. Abstract thinking is noted with ability to identify problems and form ways of solving using abstract operations
- Individuation from the family/caregiver is starting
- Social peer network becoming more important

Procedural steps
- Be aware of body image concerns
- Note affect and cooperation as part of response set
- Specific interactions with the family/caregiver important
- Talk to the patient directly
- Encourage answers from the patient
- Note sexual characteristics maturation pattern

Mid-teen—Mid-adolescence
Description
The evolution of the individual becomes more apparent as are the differences between men and women. Disparity of sexual characteristic maturation may be striking for a given age for both men and women. Peer interactions and socialization are quite strong. Fitting in with peers versus family attachment can be conflicting. Individuation from family is stronger but can have a sense of insecurity.

Key principles
- Middle school activities: engage child with what is current with the peer group
- Examiner may be seen as a parent figure
- Cooperation to examination is generally good
- Can be moody
- Sexual maturation are continuing to develop—onset of menses important part of history
- Start questions about tobacco, alcohol, drugs, self-harming behaviors, and sexual activity
- School performance may be indicative of functional abilities
- Mental health concerns: peer interactions, mood swings can be appropriate
- Consider evaluation of complaints in the context of family concerns
- School performance and family issues can be brought up such as adjustment to school such as bullying or family discord

Procedural steps
- Direct your questions to the patient; however, expect incomplete answers as well as parents answering for the patient
- Engage patient by looking at the manner of dress as well as any indications of interest

Section I: Diagnostic Considerations

Anticipated problems
- Noncooperative unless engaged
- May not give complete history
- May be self-conscious about body image

Helpful hints
- Always have another person in the room during examination

Late adolescence—Early adult
Description

Transition to independence, individuation, and self-determination are key development considerations.

Key principles
- Identity concerns may be paramount
- Parental concerns of dependence and independence may be indicative
- School performance and plans for ongoing school and independent living can be significant concerns

- Ongoing transition to adult plans important—ongoing care
- Questions about tobacco, alcohol, drugs, self-harming behaviors, and sexual activity ongoing

Procedural steps
- Anticipate independent ability to cooperate depending on developmental level/ability
- Engage directly

Helpful hints
- Transition to adult care services: primary care, OB/GYN for females, specialty care including adult PM&R services

Suggested Readings

Nickel RE, Desch LW, eds. *The Physician's Guide to Caring for Children with Disabilities and Chronic Conditions.* Baltimore, MD: PH Brookes Publishers; 2000.

Wolraich ML, Drotar DD, Dworkin PH, eds. *Developmental-Behavioral Pediatrics: Evidence and Practice.* Philadelphia, PA: Elsevier Science; 2007.

Rating Scales

Maureen R. Nelson MD

Description

There are several rating scales used frequently in evaluation and care of children with disabilities. Some of the most commonly used will be presented here, including those for evaluating strength, spasticity, coma and cognition, spinal cord injury, and movement in children with cerebral palsy.

Muscle Strength/Power

Medical Research Council Scale

0 = No contraction
1 = Flicker or trace of contraction
2 = Active movement, with gravity eliminated
3 = Active movement against gravity
4 = Active movement against gravity and resistance
5 = Normal power

Spasticity

Ashworth Scale (1964)

0 = No increase in muscle tone
1 = Slight increase in tone giving a "catch" when affected part is moved in flexion or extension
2 = More marked increase in tone but affected part is easily flexed
3 = Considerable increase in tone; passive movement difficult
4 = Affected part is rigid in flexion or extension

Modified Ashworth Scale

0 = No increase in tone
1 = Slight increase in muscle tone, manifested by a catch and release or minimal resistance at the end of the range of motion (ROM) when the affected part(s) is moved in flexion or extension
1+ = Slight increase in muscle tone, manifested by a catch, followed by minimal resistance throughout the remainder (less than half) of the ROM
2 = More marked increase in muscle tone through most of the ROM, but affected part(s) easily moved
3 = Considerable increase in muscle tone, passive movement difficult
4 = Affected part(s) rigid in flexion or extension

Tardieu Scale

This test is performed with patient in the supine position, with head in midline. Measurements take place at three velocities (V1, as slow as possible; V2, the speed of fall with gravity; and V3, as fast as possible). Responses are recorded at each velocity as X/Y, with X indicating the 0 to 5 rating, and Y indicating the degree of angle at which the muscle reaction occurs. By moving the limb at different velocities, the response to stretch can be more easily gauged since the stretch reflex responds differently to velocity.

Scoring:
0 = No resistance throughout the course of the passive movement
1 = Slight resistance throughout the course of passive movement, with no clear catch at a precise angle
2 = Clear catch at a precise angle, interrupting the passive movement, followed by release
3 = Fatigable clonus for less than 10 seconds when maintaining the pressure at the precise angle
4 = Unfatigable clonus for more than 10 seconds when maintaining the pressure and at a precise angle
5 = Joint is immovable

Adapted from Tardieu (French), by Held and Pierrot-Deseilligny, translated by Gracies et al.

Coma/Cognition

Glasgow Coma Scale (GCS) measures the motor response, verbal response, and eye opening response. The final score is determined by adding the values of these three subgroups. This number helps categorize the four possible levels for survival, with a lower number indicating a more severe injury and a poorer prognosis. Mild traumatic brain injury (TBI) is GCS 13–15, moderate is 9–12, severe is 3–8, and vegetative state is GCS less than 3.

Glasgow Coma Scale

Motor response
6 = Obeys commands fully
5 = Localizes to noxious stimuli
4 = Withdraws from noxious stimuli
3 = Abnormal flexion, that is, decorticate posturing

2 = Extensor response, that is, decerebrate posturing
1 = No response

Verbal response
5 = Alert and oriented
4 = Confused, yet coherent, speech
3 = Inappropriate words and jumbled phrases consisting of words
2 = Incomprehensible sounds
1 = No sounds

Eye opening
4 = Spontaneous eye opening
3 = Eyes open to speech
2 = Eyes open to pain
1 = No eye opening

Rancho Los Amigos levels of cognitive functioning

Level I　　= No response
Level II　　= Generalized response
Level III　　= Localized response
Level IV　　= Confused and agitated
Level V　　= Confused and inappropriate
Level VI　　= Confused and appropriate
Level VII　= Automatic and appropriate
Level VIII = Purposeful and appropriate

Rancho Los Amigos—Revised

Levels of cognitive functioning
Level I—No response: total assistance
Level II—Generalized response: total assistance
Level III—Localized response: total assistance
Level IV—Confused/agitated: maximal assistance
Level V—Confused, inappropriate nonagitated: maximal assistance
Level VI—Confused, appropriate: moderate assistance
Level VII—Automatic, appropriate: minimal assistance for daily living skills
Level VIII—Purposeful, appropriate: stand-by assistance
Level IX—Purposeful, appropriate: stand-by assistance on request
Level X—Purposeful, appropriate: modified independent
Original Scale co-authored by Chris Hagen, Ph.D., Danese Malkmus, M.A., Patricia Durham, M.A. Communication Disorders Service, Rancho Los Amigos Hospital, 1972. Revised 11/15/74 by Danese Malkmus, M.A., and Kathryn Stenderup, O.T.R. Revised scale 1997 by Chris Hagen

Galveston Orientation and Amnesia Test (GOAT)

The Galveston Orientation and Amnesia Test was developed to evaluate cognition serially during the subacute stage of recovery from closed head injury in adults. This practical scale measures orientation to person, place, and time, and memory for events preceding and following the injury. It can be administered daily. A score of 78 or more on three consecutive occasions is considered to indicate that patient is out of posttraumatic amnesia. 76–100 = Normal; 66–75 = Borderline; <66 = Impaired.

Children's Orientation and Amnesia Test (COAT)

The Children's Orientation and Amnesia Test is a standardized measure for cognitive function in children and teens recovering from TBI. It assesses general and temporal orientation as well as memory. It was designed initially to evaluate special education students.

Spinal Cord Injury

ASIA Impairment Scale

The American Spinal Injury Association (ASIA) Standard Neurological Classification of Spinal Cord Injury is a standard method of assessing the neurological status of a person after a spinal cord injury.

The ASIA impairment scale describes a person's functional impairment as a result of spinal cord injury:

Category	Description
A Complete	No motor or sensory function is preserved in the sacral segments S4–S5
B Incomplete	Sensory but not motor function is preserved below the neurological level and includes the sacral segments S4–S5
C Incomplete	Motor function is preserved below the neurological level, and more than half of key muscles below the neurological level have a muscle grade of less than 3
D Incomplete	Motor function is preserved below the neurological level, and at least half of the key muscles below the neurological level have a muscle grade of 3 or more
E Normal	Motor and sensory function are normal

Movement in Cerebral Palsy

Gross Motor Function Classification System

The Gross Motor Function Classification System (GMFCS) is a five-level classification system that differentiates children with cerebral palsy based on the child's self-initiated movement, current gross motor abilities, limitations in gross motor function, and need for assistive technology and wheeled mobility. When defining this system, the primary criterion has been that the distinctions between levels must be meaningful in daily life. The GMFCS contains four age groups: under 2 years, 2 to 4 years, 4 to 6 years, and 6 to 12 years.

Level I—Walks without limitations

Level II—Walks with limitations

Level III—Walks using a hand-held mobility device

Level IV—Self-mobility with limitations; may use powered mobility

Level V—Transported in a manual wheelchair

Developmental stages

Tanner staging measures stages of puberty. It is based on growth of pubic hair in both genders, development of genitalia in boys, and development of breasts in girls.

Tanner stage

Boys

Stage 1: No pubic hair; preadolescent testes and penis

Stage 2: Sparse, straight pubic hair; testes larger, slight increase in penis size

Stage 3: Darker hair, curls; testes larger, penis is longer

Stage 4: Adult hair, coarser; scrotum becomes pigmented; penis increases length and breadth

Stage 5: Hair spreads to thighs; adult-sized scrotum and penis

Girls

Stage 1: No pubic hair; preadolescent breasts

Stage 2: Sparse, straight pubic hair; breast buds

Stage 3: Darker hair, curls; enlargement of breasts

Stage 4: Adult hair, coarser; areola develops secondary mound above breast

Stage 5: Hair spreads to thighs; nipples project from breasts

Suggested Readings

Bohannon RW, Smith MB. Interrater reliability of a modified Ashworth scale of muscle spasticity. *Phys Ther.* 1986;67:206–207.

Ewing-Cobbs L, Levin HS, Fletcher JM, Miner ME, Eisenberg HM. The children's orientation and amnesia test: relationship to severity of acute head injury and to recovery of memory. *Neurosurgery.* 1990;27(5):683–691.

Levin HS, O'Donnell VM, Grossman RG. GOAT: The Galveston Orientation and Amnesia Test. *J Nerv Ment Dis.* 1979;167(11):675–684.

Medical Research Council of the UK. Aids to the Investigation of Peripheral Nerve Injuries. Memorandum No. 45. London, Pendragon House, 1976:6–7.

Palisano R, Rosenbaum P, Walter S, Russell D, Wood E, Galuppi B. Gross motor function classifiction system for cerebral palsy. *Dev Med Child Neurol.* 1997;39:214–223.

Testing in Pediatric Rehabilitation

Aloysia Schwabe MD

This chapter will review key items in imaging of the brain, musculoskeletal, and peripheral systems, as well as laboratory, and electrodiagnosis.

Central Nervous System Imaging

Brain computed tomography

Indications

- Acute mental status changes
- Acute focal neurological deficit with/without preceding trauma to include stroke, intracranial hemorrhage, suspected child abuse, and skull fracture
- Monitoring of increased intracranial pressure
- Surveillance study for hydrocephalus

Additional considerations

- 3D imaging for evaluation of craniosynostosis
- Temporal bone cuts for assessment of hearing loss

Brain magnetic resonance imaging

Indications

- More definitive anatomical localization in stroke, mass lesions, structural or migrational brain disorder, diffuse axonal injury after trauma, and prolonged coma
- Tumors
- Work up of global developmental delay/cerebral palsy
- Neurodegenerative and neurometabolic disorders
- Anatomical correlation in epilepsy
- Demyelinating disorders—acute disseminated encephalomyelitis, multiple sclerosis

Spine magnetic resonance imaging for cord/root pathology

Indications

- Acute neurological deficits localized to cord including sensorimotor deficit, change in bladder/bowel function or gait failure including trauma, mass lesions, hemorrhage, myelopathy, transverse myelitis, acute demyelinating encephalomyelitis, and acute inflammatory demyelinating polyneuropathy
- Suspicion of underlying neural tube defect or tethered cord

- Existing scoliosis with rapid progression in child or adolescent with normal neurological exam or superimposed on an underlying condition with risk for syrinx/tethered cord
- Congenital scoliosis—young child with curve greater than 20 degrees and normal neuro exam; abnormal neurological exam and suspicion of intraspinal pathology
- Surveillance in demyelinating disorders
- Consider in setting of existing spinal cord injury with change in strength, bowel bladder function, and spasticity to assess for syrinx

Spine ultrasound for cord pathology

Indications

- Neonatal imaging for suspected spinal dysraphism with/without lumbosacral skin findings includes assessment of sinus tracts, cord tethering, and diastatomyelia

Musculoskeletal/Peripheral Imaging

Ultrasound

- Hip
  - Developmental dysplasia of hip (DDH)—use ultrasound in infants < 4 months when abnormal hip exam and/or risk factors such as family history, breech delivery, or torticollis/clubfoot
  - Effusion—lacks determination of cause; guidance tool for aspiration.
- Superficial soft tissue masses

Plain films

- Trauma/injury for bony abnormality—Minimum two views
- Hips
  - DDH—anteroposterior (AP) view in infants 4 months and older for assessment and as followup tool
  - Subluxation/dislocation in upper motor neuron (UMN)/lower motor neuron (LMN) conditions such as cerebral palsy, myelomeningocele
  - Suspected osteonecrosis/Legg-Calve-Perthes disease—AP and frog leg lateral as initial imaging study
  - Slipped capitol femoral epiphysis

- Shoulder/humerus/clavicle
  - Consider in neonatal brachial plexus palsy if block to passive motion, abnormal alignment, and palpable callus
  - Subluxation in both UMN and LMN conditions such as stroke, brachial plexus palsy
- Spine
  - Scoliosis—initial and surveillance studies
  - Congenital malformations such as hemivertebrae, fusion, etc.
- Scanogram for leg lengths
- Congenital limb deficiency

Bone Scan
- Trauma/fracture—clinical suspicion with initial negative plain films, early stress fracture
- Infection
- Heterotopic ossification—triple phase bone scan with flow studies and blood-pool images first to become abnormal
- Metastases

Computed tomography
- Utilized when greater bony detail required than what is provided by plain films and for surgical planning
  - Spine
    Trauma/fracture, congenital abnormality, spondylolysis, and spondylolisthesis
  - Hip
    Trauma/fracture, surgical planning, and femoral anteversion

Magnetic resonance imaging
- Hips
  - Effusion
  - Infection
  - Osteonecrosis
    Utilized when initial plain films negative and then subsequently to grade severity and complications
    Include contrast, images in sagittal plane to capture anterior femoral head which is usually affected first and consider imaging contralateral hip due to increased incidence of bilateral disease
- Shoulder
  - Rotator cuff tears/impingement
  - Dysplasia of glenohumeral joint
- Spine
  - Herniated nucleus pulposus/radiculopathy
  - Ligamentous injury
- Neurography
  - Brachial plexus lesions—trauma, compression, and mass/tumor

- Terminal nerve branches—trauma, compression, and mass/tumor
- Soft tissue masses—preferred over ultrasound for deeper/complex masses

Laboratory

Hematology
Indications
- Abnormal processes affecting cell lines
  - Infection
  - Malignancy
  - Subparameters indicative of iron deficiency

Chemistries
Indications
- Electrolyte abnormalities

Inflammatory markers (erythrocyte sedimentation rate/C-reactive protein)
Indications
- Infection
- Inflammatory disorders

Markers of muscle degradation (creatine kinase, aspartate aminotransferase/alanine transaminase)
Indications
- Myositis
- Myopathy

Chromosomal microarray
Indications
- Developmental delay of unknown etiology/ regression
- Congenital anomalies/dysmorphic features

Cerebrospinal fluid/lumbar puncture
Indications
- Infection
- Neurodegenerative disease/developmental regression
- Refractory neonatal seizure
- Movement disorders

Muscle biopsy
Indications
- Muscle disease with clinical weakness
  - Inflammatory myopathies
  - Dystrophin, alpha dystroglycan, and sarcoglycan— if genetic studies inconclusive
- Neurodegenerative/mitrochondrial disease
- Document involvement of muscle in systemic disorder (sarcoid/vasculitis)

Electrodiagnosis

General indications

- Assess for focal or generalized pathology affecting LMN
  - Hypotonia/floppy
  - Plexopathies
  - Inherited and acquired neuropathies
  - Myopathies
  - Neuromuscular junction disorders
- Document evidence of neuromuscular process when initial genetic studies inconclusive
- Document severity of neuropathy and/or myopathy
- Establish electrical continuity after nerve injury
- Establish evidence of reinnervation after nerve injury

Nerve conduction studies

Indications

- Document demyelinating features
  - Prolonged onset latencies
  - Slowed nerve conduction velocities
  - Absent or prolonged F-waves
  - Increased temporal dispersion if acquired process
  - Uniform demyelinating features if inherited
- Document axonal features
  - Reduced amplitudes with axonal process or myopathy

Electromyography

Indications

- Correlate to axonal process or myopathy including
  - Abnormal rest activity with denervation potentials
  - Abnormal motor unit morphology
  - Abnormal recruitment patterns
- Assist in localization of pathology
  - Plexus lesions
  - Root pathology versus distal involvement

Single fiber electromyography

Indications

- Neuromuscular junction disorders
- Technically requires cooperation from patient

Pediatric Consideration of Drug Effects

Teresa Such-Neibar DO ■ Paul S. Carbone MD ■ Deborah Bilder MD

The evaluation and treatment of maladaptive behavior in children with neurological impairment is very complicated and, unfortunately, not straightforward. Many of the treatments suggested here have not been approved by the Food and Drug Administration in children, let alone in children with neurological impairments. We recommend careful and prudent consideration of these medications when evaluating these children, and also recommend starting medications at a low dose and increasing medications slowly with good communication with the family and caregivers.

Diagnoses That May Require Medication to Treat Maladaptive Behaviors
- Cerebral palsy (CP)
- Traumatic brain injury
- Genetic disorders/syndrome
- Autism
- Intellectual disabilities (IDs)
- Epilepsy
- Combinations of the above

Comorbidities
Children and young adults with borderline to moderate IDs experience:
- Co-occurring disorders—37%
  - Disruptive behaviors and mood disorder
  - Disruptive behaviors and anxiety disorder
- Disruptive behavior—25%
- Anxiety disorder—22%
- Mood disorder—4.4 %

Steps in Evaluating Maladaptive Behaviors in the Neurologically Impaired Child
- Rule out a medical cause
- Evaluate sleep patterns
- Identify psychiatric disorders
- Consider caregiver stress and family centered services
- Functional behavioral analysis
- Consider medications…. carefully

Differential Diagnoses of Medical Causes That May Cause Maladaptive Behaviors
- Pain—Otitis media, pharyngitis, sinusitis, dental abcess, urinary tract infection, fracture, headache, esophagitis, allergic rhinitis, constipation, hydrocephalus, feeding intolerance, reflux, and other
- Epilepsy—Prevalence of 11% to 39% in autism, pervasive developmental delay (PDD), 36% in CP, 9% in traumatic brain injury (TBI), and 30% in ID
- Consider underlying cause of disability such as a genetic disorder, that is, Down's syndrome or tuberous sclerosis, and so on
- Sleep disorders—Prevalence of 44% to 83% in PDD, 50% in CP, and 36% to 82% in TBI
- Lead intoxication—Children with PDD are more likely to have prolonged and reexposure to lead
- Iron deficiency—Children with PDD have a two- to fourfold higher prevalence
- Spasticity—Common in children with CP and TBI
- Overstimulation—Can occur in children with sensory integration deficits, CP, and TBI
- Medication side effects

Medical Workup
- History—consider the behavior, recent illness, gastrointestinal symptoms, sleep problems, review current medications, pica, family stressors, and family history of psychiatric diagnoses
- Physical examination—search for focus of infection, pain, or poor sleep

Laboratory Workup
- Guided by history and physical examination
- Complete blood count, electrolytes, calcium, lead, ferritin, thyroid stimulating hormone/Free T4, and liver function tests (LFTs)
- Further blood work, neuroimaging, electroencephalography, sleep study as indicated by history and physical examination
- Hearing and vision evaluations

Why Think About Sleep Disorders/ Disturbances?

- Sleep problems are common, prevalence rates of 36% to 82% in children with special health care needs
- Sleep problems correlate with family stress and may have significant effects on daytime function
- Good sleepers show fewer affective problems and better social interactions than poor sleepers
- Common causes of sleep disturbances are circadian rhythm disturbances, behavioral issues, and restless leg syndrome related to iron deficiency

Sleep Problems—How to Evaluate

- Sleep history will guide treatment
- Behavioral treatments can be effective
- Iron therapy may help restless sleep
- Consider referral to a sleep specialist or sleep study to rule out sleep apnea, seizures, and oxygenation deficits

Understanding Behavior

- All behaviors are responses to antecedents in the environment
- All behaviors are followed by consequences that affect that specific behavior and the probability that it will recur
- Although the behavior may seem maladaptive to caregivers, it can be serving a useful function for the child
- As long as the behavior is working for the child, it will continue

Common Antecedents of Maladaptive Behavior (Possible Contributing Factors)

- Frustration; from communication impairment
- Unexpected changes in routine; anxiety
- Transitions; anxiety
- Separation from attachment figure; anxiety
- Crowded/loud location; sensory processing deficits, anxiety
- Discomfort, pain; spasticity
- Initiation of behavior a few hours before bedtime; fatigue, sleep disorder

Consequences

Many consequences can inadvertently reinforce a maladaptive behavior such as:
- Obtaining desired item/outcome
- Receiving attention from caregiver
- Avoiding an undesirable or anxiety-provoking task

Functional Behavioral Analysis

- Systemic way of identifying the antecedents and consequences of a maladaptive behavior
- Results in a better understanding of the function of a behavior
- Leads to a strategy for intervention through behavioral techniques and environmental manipulation

Environmental Factors to Maximize Prior to Starting Medications

- Structure to decrease unexpected events
- Calm tone of voice
- Decrease stimulation
- Work on desired cause and effect
- Consistent behavior management techniques by all caregivers

Measuring Treatment Response

- Identify prominent symptoms
- Define frequency, intensity, duration of symptoms at treatment onset, so comparisons can be made at follow-up
- Use a rating scale

History is the KEY to Appropriate Treatment

- What is the behavior?
- What instigates the behavior?
- How long does the behavior last?
- What are alleviating and aggravating factors to the behavior?
- What is the impact on the child's/family's daily life?
- What has been done in the past to treat this behavior?
- What are the cultural beliefs about the behavior?

Identifying psychiatric disorders

- Anxiety/aggression
- Depression/emotional lability
- Bipolar disorder/mood disorder not otherwise specified (NOS)
- Attention deficit hyperactivity disorder (ADHD)
- Disorder of arousal regulation

Identifying anxiety/aggression precipitated by anxiety

- Behaviors that surround:
  - Changes in routine
  - Transition between activities
  - Separation from attachment figure
  - Interruption of obsessive behavior

- Increased arousal/behavior changes surrounding discrete situations that may evoke fear

Identifying depression/emotional lability
- Establish a baseline for behavior prior to the onset of disruptive behavior
- Compare the patient's current state to this baseline in regards to crying spells, enjoyment of activities, interest in being around others, sleep patterns, eating patterns, and energy level
- Note intensity, frequency, and duration
- Establish treatment targets from above list

Identifying bipolar disorder/mood disorder NOS
- Are the behaviors clustering over time in a cyclical manner?
- Do they cluster into discrete periods of manic symptoms (decreased need for sleep, increased energy, laughing for no reason, or increased vocalizations)?
- If above answer is NO, but irritable depressive symptoms are present, treat depression
- If above answer is YES, refer to child psychiatrist

Medication Selection
- Use a medication class consistent with use in a typically developing child to treat the disorder you identified
- The presence of neurological impairment does not justify use of an antipsychotic or anticonvulsant as first line treatment for anxiety, depression or for a sleep disturbance

Treatment for sleep disturbance
- Treat sleep FIRST
- Monitor for pain
- Evaluate for spasticity

Treatment options for sleep disturbances
- Melatonin effective for circadian rhythm disorder, helps initiate sleep
- Some antihistamines help with sleep without causing daytime fatigue
- Clonidine effective in reducing sleep latency and night awakenings and for impulsive, inappropriate social behavior
- Trazodone—effective to keep individual asleep longer, potential SE—priapism
- Mirtazapine—effective if anxiety and decreased appetite are also problems, keep dose low
- Zolpidem can be effective for sleep initiation for a short time

- Quetiapine if agitation and aggression are also problems, not a first line medication

Anxiety/aggression treatment—First line
- Selective serotonin reuptake inhibitors (SSRIs)
  - Sertraline—comes in a liquid
  - Citalopram—comes in a liquid
  - Fluoxetine, escitalopram, and paroxetine have more anticholinergic side-effects, and/or are more activating than the above medications, which may limit the tolerance of these medications
- Black box warning needs to be explained to caregivers

Anxiety/aggression treatment—Second line
- α 2 agonists
  - Clonidine helpful for sleep as well
    Avoid the patch unless sure patient will not remove it and put it in mouth
  - Guanfacine is less sedating and has a longer half-life
- β blockers for sympathetic storming after TBI or an anoxic event
  - Propranolol—use hypertension dosing guidelines
- Monitor blood pressure, heart rate, and check electrocardiogram prior to adding to stimulant
- May precipitate depression

Anxiety/aggression treatment— Second or third line
- Benzodiazepines
  - Advantage is quick onset of action
  - May be effective in children who do not tolerate or respond to SSRIs and α 2 agonists
  - Potential to cause disinhibition and decrease rapid eye movement sleep
  - Avoid PRNs and prescribe long-acting preparations (clonazepam) as a scheduled dose
  - Avoid if possible in individuals with TBI due to slowing of processing speed

Anxiety/aggression treatment— Third or fourth line
- Atypical antipsychotic medications
  - Use a low dose if child is activated by a SSRI and has failed clonazepam or an α 2 agonist
  - Monitor weight, fasting lipids/glucose, waist circumference
  - Monitor for extrapyramidal side effects and tardive dyskinesia (TD)—use the Abnormal Involuntary Movement Scale to detect and follow TD
  - Akathisia is a common side effect both when increasing and reducing medication dose

- Need to withdrawal these medications very slowly (over months)
- Provide appropriate informed consent (metabolic complications, TD, dystonia, and neuroleptic malignant syndrome)

Anxiety/aggression treatment

- Risperidone
  - Start on a twice a day dosing and increase after 3 to 4 weeks at each dose
  - Consider another medication or diagnosis if 1 mg twice a day is not effective addressing anxiety
  - Weight gain can be a significant problem
- Quetiapine
  - Helpful with sleep
  - Weight gain can occur but usually not as bad as with risperidone or olanzapine
  - Has a broader dosing range than many of the other atypical antipsychotics
- Aripiprazole
  - Less weight gain and sedation than above atypical antipsychotics
  - Monitor closely for akathesia

Depression/emotional lability treatment

- SSRIs as in anxiety section
- Mirtazepine
  - Helpful with sleep issues and anxiety
  - Can increase appetite
  - Increasing dose can cause less nighttime sedation and less weight gain
- Medications we avoid
  - Tricyclic antidepressants due to sleep stage interference and lowering of seizure threshold
  - Buproprion because it lowers seizure threshold

ADHD treatment

- If anxiety, depression, or sleep disturbances are also present, treat those prior to addressing the ADHD symptoms
- Treat with stimulants, more literature on methylphenidate (Ritalin), but amphetamine (Dexedrine) has also been shown to be effective
- Each class has short-acting (2–3 hour), medium-acting (6–8 hour), and long-acting (10–12 hour) preparations
- Methylphenidate comes in a patch that can be used all day if individual cannot swallow a long-acting preparation
- Monitor blood pressure, heart rate, and consider electrocardiogram
- Monitor weight and height

- Do not use if sleep is a problem until sleep disturbance is resolved
- Consider atomoxetine if side effects of stimulants are not tolerated
- Consider α 2 agonists if stimulants are not tolerated
- Avoid buproprion due to the increased risk of seizures in patients with fragile brains

Disorders of arousal (after acquired brain injury)

- Stimulants demonstrate increased activity in the cerebral cortex, caudate nucleus, and mediofrontal cortex
- Activates dopamine/norepinephrine system
- Stimulants give most consistent response
- Amantadine causes the release of dopamine and may have a NMDS receptor antagonist effect
- Modafinil demonstrated uptake in the anterior hypothalamus, hippocampus, and amygdala
- Varying treatment outcomes reported with other medications other than stimulants

Spasticity

- Oral medications
  - Baclofen
    Usually well tolerated, can be given to very young, start very slow to minimize sedation
    Monitor compounding technique
  - Diazepam
    Monitor sedation and processing speed
  - Tizanidine
    Monitor sedation
  - Dantrolene
    Monitor LFTs
  - Clonidine—second line
- Neuromuscular injections
  - Botulinum toxins
    Monitor amounts per kilogram, monitor respiratory function
    Black box warning
  - Phenol—may need sedation to identify motor point with electrical stimulation
- Consider intrathecal baclofen pump insertion for increased generalized spasticity or opisthoclonus after acquired brain injury
- Consider medications very carefully on the basis of:
  - Other medical conditions have been ruled out
  - Target symptoms are adversely affecting function or relationships
  - Suboptimal response to behavioral interventions
  - Research evidence indicates target symptoms are amenable to pharmacologic intervention

General Guidelines

- Start low, go slow
- Limit polypharmacy
- Use medications that have more than one role/function
- Monitor side effects
- Reevaluate frequently

Helpful Resource

- DM-ID: Diagnostic Manual – Intellectual Disability: A Clinical Guide for Diagnosis of Mental Disorders in Persons with Intellectual Disabilities (ID)
- Provides examples of how patients with different degrees of ID may demonstrate specific psychiatric symptoms
- Example of a functional behavioral analysis—http://psychmed.osu.edu/ncbrf.htm

Suggested Readings

Deb S, Crownshaw T. The role of pharmacotherapy in the management of behaviour disorders in traumatic brain injury patients. *Brain Inj.* 2004;18(1):1–31.

Dekker MC, Koot HM. DSM-IV disorders in children with borderline to moderate intellectual disability.

I: prevalence and impact. *J Am Acad Child Adolesc Psychiatry.* 2003;42(8):915–922.

Fadden KS, Kastner TA. Common behavioral and emotional problems in children with developmental disabilities. *Pediatr Ann.* 1995;24(5):238–241.

Fletcher R, Loschen E, Stavrakaki, C, First M. *Diagnostic Manual-Intellectual Disability: A Clinical Guide for Diagnosis of Mental Disorders in Persons with Intellectual Disability.* Kingston, USA: NADD Press; 2007

Glenn MB, Wroblewski B. Twenty years of pharmacology. *J Head Trauma Rehabil.* 2005;20(1):51–61.

Ingrassia A, Turk J. The use of clonidine for severe and intractable sleep problems in children with neurodevelopmental disorders–a case series. *Eur Child Adolesc Psychiatry.* 2005;14(1):34–40.

Jan JE, Freeman RD. Melatonin therapy for circadian rhythm sleep disorders in children with multiple disabilities: what have we learned in the last decade? *Dev Med Child Neurol.* 2004;46(11):776–782.

Levy M, Berson A, Cook T, et al. Treatment of agitation following traumatic brain injury: a review of the literature. *NeuroRehabilitation.* 2005;20(4):279–306.

Posey DJ, Erickson CA, Stigler KA, McDougle CJ. The use of selective serotonin reuptake inhibitors in autism and related disorders. *J Child Adolesc Psychopharmacol.* 2006;16(1–2):181–186.

Silver J, Arciniegas D. Pharmacotherapy of neuropsychiatric disturbances. In: Zasler, ed. *Brain Injury Medicine.* New York: Demos; 2007: 963–993

Section I: Diagnostic Considerations

Electrodiagnostic Evaluation in Pediatric Rehabilitation

Maureen R. Nelson MD

Description

In children, there are physiological and developmental considerations that must be considered in electrodiagnostic examination and interpretation. It may be beneficial to approach the study a bit differently than with adults. There are neurological differences due to maturity, growth, and development. The physical size of the infant and child requires variation in technique. Normal values vary with age (adult by 3–5 years). The common problems seen also vary.

Physiology

Neural myelination begins between the 10th and 15th week of gestation and is complete by about 5 years. At 8 to 10 years of age, axons reach the same diameter as those found in adults. Nerve conduction velocity (NCV) depends on axon length and diameter, myelin sheath thickness, internodal distance, and node of Ranvier width. The diameter of larger ulnar motor axons approaches 3.5 to 4 μm in 1 month preterm infants, 4 to 6 μm in term infants, and 9 to 13 μm in adults.

Nerve conduction changes in childhood and adolescence show different NCV maturation in boys and girls. NCVs are faster in all nerves except the median in girls than boys.

Nerve maturation is measured by age from conception, not from birth, since there is no change in the rate of acceleration of myelination at birth. This has been confirmed for the posterior tibial nerve. Since NCV is correlated with gestational age, it may be useful in the assessment of neurological maturity and evaluation of gestational age (though not very practical since physical examination may generally easily be used). There is no correlation between NCV and birth weight so that term infants who are small for gestational age have a NCV in the same range as larger term infants. Motor NCV in term newborns is faster than in premature infants and slower than in newborns of prolonged gestational age (43–44 weeks). Ulnar nerve NCV for premature infants averages 21 m/s, for term newborns it is 28 m/s; which is approximately half that of the adults studied with a value of 60 m/s. Conduction velocity at 23 to 24 weeks of fetal life is approximately 1/3 of the velocity of term newborns, with a velocity of approximately 7 to 8 m/s for a tibial or a median nerve. Normal NCV values are achieved by 3 to 5 years.

Compound muscle action potential (CMAP) amplitude is quite variable in infants and children. Median CMAP amplitude averages 4 mV at 1 month of age; increase to 14.1 mV at 6 to 11 years. Amplitude of the CMAP increases approximately 3-fold from birth to 11 years.

Sensory NCV is 50% of adult values, and achieves that level by approximately 4 years of age. The sensory response has been described as sometimes showing a bifid response with two distinct peaks, possibly representing two groups of fibers which have different maturation.

The H-reflex is easily obtained in most nerves from premature infants and term infants. It is increasingly difficult to obtain throughout the first year, and after age 1, the H-reflex is only rarely obtained, except for the tibial and median nerves.

Changes with development also occur with F-waves in children. The mean ulnar nerve F-wave is 14.6 ms from infancy to 2½ years and then gradually increases and reaches its adult value by 20 years of age, as do other nerves. The time period with no change in F-wave latency is described as the "lag time" for F-wave values. This is a period of time with a very rapid increase in conduction velocity and also of increase in arm length, occurring in the first three years of life. The balance of these two factors is reported to be responsible for the lag time. After approximately age 3, the arm length increases more than conduction velocity, so the F-wave latency increases.

The blink reflex is composed of two responses. The R1 is easily elicited in infants which is felt to be due to the fact that it is a central reflex arc and is already established at birth. The R2 is elicited in 2/3 of neonates, and is least common contralaterally, so it is not considered abnormal if it is not obtained.

Approach to Evaluation

The electrodiagnostic evaluation may present more of a challenge in a child because of technical considerations, and is potentially even more valuable because of the frequent inability to provide historical information, or to cooperate with motor exam. The approach to examining infants and children must be altered from that in the adult because of the child's behavioral characteristics. The study ideally is carefully described in a calm, matter of fact, and straight-forward manner. A useful method is to demonstrate electrical stimulation on oneself, describing the sensory response and showing a clinical motor response, and then allow the parents to feel a sensory level stimulation. Consideration may be given to calling the electrode a "wire electrode" or "pin" instead of a needle due to the emotional connotation of that word. I believe it is useful to cup the wire electrode in the examiner's hand so that neither the parent nor the child sees it. During the study, the child, parent, and examiner must be as comfortable as possible, commonly with a younger child or baby on the parent's lap. The level of discomfort is variable. It is reportedly performed with parents present 68% of the time. It has not been studied in electrodiagnosis but in other areas of pediatrics where procedures are performed, both parents and children were more satisfied with the health care system when parents are present during procedures.

Nerve conduction studies

Sensory nerve conduction studies can be performed in the usual antidromic manner, but grasp reflex may cause movement artifact to obliterate the results. This problem can be minimized by using the orthodromic technique, using ring electrodes to stimulate from the digits, with the recording electrodes over the nerve at the wrist or ankle. In both sensory and motor NCS, the reference electrode usually will be placed on a separate digit to maintain interelectrode distance, with a ring electrode a useful reference for both motor and sensory studies.

The standard stimulating distances of 8 and 14 cm are not possible for infants and small children due to their small limbs, so the traditional anatomical locations for stimulation are used and the distances used are reported with the results. It may be useful to compare nerve to nerve and side to side.

The largest source of error in NCS in infants is measurement error, which is more of a problem in infants than adults due to shorter nerve lengths. Surface measurement error of 1 cm can change the value of the infant NCV by 15%. Bony landmarks are difficult to evaluate due to adipose tissue in many youngsters. Stimulus

artifact may cause more abnormality in infants and small children due to shorter distances between the simulator and recording electrodes. This can be minimized by keeping the skin dry and by decreasing the skin impedance. Make sure that moisturizing lotion is thoroughly removed and the skin is as dry as possible. Commercially available self-sticking electrodes help to minimize this problem since electrode gel is not needed.

Repetitive stimulation

Infants differ from adults in their normal response to repetitive nerve stimulation, according to an extremely small but widely quoted study. It states that with stimulation <5 Hz CMAP is stable, at 5 to 10 Hz some normal infants show 10% or greater facilitation of CMAP, at 20 Hz most infants show a decrement of approximately 24%, with the decrement greatest in premature infants, and that at >50 Hz stimulation virtually all infants show a decrement. It was described that this demonstrates that infants have a lower normal neuromuscular junction reserve than do older individuals.

A padded IV board can be used to immobilize the wrist, hand, and fingers for repetitive stimulation. The stimulation electrodes should also be secured to the limb, not held by hand, to avoid movement error.

Electromyography

Electromyography (EMG) should be carefully planned and efficiently performed in an infant and young child. It should include proximal and distal musculature in upper and lower limbs (depending on diagnostic considerations). Frequently, the discomfort of needle insertion will allow immediate evaluation of recruitment; if not the following may be useful:

- Positive (toy or candy) or negative (sharp) stimuli
- Primitive reflexes
- Positioning of the muscle is also helpful for evaluating both recruitment and spontaneous activity of muscle
- Natural flexed positioning of infants, the biceps, iliopsoas, flexor digitorum superficialis, and anterior tibialis; recruitment; and extensor muscles for evaluating insertional and spontaneous activity

Diagnostic Considerations

Diagnostic considerations vary between adults and children—more common requests are for evaluation of floppy babies and congenital muscle or nerve diseases (not carpal tunnel syndrome, peripheral neuropathy, radiculopathy). The many advances in genetic studies are decreasing the need for electrodiagnosis in that area, though it is still useful to direct care in acute areas such as botulism, and to direct further workup in some processes. Theoretically, it may become more of an issue in children as they continue to have more potential for overuse syndromes with the popularity of videogames, computer, and texting. An example of an electrodiagnostic approach to the floppy baby follows.

Floppy baby
- Abnormality can be at the level of the brain, spinal cord, anterior horn cell, nerve, neuromuscular junction, muscle, or connective tissue
- The etiology of hypotonia in an infant is most commonly central
- Nerve conduction studies and EMG can help distinguish between possible levels of involvement and assist with diagnosis

Floppy baby etiology
- Brain: Hypoxia; ischemia; hemorrhage
- Spinal cord: Trauma; vascular compromise; congenital anomaly
- Anterior horn cell: Spinal muscular atrophy; poliomyelitis
- Peripheral nerve: Guillain-Barre Syndrome; hereditary motor sensory neuropathy (HSMN); congenital hypomyelination
- Neuromuscular junction: Myasthenia gravis (4 types); botulism
- Medications (magnesium; aminoglycosides)

- Muscle: Congenital muscular dystrophy; congenital myotonic dystrophy; congenital myopathies
- Systemic disease: Prader Willi syndrome; Down syndrome
- Metachromatic or Krabbe's leukodystrophy
- Benign congenital hypotonia

Floppy baby electrodiagnosis
- Sensory nerve conduction studies
  - >1 arm and 1 leg; abnormalities in HSMN and polyneuropathy
- Motor nerve conduction studies
  - >1 arm and 1 leg; include F-waves
- Repetitive stimulation
  - If maternal history of myasthenia gravis, baby has ptosis or constipation (honey), multiple motor responses to single stimulation, botulism, aminoglycosides, and maternal dosage of magnesium sulfate
- Somatosensory evoked potentials—consider in evaluation of spinal cord injury
- EMG—selective

Suggested Readings

Jones HR, Bolton CF, Harper CM, eds. *Pediatric Clinical Electromyography*. Philadelphia, PA: Lippincott-Raven Publishers; 1996.

Nelson MR. Electrodiagnostic evaluation of children. In: Dumitru D, Amato AA, Zwarts M, eds. *Electrodiagnostic Medicine*. 2nd ed. Philadelphia, PA: Hanley & Belfus, Inc; 2002:1433–1448.

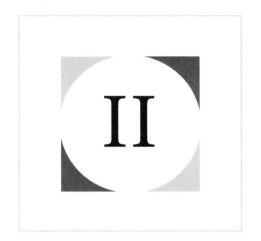

Pediatric Diseases and Complications

Amputation: Lower Extremity

Joshua Jacob Alexander MD FAAP FAAPMR ■ Brian M. Kelly DO ■ Virginia Simson Nelson MD MPH

Description
Congenital or acquired limb loss at the hip, femur, knee, tibia, ankle, or foot.

Etiology/Types
- Congenital outnumbers acquired 2:1
- Hip disarticulation
- Transfemoral
- Knee disarticulation
- Transtibial
- Ankle disarticulation: retention of calcaneal fat pad (Syme)
- Preservation of the calcaneus (Boyd)
- Chopart (removes the mid-foot and forefoot)
- The ISO/ISPO system is the standard for classifying congenital limb deficiency. In this system, transverse deficiencies are named at the segment where the limb terminates. Longitudinal deficiencies are named for the bones partially or totally affected and the fraction missing

Epidemiology
- Fibular longitudinal deficiency (fibular hemimelia) is most common
  - 25% of cases are bilateral
  - Manifests clinically as valgus foot, short leg, unstable knee, and/or unstable ankle
- Transtibial deficiency: more common than transfemoral
  - Longitudinal deficiency of tibia
- Longitudinal deficiency of femur or proximal femoral focal deficiency (PFFD)
  - Incidence 1 in 50,000 births
  - 10% to 15% cases are bilateral
- Acquired deficiencies
  - Trauma is most common cause of acquired amputation
  - Single limb loss occurs 90% of the time with 60% involving the lower extremity
  - Power tools and machines are most common cause followed by vehicular crashes, gunshot injuries, burns, and landmines (outside of United States)
  - Boys:girls ratio is 3:2
  - Childhood tumors are the most frequent cause of disease-related amputation
    - Osteogenic sarcoma and Ewing's sarcoma are the most common
    - Highest incidence of tumors between 12 and 21 years
- Infection/disease—purpura fulminans from meningococcal septicemia (may be multilimb)
- Dysvascular (uncommon in children)

Risk Factors
- High-risk behaviors
- Cancer
- Infection

Clinical Features
- Acquired amputation will affect the growth plate and may result in limb length discrepancies
- A young child may start to cry or refuse to wear the prosthesis when it is not comfortable

Natural History
- In children, limbs grow faster longitudinally than circumferentially
- Limb length discrepancies can affect posture and gait and may contribute to functional scoliosis
- Most children require a new prosthesis annually until age 5, then every 2 years between 5 and 12 years, and every 3 to 4 years until adulthood
- Phantom pain may develop, especially > 10 years old, but the incidence is less and severity is milder than in adults

Diagnosis

Differential diagnosis
- N/A

History
- Developmental and medical histories, including all trauma
- Define the functional goals of the family

Exam
- Evaluate for physical and developmental level
- Evaluate for painful terminus
- Evaluate limb for residual soft tissue (may influence suspension of prosthesis)
- Examine other areas for signs of compensation/complications
- Check for scoliosis

Testing
- X-ray and magnetic resonance imaging of involved limb can be helpful in planning surgical intervention and prosthetic rehabilitation

Pitfalls
- Hip or knee flexion contractures
- Bursa formation
- Long transfemoral amputation performed in a young child will likely result in a short residual limb, since 70% of femur growth comes from the distal femoral epiphysis
- Fitting at a later age results in a higher rate of prosthetic rejection

Red Flags
- Bony overgrowth

Treatment

Medical
- Maintain optimal postoperative pain control
- Gabapentin may be useful for children with phantom limb pain following amputation
- For infants, fit with prosthesis when ready to pull to stand

Exercises
- Range of motion, strengthening, flexibility exercises should begin as soon as possible after amputation
- Reduce residual limb edema, enhance mobility, optimize balance, and improve independence with ADLs

Modalities/prostheses hypothesize
- SACH foot is most common foot prescribed for children
- Typical prosthetic knees include single axis, polycentric, and fluid controlled
- Children often cannot control an articulated knee joint until age 2 to 3

- A transfemoral prosthesis is fit with no knee joint and a Silesian belt (an elastic suspension belt going from the front to the back of the prosthesis, around the waist) in children less than 2 years
- Suspension systems don't use suction until the child can assist with donning (age 5+)
- Suspension sleeves and silicone suction suspension sleeves are used with growth liners
- Growth liners may consist two or more layers of material to change as the child grows
- Total suction suspension for children ages 6+

Injection
- Possible for painful neuromas

Surgical
- Try to maintain maximal limb length
- Consider disarticulation over short transosseous amputation
- Consider residual limb capping to prevent recurrent bony overgrowth
- Skin grafting
- Van Ness rotational plasty for PFFD allows simulation of below knee function by rotating the foot 180° so the ankle acts as knee joint

Consults
- Prosthetist
- Orthopedic surgery

Complications of treatment
- Major causes of gait deviations are growth or worn prosthetic parts
- Approximately 12% of children with acquired limb loss will experience bony (terminal) overgrowth, an appositional overgrowth of new bone at the transected end of a long bone
- A bursa may develop over the end of the sharp bone, or the bone may protrude through the skin
- Painful neuromas
- Dermatologic problems can include stump scarring, shear injury, and/or pressure ulcer development at stump/socket interface
- Phantom pain may develop, but the incidence is lower than in adults

Prognosis
- Parental acceptance of the prosthesis is necessary for the child to accept it

- Pediatric amputees generally achieve good functional outcomes
- Increased energy expenditure for ambulation dependent upon length of residual limb and type of prosthesis used

Helpful Hints

- Benefits of saving the growth plate include reduced leg length discrepancy and fewer fitting problems
- The residual limb continues to grow until skeletal maturity is achieved
- Adjustment period with social and psychological support of patient and family is important to address sense of loss and altered body image

- Limb salvage techniques common in tumor-associated conditions

Suggested Readings

Cummings D. General prosthetic considerations. In: Smith DF, Michael JW, Bowker JH, eds. *Atlas of Amputations and Limb Deficiencies: Surgical, Prosthetic, and Rehabilitation principles.* 3rd ed. Rosemont, IL: American Academy of Orthopaedic Surgeons; 2004:789–799.

Nelson VS, Flood KM, Bryant PR, Huang ME, Pasquina PF, Roberts TL. Limb deficiency and prosthetic management. 1. Decision making in prosthetic prescription and management. *Arch Phys Med Rehabil.* 2006;87 (3 suppl 1):S3-S9.

Amputation: Upper Extremity

Virginia Simson Nelson MD MPH ▪ Brian M. Kelly DO

Description
Congenital or acquired limb loss at the finger, arm, wrist, or elbow.

Etiology/Types
- Pediatric limb deficiencies are approximately 60% congenital versus acquired
- Congenital deletions occur during the third to eighth week of gestation
- The ISO/ISPO system is the standard for classifying congenital limb deficiency. In this system, transverse deficiencies are named at the segment where the limb terminates. Longitudinal deficiencies are named for the bones partially or totally affected and the fraction missing
- Amelia: absence of limb
- Hemimelia: absence of half limb
- Phocomelia: flipper-like appendage attached to the trunk
- Acheiria: missing hand
- Adactyly: absent metacarpal or metatarsal
- Aphalangia: absent finger or toe

Epidemiology

Congenital deficiencies
- Rates of congenital limb anomalies are approximately 26 per 100,000 live births
- Upper limb deficiencies account for 58.5% of congenital limb anomalies
- Congenital conditions are the most common cause of limb deficiency in children younger than age 10
- The most common deficiency is left transradial
- There are several upper limb syndromes associated with radial deficiency, including thrombocytopenia with absent radius syndrome, Fanconi (syndrome with amputation and leukopenia), Holt-Oram (syndrome with amputation and congenital heart defects) and VACTERL (syndrome with vertebral, anal atresia, cardiac, tracheoesophageal fistula, renal, and limb anomalies)

Acquired deficiencies
- Trauma is the most common cause
- Single limb loss occurs 90% of the time with 40% involving upper extremity

- Boys:girls 3:2
- Childhood tumors are the most frequent cause of disease-related amputation
- Osteogenic sarcoma and Ewing's sarcoma occur most commonly
- Highest incidence of tumors is in the 12 to 21 year age group

Risk Factors
- High-risk behaviors
- Cancer
- Infection
- Most limb deletions are not hereditary
- Craniofacial abnormalities may be associated with upper limb deletions

Clinical Features
- Children with unilateral congenital transverse radial limb deficiency typically develop normally
- Acquired amputation will affect the growth plate so may result in shorter limb length
- A young child may start to cry or refuse to wear the prosthesis when it is not comfortable
- Children may develop bony overgrowth

Natural History
- Phantom pain may develop, especially >10-year old, but the incidence is less and the severity is milder than in adults
- Most children require a new prosthesis annually until age 5, then every 2 years between 5 and 12 years, and every 3 to 4 years until adulthood
- Scoliosis risk

Diagnosis

Differential diagnosis
- N/A

History
- Obtain developmental and medical histories; associated trauma
- Define the functional goals of the family

Exam
- Evaluate for other physical deficits
- Developmental level

- Evaluate for painful terminus
- Evaluate limb for residual soft tissue

Testing
- X-ray and magnetic resonance imaging can be helpful in planning surgeries and prosthetic rehabilitation

Pitfalls
- Fitting at a later age has been shown to result in greater rejection of the prosthesis

Red Flags
- Bony overgrowth

Treatment

Medical
- Pain management for acquired amputations
- Gabapentin may be used for phantom pain

Exercises
- General strengthening and stretching, promote age-appropriate activities of daily living

Modalities/prostheses
- Prostheses for children should have a growth liner
- Unilateral arm deficiency is fitted around 6 months (sit-to-fit)
- A passive mitt may be used initially, but these are only useful for 2 to 3 months
- For infants with transhumeral limb deletions, fit is delayed 3 months. An elbow joint is not used or is locked initially. A friction elbow is used initially that can be manually positioned in the desired position. An active elbow the child can control is initially used at 24 to 36 months. Activation of the terminal device (TD) to open should occur around 12 to 15 months
- Start with body-powered components
- Body-powered hands provide good cosmesis but weak pinch force
- A hook style TD allows improved dexterity
- A child's initial myoelectric device will be simple. The child contracts a muscle and the TD opens and will close automatically as soon as the contraction relaxes. This is referred to as a "cookie crusher system"
- Suspension system does not use suction until at least age 5 when the child can assist with donning
- A growth liner may consist of two or more layers of material. As the child grows and becomes too large for the insert, the inner layer can be removed

Surgical
- Some need revision to improve prosthetic fit or function
- Vilkke procedure: attaches a toe to the residual limb to create a pincher grip with the transferred great toe. No complication in the foot results from the procedure

Consults
- Prosthetist
- Orthopedic surgery
- Occupational therapy: children usually only need 1 to 2 sessions to learn to use UE prosthesis with a home program
- Children's Special Health Care Services (Title V agency) may provide extra insurance coverage for prosthesis and therapy

Complications of treatment
- Approximately 12% of children with acquired limb loss will experience bony overgrowth, less with congenital. The result is a distal spike-like bone that tends to grow faster than the overlying tissues and skin
- A bursa may develop over the end of the sharp bone, or the end of the bone may protrude through the skin
- Dermatologic problems include contact dermatitis, folliculitis, sebaceous cysts, excessive sweating, and scars from trauma

Prognosis
- Parental acceptance of the prosthesis is necessary for the child to accept prosthesis

Helpful Hints
- Joint disarticulation amputation is preferred before a long-bone transverse amputation
- The child with isolated limb deficiency or amputation is capable of achieving age-level skills

Suggested Readings
Jain S. Rehabilitation in limb deficiency. 2. The pediatric amputee. *Arch Phys Med Rehabil.* 1996;77(3 suppl):S9-S13.

Nelson VS, Flood KM, Bryant PR, Huang ME, Pasquina PF, Roberts TL. Limb deficiency and prosthetic management. 1. Decision making in prosthetic prescription and management. *Arch Phys Med Rehabil.* 2006;87(3 suppl 1):S3–S9.

Arthrogryposis

Kenneth M. Jaffe MD

Description

More than 300 clinical entities have been identified with multiple congenital joint contractures, so-called arthrogryposis multiplex congenita. Amyoplasia is the most prevalent form of this heterogeneous group of disorders. The term means *a*, no; *myo*, muscle; and *plasia*, growth.

Etiology/Types

- Amyoplasia is a sporadic disorder
- Cause is unknown, but thought to be multifactorial
- Three principal groups:
  - Mainly limb involvement (amyoplasia and distal forms of arthrogryposis)
  - Involvement of the limb and other body structures
  - Limb involvement and central nervous system dysfunction. (Up to 50% of these children die as newborns, accounting for the increased prevalence of those with limb involvement)

Epidemiology

- Approximately 1 in 200 infants is born with some form of joint contracture or joint stiffness [isolated clubfoot (1/500), congenital dislocated hip (1/200–1/500) or multiple contractures (1/3000)]
- Incidence of amyoplasia is 1/10,000 live births (one-third of all cases of liveborns with arthrogryposis)

Pathogenesis

- Intrauterine joint formation during embryogenesis is normal
- Subsequent lack of fetal joint movement leads to contracture through multiple causes:
  - Neurologic deficits
  - Fetal crowding
  - Maternal illness
  - Connective tissue or skeletal defects
  - Vascular compromise
  - Muscle defects

Risk Factors

- Twins/multiples

Clinical Features

- Normal intelligence
- Limb involvement: typically symmetrical (all limbs 84%, legs only 11%, arms only 5%)
- Upper limbs: internally rotated, down sloping shoulders; extended elbows; pronated forearms; flexed wrists and fingers
- Lower limbs: variable, with hips commonly flexed, abducted, and externally rotated, or extended and subluxated or dislocated; flexed or extended knees; equinovarus foot deformities
- Skin; midline facial hemangioma (flame nevus)
- Spine: approximately one-third with scoliosis
- Other: micrognathia, abdominal wall defects (i.e., gastroschisis), bowel atresia, genital abnormalities (cryptorchidism in males, labial abnormalities in females), poor enteral intake, constipation, poor weight gain, and failure to thrive

Natural History

- Worst contractures present at birth—respond to early stretching, casting, and splinting
- Potential for excellent functional outcomes with proper management
- Ambulation: 50% to 85% household or community ambulators (decreases into adulthood)
- Maximal function achieved by age 10 years (dependent on appropriately timed orthopedic surgery and rehabilitation)
- Lower levels of physical activity than typically developing peers
- ADL's: 75% independent for feeding, 35% for toileting, 25% for bathing, 20% for grooming, and 10% for dressing
- Poorly documented functional skills in adulthood

Diagnosis

Differential diagnosis

- Distal arthrogryposis type I
- Bony abnormalities such as fusions (i.e., symphalangism)
- Contractural arachnodactly (Beals syndrome)
- Multiple pterygium syndromes
- Osteochondrodysplasia (dwarfing conditions)

History
- Intrauterine restriction/reduced fetal movement
- Delayed motor milestones
- Normal intellectual development
- Neuromuscular disease

Exam
- Limb range of motion (ROM) and strength
- Spine
- See Clinical Features

Testing
- Extensive diagnostic workup (i.e., electrodiagnostics, nerve or muscle biopsy, and genetic testing) is unnecessary without specific clinical indications

Treatment

Medical
- Monitor growth and maximize nutrition
- Manage constipation

Exercises
- Passive ROM beginning shortly after birth

Modalities
- Splinting and casting
- Developmentally appropriate mobility aids and adaptive equipment

Injections
- N/A

Surgical
- Orthopedic management for correction of clubfoot deformities
- Correction of unilateral hip dislocation (correction of bilateral dislocations is controversial); management of hip contractures
- Management of knee abnormalities for successful ambulation or sitting

Consults
- Orthopedic surgery

Prognosis
- Potential ambulators have grade 4 or greater hip extensor strength, hip contractures less than 20°, and grade 3 or 4 quadriceps strength, with less than 20° knee flexion contracture, good torso strength and sitting balance, and the ability to knee walk

Helpful Hints
- Surgery places joint arc of motion in functional position—it does not change the arc of that joint

Suggested Readings
Bevan WP, Hall JG, Bamshad M, Staheli LT, Jaffe KM, Song K. Arthrogryposis multiplex congenita (amyoplasia): an orthopaedic perspective. *J Pediatr Orthop*. 2007;27(5):594–600.

Staheli LS, Hall JG, Jaffe KM, Paholke DO, eds. *Arthrogryposis: A Text Atlas*. New York, NY: Cambridge University Press; 1998.

Attention Deficit Hyperactivity Disorder

James R. Christensen MD

Description

Neurodevelopmental disorder with impaired executive function, self-regulation, and in some cases inhibition; results in impulsiveness, hyperactivity, and inattention.

Etiology/Types

- Three forms of attention-deficit hyperactivity disorder (ADHD)
  - ADHD-CT (combined type)
  - ADHD-PI (predominantly inattentive type)
  - ADHD-PH/I (predominantly hyperactive-impulsive type)
- Secondary "ADHD" due to known etiology (TBI, CNS infections, etc.)

Epidemiology

- Prevalence is from 8% to 12%
- Two to three times more common in males
- Girls more likely to have ADHD-PI, boys ADHD-CT

Pathogenesis

- Dysfunction in the fronto-subcortical-cerebellar catecholaminergic circuits
- Neuroimaging: structural differences in frontal lobes, basal ganglia, corpus callosum, and cerebellum; reduced gray and white matter volume; functional magnetic resonance imaging shows hypoactivation of fronto-striatal and fronto-parietal networks
- Genes implicated include those associated with multiple neurotransmitters

Risk Factors

- Polygenic inheritance (heritability estimated at 65%–90%)
- Increased adverse perinatal factors, toxins (fetal alcohol exposure, maternal cigarette smoking, and elevated lead levels), environmental exposures, stress, sleep disorders, and nutritional deficiencies

Clinical Features

- Executive dysfunction
- Inattention ± hyperactivity/impulsivity
- Significant intraindividual variability
- Common comorbidities: learning disabilities, adaptive dysfunction, developmental coordination disorder, oppositional defiant disorder, conduct disorder, tic disorders, depression, anxiety, sleep difficulties, and voiding disorders

Natural History

- ADHD-CT: the most common and persistent type
- ADHD-PH/I: often transforms into ADHD-CT
- Majority still meet criteria and require care for ADHD as adolescents and adults
- Pharmacotherapy of ADHD decreases risk of substance-use disorder by 50%

Diagnosis

Differential diagnosis

- Vision and hearing problems
- Poor nutrition
- Sleep disorder
- Thyroid disease
- Seizure disorder (absence seizures)
- Syndromes (fragile X, fetal alcohol, Williams)
- Social stressors
- Learning or intellectual disabilities
- Pervasive developmental disorder (PDD)
- Anxiety
- Depression

History

- Maladaptive and developmentally inappropriate symptoms of inattention, hyperactivity, and impulsivity
- Onset before 7 years
- Impairment present in at least two settings (eg, school, work, and home)
- Interference with social, academic, or occupational functioning
- Persistence for at least 6 months
- Cannot be better attributed to another mental disorder, PDD or psychosis

Exam

- Signs of inattention, hyperactivity, and impulsivity
- Possible impaired or delayed fine and gross motor coordination, especially in boys

Testing

- Clinical diagnosis. Medical tests often not required (dictated by differential diagnoses)
- Rating scales from parents and teachers useful for supporting diagnosis, screening for other behavioral issues, and for monitoring
- Broadband rating scales include the Child Behavior Checklist (Achenbach) or Conners' Rating Scales
- Narrowband rating scales specific to ADHD include Vanderbilt scales

Pitfalls

- Child interview essential to distinguish ADHD from internalizing disorders (anxiety, depression)
- Failure to recognize inattention
- Inattention related to other conditions such as PDD
- Inappropriate expectations for child with intellectual disabilities

Red Flags

- Late or abrupt onset of symptoms is likely not ADHD
- Deteriorating neurological function
- Parent with psychiatric disorder or ADHD, or parental disagreement on management

Treatment

Medical

- Medications: First choice are stimulants (short- or long-acting forms of methylphenidate or dextroamphetamine); second choice are nonstimulants
- Monitor with feedback from home and school (rating scales for symptoms and medication side effects)
- Recommend appropriate classroom accommodations (preferential seating, nonverbal cues for off-task behavior, unlimited time for test completion, tailored assignments so that work may be completed in a reasonable time frame, organizational aids, and a positive reward system)

Exercises

- Attention training

Consults

- Behavioral therapy/parent training for significant child-parental discord, continuing oppositional behavior, children younger than 5 years of age
- Neuropsychology and/or education
- Speech therapy evaluation and treatment for communication disorders
- Occupational therapy for fine motor and ADL deficits, dysgraphia
- Physical therapy for coordination deficits
- Mental health for psychiatric comorbidity
- Executive coach

Complications of treatment

- Common medication side effects: poor appetite, headache and stomach ache, delayed sleep onset, and weight loss

Prognosis

- Medication and parent training result in significant clinical improvement
- Chronic course: symptoms usually persist in modified fashion over time
- Risk factors for poor outcome: poverty, family discord, and family psychopathology

Helpful Hints

- Medications must be titrated upward until no further benefits are seen, as long as side effects are tolerable. Don't stop too early
- To assess treatment of inattention, have family measure target behaviors (eg, length of time required for task completion, number of calls from teacher)
- Secondary ADHD may not respond as well to mono-medication therapy and will usually require multidisciplinary evaluations and interventions

Suggested Readings

Biederman J, Faraone SV. Attention-deficit hyperactivity disorder. *Lancet.* 2005;366(9481):237–248.

Rappley MD. Clinical practice. Attention deficit-hyperactivity disorder. *N Engl J Med.* 2005;13;352(2):165–173.

Autism

Rajashree Srinivasan MD

Description

Autism is a neurodevelopmental disorder of the brain presenting with impairment in social interaction, communication, and imaginative play. Children have stereotypic and ritualistic behaviors. Signs and symptoms present at 18 months to 2 years of age.

Etiology/Types

- Thought to be multifactorial
- Genetic—seen in twins, family history
- Environment—prenatal and postnatal—maternal infection, teratogens, pesticides, thyroid problems, folic acid, lead poisoning, and mercury exposure all theorized to be involved but not proven etiologies
- Autistic spectrum disorders (ASD) comprise Autism, Asperger's syndrome, Rett's disorder, Childhood disintegrative disorder, and Pervasive developmental disorder

Epidemiology

- In the United States, the prevalence of autism is 1 to 2 per 1000
- Prevalence of ASD is 6 per 1000
- The increase in the prevalence and incidence from the 1980s to current values is likely due to better diagnosis and increased awareness, or there may be different environmental influences
- Boys affected more than girls, 4:1

Pathogenesis

- No clear mechanism defining pathophysiology
- Thought possibly due to abnormal local overconnectivity and abnormal formation of synapses and dendritic spines

Risk Factors

- Familial
- Environmental theorized

Clinical Features

- Typical history of problems with language, communication, and behavior emerges at about age 2
- May have a lack of eye contact, difficulty playing with others

- No response to name when called
- Delayed speech
- IQ varies from impaired to high range
- Due to associated sensory integration disorder, nutrition may be affected

Natural History

- Variable

Diagnosis

- Based on Autism Diagnostic Observation Scale (ADOS) which evaluates social interaction and play

Differential diagnosis

- Hearing loss
- Cerebral palsy (CP)—10% of patients with CP have autistic features
- Fragile X syndrome—DNA testing for mutation of FMR1 gene on X chromosome
- Angelman's syndrome—Chromosomal tests
- Metabolic diseases
- Asperger's—is a developmental disorder which is part of autism spectrum disorder, presenting with difficulties in social interaction, language delay, one-sided conversation, and problems with cognitive development; problems with nonverbal communication, clumsiness, and decreased empathy

History

- Usually significant for lack of eye contact early on, incessant crying, difficulty soothing, and impaired pretend play

Exam

- Based on behavior

Testing

- ADOS is the gold standard. It is a standardized behavioral observation protocol to objectively assess social and communicative behavior associated with autism, giving scores for autism, and autism spectrum disorder

Pitfalls

- Difficult to recognize early on as parallel play is a normal phenomenon

Red Flags

- Speech delay
- Difficulties in playing with other children

Treatment

- Focus on behavioral training, positive reinforcement of DESIRED behavior
- Early intervention as soon as possible
- Focus on improving language, communication, and social interaction
- ABA—Applied behavior analysis
- TEECCH—Treatment and Education of Autistic and Related Communication Handicapped Children
- Physical therapy focus on gross motor skills
- Occupational therapy focus on arm strengthening, fine motor coordination skills, and sensory integration
- Speech therapy focuses on language and speech; pragmatic skills
- Medications to treat anxiety, depression, attention deficit, and hyperactivity often prescribed, though not proven to help autism
- Family psychological support for stress
- Visual therapies often helpful as some think well with pictures
- Parents often try different unproven approaches, including chelation, to attempt to treat heavy metal disturbance; along with mega-vitamin doses, and mineral supplements, though unproven
- Music therapy, animal assisted therapy, and vest therapy are also commonly tried but unproven

Consults

- Developmental pediatrics
- Child psychiatry
- Pediatric neurology

Prognosis

- Variable

Helpful Hints

- Listen to parents with concerns of social deficiencies
- A.L.A.R.M fact sheet
  - **A**—Autism is prevalent
  - **L**—Listen to parents
  - **A**—Act early
  - **R**—Refer
  - **M**—Monitor

Suggested Readings

Carr JE, LeBlanc LA. Autism spectrum disorders in early childhood: an overview for practicing physicians. *Prim Care.* 2007;34(2):343–359.

Myers SM, Johnson CP. Management of children with autism spectrum disorders. *Pediatrics.* 2007;120(5):1162–1182.

Blount's Disease

Maurice Sholas MD PhD

Description

A progressive and excessive varus alignment and shortening of the legs due to partial fusion of the medial portion of the proximal tibia. There is a depression of the medial tibial plateau, causing joint incongruity and instability.

Etiology/Types

- The result of a focal growth arrest of the medial proximal tibial physis
- Progressively, this leads to internal rotation and varus deformity of the knee
- Other names used to describe this condition include osteochondrosis deformans tibiae and tibia vara
- Most commonly, this is a disease of adolescence and preadolescence, but there is an infantile presentation at 9 to 36 months

Epidemiology

- Uncommon growth disorder
- Less than 1% prevalence in the general population
- Increased incidence in obese, black males (except in infantile type) where the prevalence is 2.5%
- Infantile presentation is more prevalent in females unlike the more typical presentation in preadolescence

Pathogenesis

- Multifactorial process
- Weight bearing is a prerequisite as this does not occur in nonambulatory children
- There is believed to be an alteration in endochondral bone formation that is exacerbated by compressive forces
- The pathogenesis represents an extreme of Volkmann's law where compressive forces inhibit physeal bone growth and distraction forces stimulate it
- There is also believed to be an element of cartilaginous damage that results in slowed ossification and growth limitation
- The progressive nature of this process is likely related to cyclical growth arrest, varus deformity, and additional arrest

Risk Factors

- No proof of genetic inheritance
- Not associated with trauma or infection
- Some have a prior family history
- Obesity
- Male
- Black

Clinical Features

- Progressive bowing of the legs
- Medial knee pain
- Can be unilateral with significant leg length discrepancy

Natural History

- Infantile presentation is at 9 to 10 months and is more severely progressive
- Infantile presentation is more commonly bilateral
- Standard presentation starts in the second decade
- Initially there is progressive tibia vara with medial knee pain. Subsequently, there can be distal femoral deformities as well
- Long term, there is an increased risk of osteoarthritis due to abnormal distribution of forces across nearby joints

Diagnosis

Differential diagnosis

- Tibial plateau fracture
- Osteochondritis dessicans
- Osteoarthritis
- Tendonitis
- Physiological genu varus
- Growth plate fracture

History

- History of medial knee pain
- Medial, proximal tibial tenderness
- Leg length discrepancy
- Clumsiness with walking and gross motor skills

Exam

- Point tenderness at medial aspect of the tibia distal to the plateau
- Genu varus
- Leg length discrepancy

Testing
- X-rays demonstrate the early focal closure of the proximal tibial growth plate
- X-rays also allow quantification of the degree of angulation

Pitfalls
- Over interpretation of imaging studies

Red Flags
- Rapidly progressive bowing of the lower extremities
- Genu varum with leg length discrepancy

Treatment

Medical
- Analgesics
- Quarterly imaging to document progression
- No required monitoring beyond skeletal maturity

Exercises
- Maintain quadriceps strength
- Maintain foot dorsiflexor and plantiflexor strength
- Maintain passive and active range of motion about the knee

Modalities
- Cryotherapy

Orthotics
- Brace worn during active play and at nighttime
- Medial knee offloading device
- KAFO (knee-ankle-foot orthosis)
- HKAFO (hip-knee-ankle-foot orthosis)

Surgical
- Osteotomy ± pin fixation
- External fixation
- Epiphyseodesis
- Osteotomies are performed before age 4 if possible
- Surgical interventions in older children are often complicated by obesity

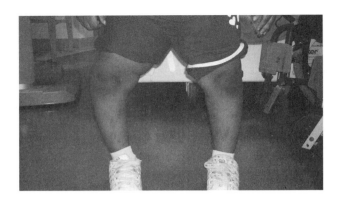

Six-year-old African American female child with Blount's disease.

Consults
- Orthopedic surgery for painful, rapidly progressing or debilitating angulation

Complications of Surgery
- Saphenous nerve (infrapatellar branch) injury
- Anterior tibial artery injury
- Overcorrection
- Total growth arrest

Prognosis
- Highly variable

Helpful Hints
- Can see this in preparticipation physicals for sports in otherwise healthy boys. Sports that emphasize girth and size select for the population in which this condition is most prevalent

Suggested Readings
Staheli LT. *Practice of Pediatric Orthpedics*. Philadelphia, PA: Lippincot Williams & Wilkins; 2001.

Wenger DR, Mickelson M, Maynard JA. The evolution and histopathology of adolescent tibia vara. *J Pediatr Ortho*. 1984;4(1):78–88.

Botulism

Joyce Oleszek MD

Description

Infantile botulism is an uncommon disease that occurs when ingested spores of the *Clostridium botulinum* (a common soil-dwelling bacterium) germinate and produce botulinum neurotoxin in the colon. The resulting illness varies from mild hypotonia to severe systemic flaccid paralysis to sudden unexpected death.

Etiology/Types

- Infantile botulism: continued intraintestinal production of toxin after ingestion of spores
- Foodborne botulism: preformed toxin is ingested in a single episode
- Wound botulism
- Types of toxins: A, Ab, B, Bf, C, Ec, F, A and Ba, A and Eb

Epidemiology

- Approximately 98% of infants affected present between ages 1 and 6 months, but cases have been reported as early as first week of life and as late as 12 months
- >90% from type A (especially western US) or type B (usually eastern US)
- Annual incidence is 1.9/100,000 live births in US
- The United States, Argentina, Australia, Canada, Italy, and Japan, in this order, report the largest number of cases
- California has the highest reported incidence followed by eastern Pennsylvania and Utah
- Type A toxin is the predominant type in the Western United States. Type B toxin is more commonly reported in the Eastern United States
- Males and females are equally affected

Pathogenesis

- The infant intestinal tract has low oxygen and low acid due to a lack of protective bacterial flora of *Clostridium*-inhibiting bile acids of older individuals so that the *C botulinum* can flourish and produce the toxin that causes the disease
- The enteric toxin of *C botulinum* causes intestinal immotility and progressive paralysis due to the effect on acetylcholine release at the neuromuscular junction (NMJ) and other cholinergic nerve terminals, particularly in the gastrointestinal tract
- NMJs have a large margin of safety; before weakness is detected clinically, 75% of receptors need to be blocked by toxin
- Diaphragmatic function will be affected at 90% to 95% blockage of NMJs

Risk Factors

- Honey consumption in infants
- Weaning from breast feeding and introducing non-human sources of nourishment (this creates changes in normal gut florae)
- Season: higher occurrence between March and November (more south winds and absence of snow cover)
- Aminoglycoside antibiotics can potentiate weakness at NMJ
- Exposure to environmental sources of spores (near active construction)

Clinical Features

- Constipation
- Bulbar and extremity weakness
- Dysphagia
- Weak cry
- Respiratory compromise

Natural History

- Blocking of receptors occurs regardless of the route of exposure
- Onset is 18 to 36 hours after food consumption
- Complete resolution after weeks/months with supportive care
- Rarely, poor outcomes or death occur with delayed diagnosis or medical care

Diagnosis

Differential diagnosis

- Sepsis or dehydration
- Guillain Barre syndrome
- Spinal muscular atrophy
- Polio

- Myasthenia gravis
- Failure to thrive
- Encephalitis/meningitis
- Metabolic disease

History
- Less than 1-year-old infant
- Constipation
- Poor suck
- Weak cry/hypophonia
- Dysphagia
- Dehydration
- Loss of motor milestones

Physical exam
- Diminished gag
- Drooling
- Ptosis
- Sluggish pupillary light reflexes
- Ophthalmoplegia
- Facial weakness
- Decreased head control
- Shoulder-girdle weakness
- Descending symmetric flaccid paralysis
- Generalized hypotonia
- Decreased or absent muscle stretch reflexes

Testing
- Identification of toxin in stools
- Electromyography shows reduced amplitudes, increased positive sharp waves, and fibrillations
- Nerve conduction studies show reduced compound motor amplitude
- Repetitive stimulation shows decrement with low rate stimulation and increment with high rate repetitive stimulation.
- Single-fiber EMG shows increased jitter and blocking

Pitfalls
- Stool toxin confirmation is time consuming and not an absolute requirement for diagnosis
- Electrodiagnosis can have false-positive and false-negative results, which are nonspecific

Red Flags
- Rapid rate and severity of progression

Treatment
Medical
- Single dose of Botulism Immune Globulin Intravenous (BIG-IV) at 50 mg/kg when diagnosis made (start within 7–10 days)
- Supportive care, including ventilatory support and tube feeding, if needed

Exercises
- Frequent repositioning
- Passive range of motion
- General strengthening

Injections
- N/A

Surgical
- Tracheostomy
- Gastrostomy

Complications of treatment
- BIG-IV: transient blush-like rash (most common)
- Anaphylaxis and hypotension (uncommon)

Prognosis
- Most infants recover without residual sequelae

Helpful Hints
Early suspicion of infantile botulism is important to provide:
- Appropriate early supportive care
- Early treatment with BIG-IV
  - Shortens pediatric intensive care unit stay
  - Decreases length of mechanical ventilation
  - Reduces costs of hospitalization
  - Decreases psychosocial impact
  - Allows more rapid improvement

Suggested Readings
Thompson JA, Filloux FM, Van Orman CB et al. Infant botulism in the age of botulism immune globulin. *Neurology.* 2005;64: 2029–2032.

Underwood K, Rubin S, Deakers T, Newth C. Infant botulism: a 30-year experience spanning the introduction of botulism immune globulin intravenous in the intensive care unit at Children's Hospital Los Angeles. *Pediatrics.* 2007;120:e1380-e1385.

Brachial Plexus Palsy

Maureen R. Nelson MD

Description

Birth brachial plexus palsy (BBPP) is an injury to the nerves that control movement and sensation of the arm. It was first described in 1768, with the first nerve grafting for treatment published in 1903.

Etiology/Types

- Lateral stretch
- Congenital anatomical variation
- Erb's palsy, C5–6, upper plexus
- Klumpke's palsy, C8-T1, lower plexus, controversial if exists in BBPP unless significant congenital variation
- Combination of levels

Epidemiology

- 1 to 2/1000 live births
- Congenital variation exists

Pathogenesis

- Neurapraxia is a reversible loss of nerve conduction; will have recovery; no physical disruption
- Axonotmesis has variable severity; physical disruption of nerves but preserved endoneurium around axons
- Neurotmesis is the most severe; complete physical disruption of nerve fibers
- Avulsion is a preganglionic neurotmesis
- Rupture is a postganglionic neurotmesis
- Described as most commonly seen with a lateral stretch during the birth process
- Rarely, intrauterine process such as anomalous ribs may cause compression of nerve fibers

Risk Factors

- Shoulder dystocia
- Multiparous mother
- Large birth weight (>4500 g)
- Prior infant with BBPP

Clinical Features

- Lack of active movement in arm
- Lack of sensation in arm
- Contractures are common

Natural History

- 75% have spontaneous functional recovery
- The elbow by 3 to 4 months may show full recovery; but if not, expect need for surgery for functional arm
- Commonly see asymmetry of shoulder joint development if not resolved early

Diagnosis

Differential Diagnosis

- Fracture of humerus or clavicle
- Osteomyelitis
- Spinal cord injury
- Tumor

History

- Birth weight
- Parity of mother
- Shoulder dystocia
- Flaccid arm/portion of arm at delivery
- Lack of feeling in the arm
- Early pain with shoulder range of motion (ROM)/ clothing changes
- Changes over time in movement

Exam

- Absent reflex in involved distribution
- Absent motor function
- Absent sensation
- Moro reflex asymmetry
- ROM/contractures
- Decreased muscle bulk
- Size of the arm
- Temperature of the arm
- Torticollis

Testing

- Magnetic Resonance Imaging
- Plain radiographs to rule out other etiologies
- Electrodiagnosis including H reflexes and F waves to look at proximal function
- Cannot use standard distance measurements for nerve conduction studies (NCS) because of the size of child and so must list measurement used

- NCS with conduction velocity; maturational changes with age; so check reference values
- Sensory NCS important in areas of sensory loss: if response is present, it indicates preganglionic lesion
- Somatosensory evoked potential—not usually done diagnostically as must sedate (so no movement), and findings are overlapping, but helpful intraoperatively

Pitfalls
- Lack of awareness of arm

Red Flags
- Phrenic nerve C3, 4, 5, may be injured

Treatment

Medical
- Education of parents regarding awareness of the arm and future delivery risks

Exercises
- ROM, gentle, especially shoulder external rotation and abduction, wrist and elbow flexion/extension, and forearm supination
- Focus on baby's awareness of the arm
- Splinting: early wrist extensor splints; later supinator straps also

Modalities
- Electrical stimulation(Neuromuscular electrical stimulation)
- Taping

Injection
- Botulinum toxin for contractures occasionally

Surgical
- Nerve grafting in early stages: neurolysis to remove scar (no longer recommended by itself); nerve grafts with donor fibers, commonly sural nerve, for fascicles to give path for axonal fiber regrowth; direct end-to-end fascicle anastomosis rarely an option but optimal if possible; later localized neurolysis, partial grafts such as Oberlin
- Muscle, tendon, bony procedures
- Shoulder capsule procedure
- Steindler flexorplasty: surgically move the flexor/pronator muscles from the medial epicondyle to more proximally on the humerus to flex elbow
- Osteotomies

Consults
- Usually neurosurgeon or plastic surgeon/microsurgeon for nerve procedures
- Orthopedic surgeon or plastic surgeon for muscle, tendon, or bony procedures

Complications
- Contractures
- Shoulder dysplasia/subluxation
- Lack of awareness of arm
- Altered development of body image
- Altered child development

Prognosis
- If flexing the elbow by 3 to 4 months may show full recovery; if not, expect need for surgery for function
- Contractures may cause shoulder problems

Helpful Hints
- Primitive reflexes useful in eliciting active movement in infants
- Discuss with parents to consider discussion with obstetrician for scheduled C-section prior to labor for any future pregnancies

Suggested Readings
Hale HB, Bae DS, Waters PM. Current concepts in the management of brachial plexus birth palsy. J Hand Surg 2010; 35A: 322–331.

Waters PM. Comparison of the natural history, the outcome of microsurgical repair, and the outcome of operative reconstruction in brachial plexus birth palsy. *J Bone Joint Surg Am.* 1999;(81):649–659.

Burns

Susan Quigley MD

Description

A burn is a permanent destruction of tissue proteins by an external agent.

Etiology/Types

- Thermal, electrical, chemical, and radiation energy cause burns
- Thermal injuries
  - Scald burns result from contact with hot liquid or gas
  - Direct-flame exposure causes flame burns, resulting from ignition of clothing
  - Contact burns occur in children who come in contact with a hot object
  - Explosions may cause flash burns
- Electrical burns occur as a result of electrical current passing through the skin and tissue structures of the body

Epidemiology

- Burns are the most common cause of unintentional deaths in children younger than age 2, the second most common cause for those younger than age 4, and the third leading cause for all those younger than age 19
- Burns are second only to motor vehicle crashes as a cause of death in children
- Approximately 100,000 children in the United States are hospitalized annually for the treatment of burn injuries
- Approximately 3000 deaths in children occur annually due to burns, and three to four times this number suffer severe and prolonged disability
- Male:female 2:1

Pathogenesis

- The mechanism of heat transfer to the skin influences the type and severity of thermal burns
- In the deepest burns, protein coagulation causes cell death
- Lesser burned tissue has a surrounding area of stasis and potentially reversible changes

- Very superficial burns have an area of hyperemia with little cellular compromise

Risk Factors

- Very young age
- Male
- Associated injuries
- Children with disabilities
- Infants are more susceptible than older children to severe burn injuries because of their thinner epidermal layer

Clinical Features

Burn Classifications

Class	Tissues involved	Clinical presentation	Prognosis
First degree	Superficial epidermis	Redness, no blistering; painful 1–3 days	No scarring
Second degree	Superficial dermis; superficial partial thickness	Painful; red; blisters	Heals 7–14 days; possible permanent scarring
	Deep reticular dermis deep partial thickness	Painful; red; blisters; possible white eschar	Hyperemia; scarring likely; 3–4 weeks
Third degree	Full thickness; muscle, tendon, or bone	Non-painful; white, brown, black or red	Possible amputation; severe scarring; grafting required; heals weeks to months

- The percentage of total body surface area (TBSA) burned is estimated by the rule of nines: 9% for each arm and head; 18% for each leg, anterior trunk, and posterior trunk for teens

- Modified for smaller children to estimate body surface area because differing body proportions with larger head and smaller limbs so that the surface of a child's palm represents about 1% TBSA

Diagnosis

Differential diagnosis
- Sepsis

History
- Tetanus/immunization status
- Mechanism of burn
- Inhalation injury
- Time of initial injury
- Edema
- Assess for other possible injuries and allergies
- Premorbid health factors

Exam
- Severity
- Additional injuries, including fracture or brain injury
- Utilize modified rule of nines formula to calculate TBSA of burn or adaptation described above

Testing
- Lab: complete blood count, electrolytes, albumin, and total protein
- Chest x-ray and x-rays of other potential injuries

Pitfalls
- Infection
- Inadequate pain medication/pain control
- Poor positioning

Red Flags
- Signs of suspected child abuse (i.e., scald pattern not consistent with child's developmental level/mobility)
- Circumferential burns can compromise chest expansion and compromise breathing or peripheral perfusion and may need an escharotomy emergently.

Treatment

Medical
- Minimize risks for infection
- Pain management

- Burn site coverage by artificial membranes, or with skin grafting is an ongoing process; silvadene has been a mainstay of topical therapy, but new options continue to be developed
- Burn patients lose heat through their compromised skin barrier and insensible losses, so ambient temperature of the room is important
- Burn injuries that warrant hospitalization due to serious prognosis:
  - Second-degree burns covering > 10% of BSA
  - Third-degree burns covering >2% of BSA
  - Significant burns involving hands, feet, face, joints, or perineum
  - Self-inflicted burns
  - Burns resulting from suspected child abuse
  - Electrical or inhalation burns
- Circumferential burns may predispose to vascular compromise
- Explosion, inhalation, or chemical burns may have other organ trauma involvement

Exercise
- Positioning/passive range of motion/active range of motion
- Strengthening exercises
- Postural exercises
- Pool therapy

Modalities
- Splinting
- Pressure garments for reduction of hypertrophic scarring
- Continuous passive motion machines

Surgical
- Escharotomy for circumferential burns
- Skin grafting
- Scar revisions
- Amputation/limb salvage surgery
- Gastrostomy tube placement

Consults
- Plastic surgery
- Orthopedic surgery
- Infectious disease
- Psychiatry

Complications
- Hypertrophic scarring
- Contractures
- Limb loss/amputation

- Disfigurement/cosmesis issues
- Heterotopic ossification
- Cataract development
- Neuropathies
- Posttraumatic stress disorder and/or depression
- Impaired bone growth/development
- Infection risks

Prognosis

- Poor prognosis in significant burns in children with chronic metabolic or connective tissue diseases (in whom healing may be compromised with the increased risk of secondary infection) or in children younger than 2 years

Helpful Hints

- Patients attempt to adopt a flexed protective position, due to pain; therefore, positioning must counteract that position
- Classic desired position: neck extended, shoulders abducted 90°, elbows extended, forearms supinated, wrists 15° to 20° extension, palms up, fingers extended, hips abducted 10° to 15°, knees extended, and ankles dorsiflexed

Suggested Readings

Behrman RE, Kliegman R, Nelson WE, eds. *Textbook of Pediatrics.* 15th ed. Philadelphia, PA: W.B. Saunders Company; 1996.

Parish RA. Thermal burns. In: Barkin RM, ed. *Pediatric Emergency Medicine: Concepts and Clinical Practice.* St Louis, MO: Mosby-Year Book; 1992.

Cancer: Bone/Limb

Marcie Ward MD

Description

Long bone tumors of the pediatric patient resulting in varying levels of disability depending on their location and the necessary treatment.

Etiology/Types

- Osteosarcoma
- Ewing sarcoma

Epidemiology

- Osteosarcoma
  - 5.6 cases per million children
  - Typically affects children in 2nd decade
  - Most commonly seen in the femur, tibia, and humerus (can be found in the skull, jaw, or pelvis)
- Ewing sarcoma
  - 2.1 cases per million children
  - Typically children between 5 and 25 years of age
  - Predominantly affects teenage boys

Pathogenesis

- Aggressive tumors that metastasize quickly (to lungs and bone)
- ~25% of patients have metastases at presentation
- 90% of osteosarcomas involve the metaphysis

Risk Factors

- Osteosarcoma
  - Rapid bone growth
  - History of retinoblastoma
  - Ionizing radiation exposure
  - Genetic risk factors
- Ewing sarcoma
  - Rapid bone growth
  - Caucasian race

Clinical Features

- Pain and swelling
- Mass is almost always present initially in Ewing's and 40% of the time with Osteosarcoma
- ± Pathologic fracture

Natural History

- If untreated, rapid progression to death

Diagnosis

Differential diagnosis

- Osteomyelitis
- Benign bone tumors of children
- Rhabdomyosarcoma
- Giant cell tumor
- Nonrhabdomyosarcoma soft tissue sarcoma
- Fibrosarcoma
- Chondrosarcoma

History

- Pain/swelling/mass
- Often at presentation patient incidentally reports a history of trauma
- Fever
- Weight loss

Exam

- Palpable mass
- Warmth
- Tenderness
- Erythema
- Gait changes/antalgia
- Decreased range of motion

Testing

- Complete blood count, erythrocyte sedimentation rate, c-reactive protein, alkaline phosphate, lactate dehydrogenase
- Plain radiographs in two planes:
  - 90% of osteosarcomas involve the metaphysis
  - Medullary destruction with poorly defined margins
  - Cortical destruction
  - Reactive periosteal bone
- Magnetic resonance imaging
- Computed tomography, Positron emission tomography, or bone scan to evaluate metastases
- Biopsy

Pitfalls

- Delay in diagnosis means decrease in survival rate
- Biopsy must be performed by a qualified orthopedic oncologist

Red Flags

- Metastases
- Recurrence

Treatment

Medical
- Chemotherapy
- Radiation therapy in limited cases of Ewing's
- Oral medications for pain

Exercises
- Early mobilization with range of motion
- General conditioning exercises for fatigue as tolerated
- Strength and balance activities
- Gait retraining after limb surgery
- Upper extremity strengthening and modified activities of daily living
- Limb salvage patients are restricted from high impact and high coordination sports
- Modified physical education classes

Modalities
- Prosthesis if amputation performed
- Orthoses for weak limb support
  - Consider orthotic support of the knee
  - Consider shoe lifts as needed for leg length discrepancies
- Desensitization of residual limb

Surgical
- Osteosarcomas need total resection of primary tumor and metastases
- Surgical resection of Ewing sarcoma is preferable to radiation (due to high risk of second cancers after radiation exposure)
- Limb salvage (surgery to remove cancer and avoid amputation, while maintaining maximal function) is often considered to produce a cosmetically superior result
- Amputation if patient at high risk for recurrence
- Surgical resection of metastases is necessary

Consults
- Oncology
- Orthopedic oncologist
- Prosthetist /Orthotist
- Psychology and Social Work
- Peer mentor

Complications of treatment
- Infection
- Neurovascular injury
- Limb length discrepancy/slowed growth
- Tumor bed contamination/second neoplasm
- Ototoxicity, liver, renal, or cardiac toxicity, and sterility from chemotherapy
- Osteonecrosis

Prognosis
- Osteosarcoma 3- to 5-year survival rate
  - Without metastases is ~ 58% to 76%
  - With metastases is ~ 14% to 50%
- Ewing sarcoma 3- to 5-year survival rate
  - Without metastases is ~ 50% to 70%
  - With metastases is ~ 19% to 30%
- Axial and pelvic lesions carry a poorer prognosis

Helpful Hints
- Best outcomes result from early identification and referral to a center capable of managing the entire course of the disease
- Biopsy and incision selection are critical to the success of subsequent limb sparing surgery
- Early mobilization and adherence to a home-exercise program to maintain range of motion is crucial to avoiding contractures

Suggested Readings

Carola AS, William MC. Common musculoskeletal tumors of childhood and adolescence. *N Engl J Med.* 1999;341(5):342–352.

Frieden RA, Ryniker D, Kenan S, Lewis MM. Assessment of patient function after limb-sparing surgery. *Arch Phys Med Rehabil.* 1993;74:38–43.

Cancer: Brain

Maurice Sholas MD PhD

Description

Brain tumors are the most common solid tumors in children and the second most common malignancy. Nearly two-thirds are infratentorial. Neurologic symptoms vary depending on the size, location, and spread of the tumor.

Etiology/Types

- Tumors of the brain in children are most often primary, rather than metastatic
- Classification depends on the type of tissue involved, how invasive the tumor cells are into surrounding tissues and the location of the growth
- Most tumors are rare in the first year of life
- Some common types include astrocytomas, ependymomas, and medulloblastomas

Epidemiology

- Multifactorial risk factors
- Most occur in children older than 12 months

Pathogenesis

- Brain tissue loses the ability to regulate growth and differentiation normally
- The abnormal tissue grows in a way that compresses or negatively affects the nearby tissues
- Symptoms are directly related to the size and location of the tumorous growth

Risk Factors

- Genetic inheritance
- Exposure to oncogenic chemicals
- Exposure to excessive radiation

Clinical Features

In order of most to least common:
- Seizures
- Malaise
- Headache
- Nausea
- Vomiting
- Mental status changes
- Speech problems
- Weakness or paralysis
- Increased muscle tone
- Lethargy
- Bulging fontanelles (young children)
- Increased head circumference (young children)
- Memory loss
- Impaired judgment
- Loss of red reflex in eye
- Vision changes
- Movement disorder
- Weight gain or loss
- Dysphagia
- Hearing acuity changes
- Decorticate or cerebrate posturing
- Decreased coordination and falls
- Delayed or precocious puberty
- Hiccups

Natural History

- Meduloblastomas are the most common malignant brain tumor in children; 20%. They are in the cerebellum most frequently. There may be postoperative cerebellar mutism from 48 hours to weeks or months.
- Ependymomas generate from within the ventricles. They can behave aggressively, but tend to be differentiated and benign. Treat these with surgery.
- Brain stem gliomas can be fast or slow growing; they tend not to be resectable and require radiation and chemotherapy. Glioblastoma mutliforme are high-grade gliomas and have a poor prognosis.
- Gangliogliomas are low-grade gliomas; slow growing and most often benign.
- Pilocytic astrocytomas are the most common low-grade glioma. They are cytic and treated with resection.
- Craniopharyngiomas are congenital tumors that are typically benign. Hydrocephalus and endocrine symptoms are common, with 93% growth failure.
- Pineal tumors are near the posterior portion of the third ventricle. They are most often germinomas, but teratomas, pineocytomas, and pineoblastomas occur in this area as well.

Diagnosis

Differential diagnosis

- Seizure disorder
- Infectious process
- Hydrocephalus
- Encephalitis
- Chemical/medication toxicity

- Neurodegenerative disorder
- Anoxic or traumatic brain injury
- Intracranial hemorrhage
- Congenital malformation

History
- Headache or vision changes
- Gross motor skill decline or clumsiness
- New onset of seizures
- Mental status changes
- Loss of developmental milestones

Exam
- Visual field evaluation
- Evaluate for weakness/hemiparesis
- Mental status evaluation
- Red reflex in the eyes
- Optic discs may bulge
- Coordination testing
- Communication and cognitive tests
- Dysphagia evaluation
- Pathologic reflexes, depending on lesion

Testing
- Computed tomography of the head is the most common method of screening
- Magnetic resonance imaging (MRI) of the head is useful to gain additional information on tumor size and type
- Biopsy is useful for tissue diagnosis of a suspicious mass
- Functional brain scans (*Positron emission tomography* scan and functional MRI) are secondary survey tools for monitoring tumor characteristics and response to treatment
- Electroencephalography to evaluate seizure activity
- Lumbar puncture (limited circumstance) to see if tumor material is in the cerebral spinal fluid

Pitfalls
- Over interpretation of imaging studies

Red Flags
- New onset focal neurological dysfunction
- New onset seizures
- Uncontrolled emesis
- Progressive mental status depression
- Loss of red reflex in eye exam

Treatment

Medical
- Often in concert with surgical treatment
- Corticosteroids
- Chemotherapy is often very specific in composition, duration, and initiation to each tumor identified

- Radiation
- Anticonvulsant medication
- Pain medication

Exercises
- Exercise is relatively contraindicated if platelet count is below 30,000. If the child has inadequate neutrophils they may not do therapies in a communal setting.

Modalities
- Transcutaneous electrical nerve stimulation and ultrasound are contraindicated over tumor site

Surgical
- Biopsy
- Decompression
- Craniectomy
- Craniotomy
- Tumor resection—total or subtotal
- CSF shunts
- Gamma knife

Consults
- Neurology
- Neurosurgery
- Hematology/Oncology
- Radiation oncology

Complications
- Weakness
- Cognitive deficits
- Abnormal muscle tone
- Dysphagia
- Dysarthria
- Poor balance and coordination
- Seizures
- Loss of developmental milestones
- Side effects of chemotherapeutics
- Death

Prognosis
- Noninvasive tumors like gliomas are curable with simple surgery
- More invasive tumors like glioblastoma multiformae have a more guarded prognosis
- In general 5-year survival with chemotherapy, radiation, and surgery is 40% to 80%.

Suggested Readings
Buckner JC, Brown PD, O'Neill BP, et al. Central nervous system tumors. *Mayo Clin Proc.* 2007;82(10):1271–1286.
Grondin RT, Scott RM, Smith ER. Pediatric brain tumors. *Adv Pediatr.* 2009;56:249–269.

Cerebral Palsy: Dyskinetic

Rita Ayyangar MBBS ■ Liza Green MD MS ■ Edward A. Hurvitz MD

Description
Dyskinetic cerebral palsy (CP) is one of the most disabling forms of CP and is characterized by a predominance of stereotyped, involuntary movements that are accentuated with effort.

Etiology/Types
Seen with injury to the extrapyramidal system (mainly the basal ganglia and thalamus) while the more common spastic form is associated with pyramidal tract involvement.

Classified as given below:
■ Dystonic
■ Hyperkinetic
  – Slow movements: Athetosis
  – Fast movements: Chorea, Ballismus, Tremors

Five percent of children with CP may have ataxic type of CP. This is seen with injury to the cerebellum or cerebellar pathways and children are often hypotonic. This chapter will focus primarily on the dyskinetic form and the spastic and ataxic forms will be covered elsewhere.

Epidemiology
■ Lack of a standard classification system makes it difficult to determine the exact worldwide prevalence
■ The prevalence of dyskinetic CP per 1000 live births increased from 0.08 in the 1970s to 0.14 in the 1990s
■ 3% to 15% of children with CP have dyskinetic type
■ Dyskinetic CP is more commonly seen in term infants with only a third occurring in preterm infants

Pathogenesis
■ Outstanding neuropathological feature of dystonia is bilateral sclerosis of the globus pallidus
■ Dystonia is seen with lesions involving the thalamus and basal ganglia, particularly the striatopallidal tracts
■ Athetosis due to asphyxia is seen with lesions of the caudate nucleus and putamen
■ Athetosis from kernicterus is seen in lesions of the globus pallidus and subthalamic nuclei as well as cranial nerve nuclei in the floor of the fourth ventricle

Risk Factors
■ Perinatal adverse events account for more than two-thirds of those with dyskinetic CP; prenatal events in 20%
■ Term infants and those weighing >2500 g at birth
■ Low Apgar scores (0–3) at 1 and 5 min. The lower the score, the more severe the functional impairments noted
■ Neonatal jaundice and kernicterus are risk factors for dyskinetic CP, particularly athetosis, but are not as common now as in the days of Rh incompatibility

Clinical Features
■ Dystonia: abnormal postures from sustained muscle contractions; usually combined with some spasticity
■ Athetosis: slow writhing movements
■ Chorea: rapid, jerky, and dancing movements
■ Athetosis and chorea are usually seen together as choreo-athetoid CP
■ While visual impairments are common findings in spastic CP, hearing impairments may be seen more frequently with dyskinetic CP
■ Motor control, communication, and learning may be affected
■ The motor limitations and dysarthria from dyskinetic CP may cause individuals to appear as if they are cognitively impaired even when in reality they may be of higher than normal intelligence
■ Movements may be accentuated by effort and excitement, and are frequently abolished by sleep
■ Hands are well developed and appear relatively large as compared to children with predominantly spastic forms of CP

Natural History
■ Infants at risk for the development of dyskinetic CP show fewer spontaneous "fidgety" movements than normal in the first few months. They show arm movement patterns that differentiate them from those at risk for spastic CP
■ Postural impairments of head and trunk control are the earliest signs; dyskinesias develop by the end of the first year or later
■ Dyskinesias may worsen over time

Diagnosis

Differential diagnosis

- Glutaric aciduria type I (a condition where the infant is usually normal at birth, may have sudden onset of vomiting, hypotonia, and neurological problems after a period of normal development, may have intracranial bleeds and is often mistaken for child abuse) and other amino acid disorders
- Primary and dopa responsive dystonia, which shows a diurnal variation in gait disturbance
- Metabolic disorders including mitochondrial disorders and biopterin deficiency
- Lipid disorders such as metachromatic leukodystrophy
- Inherited disorders such as neurodegeneration with brain iron accumulation (NBIA) previously known as Hallervorden-Spatz disease and Rett syndrome

History

- Perinatal adverse event history suggests CP
- Age at onset of concerns and at onset of dyskinesia may help differentiate between CP and glutaric aciduria I (GTA1 macrocephaly)
- No relationship of onset of symptoms to illnesses (as seen in Sydenham's chorea)
- No response to a trial of low dose Levodopa in CP (as seen in dopa responsive dystonia)
- Cognitive regression goes against a diagnosis of CP
- Consanguinity or Jewish ancestry

Exam

- Growth chart—head circumference may be small (macrocephaly is associated with GTA1 and the leukodystrophies
- Hand wringing and stereotypic behavior (Rett syndrome)
- Ophthalmalogic evaluation for Kayser-Fleischer rings (Wilson's disease) or retinitis pigmentosa seen with NBIA
- Focal versus generalized dystonia has implications for treatment and prognosis. DYT1 dystonia that starts focally in arm has a 50% chance of becoming generalized while that starting in the foot has a 90% chance of becoming generalized

Testing

- Lateral and flexion/extension views of cervical spine to assess for disc degeneration, listhetic instability and narrowing of the cervical spinal canal in adulthood or if complaining of neck pain
- Somatosensory evoked potential may be used to assess cervical cord compression if complaining of new onset sensory or motor changes

- Neuroimaging with magnetic resonance imaging to assess for brain maldevelopment and identify lesions in basal ganglia and thalamus and other nearby structures
- Gene and DNA testing: MECP2 mutation on X chromosome in Rett syndrome, DYT1 gene mutation for primary dystonias
- Trial of oral carbidopa-levodopa—Response to a trial of low dose Levodopa suggests dopa responsive dystonia or Segawa's disease

Pitfalls

- Missing a treatable cause such as DOPA responsive dystonia or glutaric aciduria I

Red Flags

- Neck pain with progressive weakness in an individual with dyskinetic CP may indicate compression of the cervical nerves or cord from disc degeneration, listhetic instability, or cervical stenosis.

Treatment

Medical

- Trihexyphenidyl—an anticholinergic antiparkinsonian agent that is useful in treatment of dystonia
- Levodopa—particularly useful in dopa responsive dystonia
- Levetiracetam—may be helpful in the management of choreoathetosis
- Tetrabenazine—is a dopamine depleting agent and is reportedly useful in the treatment of hyperkinesias, particularly chorea associated with Huntington's disease

Exercises

- General strengthening and stretching of the dystonic muscles
- Truncal strengthening for stability in sitting

Modalities

- Heat
- Cold
- Transcutaneous electrical nerve stimulation

Injection

- Focal botulinum toxin injections
- Phenol injections

Surgical

- Deep brain stimulation
- Intrathecal baclofen therapy is helpful in treating dystonia

Consults

- Neurology or developmental pediatrician early in course to aid with diagnosis in infant with developmental delay and dyskinesia

Complications

- Cervical disc degeneration starts earlier and progresses more rapidly, often starting in late adolescence or early adulthood and is generally present in over 97% of patients beyond 35 years of age
- Listhetic instability and narrowing of the cervical canal are a common occurrence and combined with the disc degeneration predisposes individuals with athetoid CP to rapidly progressive devastating neurological deficits

Prognosis

- Although the brain lesion is considered "nonprogressive" in CP, dyskinesia may progressively worsen, especially in late adosecence or adulthood.

Helpful Hints

- Dyskinetic movements are often accentuated by effort and abolished by sleep

Suggested Readings

Himmelman K, McManus V, Hagberg G, et al. Dyskinetic cerebral palsy in Europe: trends in prevalence and severity. *Arch Dis Child*. 2009;94:921–926.

Hyperkinetic syndromes. In: Goetz CG. *Textbook of Clinical Neurology*, 3rd ed. Philadelphia, PA: Saunders; 2007.

Cerebral Palsy: Gross Motor Function Classification System I–III

Edward A. Hurvitz MD ■ Rita Ayyangar MBBS ■ Liza Green MD MS

Description
Cerebral Palsy (CP) is a group of disorders affecting the development of movement and posture. They affect the developing fetal or infant brain and are generally nonprogressive. Gross Motor Function Classification (GMFCS) I–III individuals have more motor function than those who are IV–V, and can ambulate.

Etiology/Types
- GMFCS I—Walking mildly delayed, eventually moves around independently in environment without assistive devices
- GMFCS II—More difficulty with stairs, outdoors; high level gross motor skills but can still walk without assistive device
- GMFCS III—Walk with walker or other assistive device. May use wheelchair.
- Topology: Most children in this group are hemiplegic or diplegic, rarely quadriplegic
- Tone disorder: Spasticity is most common (>90%), often combined with some dystonia

Epidemiology
- CP occurs in 2 to 3 of 1000 births

Pathogenesis
- White matter damage (periventricular leukomalacia) most common

Risk Factors
- Prematurity
- Multiple pregnancy
- Intrauterine infection
- Other prenatal problems (thyroid deficiency and coagulopathy)
- Postbirth trauma, such as stroke or traumatic brain injury in first few years of life can technically be called CP

Clinical Features
- Developmental delay
- Can be floppy at birth
- Motor impairment—spasticity, dystonia, weakness, truncal hypotonia, and lack of selective motor control
- Sensory impairment—proprioception, stereognosis, 2-point discrimination
- Cognitive impairment—less common than in GMFCS IV–V

Natural History
- Nonprogressive (although some question about "early aging")
- Growth is associated with contracture and joint dislocation, leading to increased functional deficit if not treated

Diagnosis

Differential diagnosis
- Brain tumor
- Dopamine dependent dystonia
- Familial spastic paraparesis
- Muscular dystrophies
- Brachial plexus palsy

History
- Premature birth with complications
- Maternal infection
- Delay in gross motor and fine motor skills
- Learning deficits, cognitive impairment common
- Asymmetric hand or leg use
- Tight muscles in arms and legs
- Urinary incontinence may be seen

Exam
- Asymmetry of use, tone, and/or growth of limbs (by side or legs vs arms)
- Spasticity—spastic catch + velocity dependent increased resistance to stretch, seen particularly in:
  - Upper extremity: shoulder internal rotators, elbow and wrist flexors
  - Lower extremity: hip flexors, hamstrings, gastrocnemius soleus, posterior tibialis
- Gait pattern—excessive hip and knee flexion; and may see scissoring

Testing

- Cranial ultrasound in newborn
- Magnetic resonance imaging (MRI) of brain
  - Abnormal findings in 83%
  - White matter damage around ventricles (periventricular leukomalacia), or white matter combined with gray matter (especially hemiplegia)
  - Greater indication if progression of symptoms
- Metabolic and thyroid workup
- Genetic test

Pitfalls

- MRI is overused—repeat studies rarely indicated, though often requested

Red Flags

- Changing neurologic picture—NOT CP

Treatment

Medical

- Antispasticity medications such as baclofen, dantrolene, zanaflex, and diazepam
- Medications for attention and concentration
- Seizure medications

Exercises

- Constraint induced therapy or bilateral training therapy for upper extremity function
- Range of motion
- Strengthening
- Gait training
- Developmental stimulation
- Speech and language therapy for communication and cognition
- Swallowing therapy

Modalities

- Ankle-foot orthoses and other orthoses
- Hippotherapy, aquatherapy, and massage are all popular but unproven
- Complementary and alternative medicine chosen by more than 50% of families, though unproven benefit

Injection

- Botulinum toxin or phenol to reduce spasticity

Surgical

- Orthopedic muscle releases, tendon transfers
- Bony reconstruction of hip joint and ankle fusions
- Selective dorsal rhizotomy decreases tone, improves gait—indicated for GMFCS I–III more so than IV–V
- Intrathecal baclofen pump allows adjustable tone treatment

Consults

- Rehabilitation psychology to address learning, attention, and emotional issues
- Orthopedic surgery
- Neurosurgery for rhizotomy, intrathecal baclofen pump
- Ophthalmalogy for strabismus
- Urology to optimize continence

Prognosis

- Long term effects of treatments not well understood
- Recent studies suggest obesity and poor fitness levels is a concern in this group
- Normal lifespan, but face problems with loss of function, chronic pain, and "early aging" in adulthood

Helpful Hints

- Families tend to focus on walking; we should focus on fitness, cognition, participation, and overall function
- Provide early information about treatment options, including "alternative" therapies (prevalent on the web) and about transition to adulthood
- CP does not "get worse." The early brain injury combines with growth and development to produce problems of function and of the neuromusculoskeletal and other systems which should be addressed as treatable challenges.

Suggested Readings

Bax M, Goldstein M, Rosenbaum P, Leviton A, Paneth N. Proposed definition and classification of cerebral palsy. *Dev Med Child Neur.* 2005;47:571–576.

Green LB, Hurvitz EA. Cerebral palsy. *Phys Med Rehabil Clin N Am.* 2007;18:859–882.

Cerebral Palsy: Gross Motor Function Classification System IV–V

Liza Green MD MS ■ Edward A. Hurvitz MD ■ Rita Ayyangar MBBS

Description
Cerebral Palsy (CP) is a group of disorders affecting the development of movement and posture that are generally nonprogressive and affect the developing fetal or infant brain. Gross motor classification IV–V individuals have very limited functional mobility.

Etiology/Types
- GMFCS IV—some evidence of head and trunk control, powered mobility possible
- GMFCS V—Very limited head and trunk control, usually no independent mobility
- Topology—Most are quadriplegic, one side of the body can be more affected
- Tone disorder—Spasticity usually combined with some dystonia/dyskinesia

Epidemiology
- CP occurs in 2 to 3 of 1000 births

Pathogenesis
- Damage is more global and anoxia is a frequent cause

Risk Factors
- Extreme prematurity
- Multiple pregnancy, especially with twin-twin transfusion
- Intrauterine infection
- Birth trauma resulting in anoxia (i.e., placental abruption and severe pre-eclampsia)
- Postbirth trauma, that is, traumatic brain injury and shaken baby, early episodes of meningitis

Clinical Features
- Often floppy at birth
- Characterized by persistent primitive reflexes (i.e., asymmetric tonic neck reflex, exaggerated and persistent startle reflex, and persistent palmar/plantar grasp reflexes)
- Motor impairment—spasticity usually in the flexor muscle groups of the extremities; may have hypotonia in the trunk; lack of selective motor control; dystonia is common
- Sensory impairment—involving all types of sensation, sight is also commonly impaired
- Cognitive impairment—common but by no means universal

Natural History
- Nonprogressive, (although some question about "early aging")
- Growth is commonly associated with contracture, joint dislocation, and scoliosis, leading to increased functional deficit and discomfort if not treated
- There are a number of medical issues that can result in early death

Diagnosis

Differential diagnosis
- Brain tumor
- Dopamine dependent dystonia
- Familial spastic paraparesis
- Muscular dystrophies
- Genetic disorders
- Metabolic disorders

History
- Premature birth with complications
- Maternal or infant infection
- Severe delay in gross motor and fine motor skills
- History of a seizure disorder, failure to thrive, decreased pulmonary function, strabismus, constipation, and dysphagia

Exam
- Persistent reflexes
- Spasticity in the limbs with severe truncal hypotonia or extensor thrust of the trunk
- Microcephaly
- Strabismus

Section II: Pediatric Diseases and Complications

- Limited functional mobility
- Sialorrhea
- Joint contractures/scoliosis

Testing
- Cranial ultrasound in newborn often shows grade III–VI intraventricular hemorrhage
- Magnetic resonance imaging of the brain commonly shows diffuse damage and evidence of atrophy
- Metabolic and thyroid workup to look for treatable causes
- Genetic testing to look for cause, expected course, and future risk

Red Flags
- Changing neurologic picture—NOT CP

Treatment

Medical/Surgical
- Spasticity
  - Medications commonly used include baclofen, dantrolene, zanaflex, and valium
  - Intrathecal baclofen useful for increasing comfort and ease of care, but complication rate increased in children who undergo multiple hip and spine surgeries
  - Injection therapy with botulinum toxin and/or phenol can be targeted to improve function of the less involved arm to allow for powered mobility, or to improve ease of care for dressing and hygiene
  - Selective dorsal rhizotomy surgery can be used in this population
- Seizures
  - Often difficult to control, requiring multiple medications
  - Ketogenic diet often used and can be an easier option for tube fed children
  - Vagal nerve stimulator also used
- Pulmonary issues
  - Reactive airway disease, especially with children who were premature
  - Obstructive lung disease also common and can lead to sleep apnea
  - Restrictive lung disease develops in children with scoliosis or severely decreased chest wall expansion due to truncal hypotonia
  - Pneumonia is a frequent cause of death in severely involved individuals
- Gastrointestinal issues
  - Failure to thrive develops in infants due to poor oral motor function and often necessitates G-tube

  - Gastroesophageal reflux disease requires medications or a Nissen fundoplication (often done in combination with G-tube)
  - Constipation requires management with stool softeners, laxatives, suppositories, and/or enemas
- Orthopedic issues
  - Joint contractures treated with tendon releases
  - Hip subluxation initially treated with tendon releases and bony reconstruction, persistent subluxation may be treated with girdlestone procedure
  - Scoliosis usually treated surgically when the curve reaches 60°. Thoracic lumbosacral orthosis (TLSO) bracing not usually helpful in decreasing curvature. Vertical expandable prosthetic titanium rib (VEPTR) is an option for very young children with bad curves by expanding and supporting a deformed thorax using telescoping rods

Exercises
- Range of motion is the mainstay of therapy
- Strengthening may be possible
- Weight bearing in standers or limited ambulation in supportive gait trainers
- Developmental stimulation
- Speech and language therapy for adaptive communication
- Swallowing therapy

Equipment
- Small children
  - adaptive seating systems can often be transferred from an immobile base for use at home to a stroller for use in the community
  - adaptive high chairs
  - adaptive car seats
  - standers
  - gait trainers
  - bracing including ankle-foot orthoses, thumb splints, and wrist extension splints
  - trunk supports such as neoprene vests or TLSOs to improve trunk stability
- Older children
  - wheelchairs—manual or electric
  - seating either with customized lateral supports or custom molded seating
  - must be safe to tie down for transportation on school bus
  - wheelchair ramps and accessible vans
  - lifts

Consults
- Orthopedic surgery
- Neurosurgery
- Ophthamology for strabismus
- Gastroenterology/surgery
- Neurology
- Sleep specialist
- Pulmonology
- ENT
- Psychology

Prognosis
- Survival into adulthood is the norm, with improved survival over the past 20 years.

- Early death often due to pneumonia, intractable seizures

Helpful Hints
- Remember to advocate for these children to get the different types of therapy services that they are eligible for through the school districts under the Individuals with Disabilities Education Act.

Suggested Readings
Green LB, Hurvitz EA. Cerebral palsy. *Phys Med Rehabil Clin N Am.* 2007;18:859–882.

Strauss D, Shavelle R, Reynolds R, Rosenbloom L, Day S. Survival in cerebral palsy in the last 20 years: signs of improvement? *Dev Med Child Neuro.* 2007;49;86–92.

Section II: Pediatric Diseases and Complications

Clubfoot

Heakyung Kim MD

Description

Clubfoot is a congenital deformity of the foot, which includes equinus, varus, adduction, rotational, and cavus deformities.

Etiology/Types

- Multifactorial; may be associated with a specific (eg, Edward's syndrome, teratogenic agents such as sodium aminopterin, congenital talipes equinovarus [CTEV]), or generalized disorder (eg, growth arrest, arthrogryposis, muscular dystrophies).
- Majority are idiopathic.
- Multiple classification schemes exist
  - Extrinsic vs. intrinsic causes (intrauterine compression vs anatomic deformities)
  - Postural/positional vs. fixed/rigid
  - Correctable vs resistant (based on the basis of therapeutic modality)
  - Other formal schemes include Pirani, Goldner, Di Miglio, Hospital for Joint Diseases (HJD), and Walker classifications.

Epidemiology

- Occurs in approximately 1 out of 1,000 births.
- 30–50% of cases present with bilateral involvement.
- There is a 2:1 male-to-female ratio.

Pathogenesis

- Intrauterine neurogenic events (stroke, spina bifida) leading to altered innervation patterns in posteromedial and peroneal muscle groups
- Arrest of fetal development at fibular stage
- Retracting fibrosis due to increased presence of fibrous tissue in muscle/ligaments.
- Anomalous tendon insertions

Risk Factors

- Familial: 2% incidence in first-degree relatives
- CTEV can be seen in syndromes involving chromosomal deletion.

Clinical Features

- Heel inverted (varus) and internally rotated.
- Forefoot inverted and adducted, with medial foot concave, lateral foot convex, foot inverted, and deep medial and posterior creases in severe deformities
- Plantar flexion with inability to dorsiflex. Equinus with tight heel cord.
- Tibial torsion may be present.

Natural History

- Present at birth
- Worsens over time if untreated
- Treated conservatively with serial manipulation/casting.
- More difficult cases (eg, teratological etiology) may require surgical release

Diagnosis

Differential diagnosis

- Metatarsus adductus

History

- Seek a detailed family history of clubfoot or neuromuscular disorders

Exam

- Examine feet with child prone, with plantar aspect visible, as well as supine, to evaluate internal rotation and varus.
- Ankle seen in equinus, foot supinated (varus), and adducted
- Dorsiflexion beyond 90 degrees not possible
- Cavus (high arch) deformity
  - Navicular and cuboid displaced medially
  - Talar neck easily palpable
  - Medial plantar soft tissue contractions present (triceps surae, flexor digitorum longus, flexor hallucis longus)
- Heel small and soft
- Tibia may exhibit internal torsion
- If child can stand, test for: plantigrade foot, foot/ankle position, and weight bearing heel

Testing

- Although imaging is not necessary to diagnose nature or severity of clubfoot, x-rays may be useful for monitoring response to treatment.

- Anteroposterior (AP) and lateral views used to calculate talocalcaneal angles (TCA) and index.
- Talocalcaneal parallelism is the radiographic feature of clubfoot.

Pitfalls
- Starting treatment late
- Overaggressive surgery

Red Flags
- Don't use force to correct equinus, as this may break the foot and result in rockerbottom foot.

Treatment

Medical
- N/A

Modalities
- Stretching/manipulation followed by serial casting, most often by Ponseti method. The **Ponseti method** is a manipulative technique that corrects congenital clubfoot by gradually rotating the foot around the head of the talus over a period of weeks during cast correction. It is recommended that this modality be started soon after birth (7 to 10 days)
- Order of correction: forefoot adduction, forefoot supination, then equinus
- Splints/braces (i.e., ankle-foot orthoses, Denis-Browne Bar, a corrective device in which straight last boots are locked in position by a metal bar, which promotes ankle dorsiflexion and relative foot external rotation.)

Injection
- Botulinum toxin applied to muscular contractures in conjunction with above modalities.

Surgical
- Achilles tenotomy
- Anterior tibial tendon transfer if dynamic supination deformity

Consults
- Orthopedic surgery

Complications/side effects
- Under-correction following conservative treatment or in cases of difficult teratological origin
- Overcorrection resulting in calcaneus deformity, hypermobility, or other problems
- Recurrence
- Scar tissue resulting in functional, growth, or aesthetic issues following extensive surgery
  - Persistent intoeing due to insufficient external rotation correction.

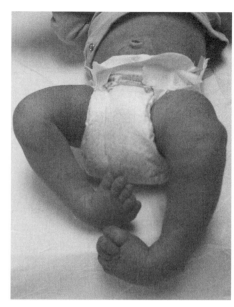

Baby with bilateral clubfeet, demonstrates varus heel, forefoot inversion and adduction, and concave medial foot.

Prognosis
- Uncorrected prognosis is poor, with sequelae including:
  - Aesthetic impairments
  - Secondary bone changes
  - Breakdown, ulceration, and infection of inadequately keratinized skin not meant to be weight bearing
- With treatment, prognosis is good to excellent; with Ponseti method correction, 90–95% success rates have been reported.
- A discrepancy in range of motion and muscularity may persist.
- Pain may occur at site of deformity later in life necessitating shoe modifications or additional corrective surgery

Helpful Hints
- Start early (traditional nonoperative treatment begins 2–3 days after birth)

Suggested Readings
Churgay CA. Diagnosis and treatment of pediatric foot deformities. *Am Fam Physician.* 1993 Mar;47(4):883–9.
Hulme A. The management of congenital talipes equinovarus. *Early Hum Dev.* 2005 Oct;81(10):797–802. Epub 2005 Nov 2. Review.

Section II: Pediatric Diseases and Complications

Connective Tissue Disease: Benign Joint Disease

Charles E. Sisung MD

Description

Benign joint hypermobility syndrome is a connective tissue disorder with joint hypermobility and musculoskeletal symptoms in the absence of a systemic rheumatologic process.

Etiology/Types

- A strong autosomal dominant pattern, with first-degree relatives affected in up to 50% of cases
- Thought to be a not yet fully defined abnormality in collagen or collagen ratio subtypes
- Joint hypermobility may be a single phenotypic manifestation of a more systemic collagen-related problem

Epidemiology

- Hypermobility not associated with systemic disease occurs in about 4% to 15% of the population
- General joint laxity increases to a maximum at adolescence, diminishes with age, and especially manifest at growth spurts
- More common in women than men, and more common in those of African, Asian, and Middle Eastern descent

Pathogenesis

Possible contributing factors to joint pain with hypermobile joints are as follows:
- Collagen structure
- Bony structure and articulating surface
- Neuromuscular tone and strength
- Joint propricoception

Risk Factors

- Familial inheritance of hypermobility
- Activity related to stress, resulting in joint/connective tissue overuse

Clinical Features

- Patients may give a history at being "double-jointed"
- Can begin at any age, child or adult
- Early on, activity-related joint pain in one or more joints
- Pain usually later in the day, with joint use
- Less common joint stiffness, myalgia
- Pain with joint manipulation

Natural History

- Pain may progress to more persistent or prolonged periods in adolescence or young adulthood
- Other progressive signs of laxity in connective tissue are as follows:
  - Pes planus
  - Genu valgum
  - Lordosis
  - Scoliosis
  - Patellar/shoulder dislocation
  - Recurrent joint effusions
  - Sprains

Diagnosis

Differential diagnosis

- Diagnosis of exclusion
- JRA/inflammatory joint disease
- Marfans syndrome
- Ehlers-Danlos syndrome

History

- Activity-related joint pain in one or multiple joints
- Brighton criteria for the diagnosis:
  - Major criteria
    - A Beighton score of 4/9 or greater (either joints currently or historically); the Beighton score is a simple system to quantify joint hypermobility
    - Arthralgia for more than 3 months in 4 or more joints
  - Minor criteria
    - A Beighton score of 1, 2, or 3/9
    - Arthralgia (>3 months) in one to three joints or back pain (>3 months), spondylosis, spondylolysis/spondylolisthesis
    - Dislocation/subluxation in more than one joint, or in one joint on more than one occasion
    - Soft tissue rheumatism >3 lesions (eg, epicondylitis, tenosynovitis, and bursitis)

○ Marfanoid habitus (tall, slim, arm span/height ratio >1.03, upper:lower segment (top of head to pubic ramus:pubic ramus to floor) ratio less than 0.89, arachnodactyly (positive Steinberg [thumb goes beyond ulnar border while opposed in a clenched fist]/wrist signs[distal phalanges of first and fifth fingers overlap when wrapped around the other wrist])

○ Abnormal skin: striae, hyperextensibility, thin skin, papyraceous scarring

○ Eye signs: drooping eyelids, myopia, or antimongoloid slant

○ Varicose veins, hernia, or uterine/rectal prolapse

○ Diagnose in the presence of two major, one major and two minor, or four minor criteria

Exam

- Evidence of joint hypermobility based upon flexibility maneuvers of Carter-Wilkinson or a Beighton score ≥4 indicating generalized joint laxity
- Beighton score to assess hypermobility at the elbows, thumbs, fingers, knees, and trunk/spine (see drawings)

Testing

- With painful swollen joints important to rule out inflammatory arthritis: complete blood count, erythrocyte sedimentation rate, rheumatoid factor, antinuclear antibody

Pitfalls

- Eliminating all activity to decrease pain leads to deconditioning

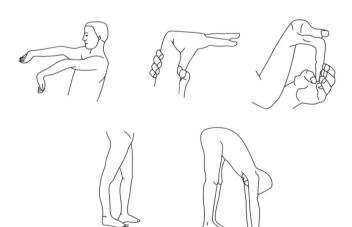

Red Flags

- More global chronic pain complaints overlapping with psychosomatic pain disorders: fibromyalgia and complex regional pain syndrome

Treatment

Medical

- Modification of activities to not exacerbate symptoms
- Nonsteroidal anti-inflammatory drug, acetaminophen

Exercise

- Joint strengthening/protective program
- Joint stretching/muscle balance
- Joint proprioceptive training, for example, wobble board

Modalities

- Heat
- Cold
- Supportive footwear
- Splinting or joint taping
- Massage
- Mobilization/counter strain

Consults

- Rheumatology
- Orthotist

Complications

- Potential for early onset osteoarthritis

Prognosis

- Symptoms generally nonprogressive as joint laxity decreases with age
- Good

Helpful Hints

- Maintain good physical fitness by program modification and elimination

Suggested Readings

Bird HA. Joint hypermobility. Patient information booklet for the Arthritic Research Campaign; 2000.

Grahame R. The revised (Brighton 1998) criteria for the diagnosis of benign joint hypermobility syndrome (BJHS). *J Rheumatol.* 2000;27:1777–1779.

Mishra MB, Ryan P, Atkinson P, et al. Extra-articular features of benign joint hypermobility syndrome. *Br J Rheumatol.* 1996;35(9);861–866.

Connective Tissue Disease: Dermatomyositis

Colleen A. Wunderlich MD

Description

Dermatomyositis is an inflammatory myopathy with characteristic skin rashes.

Etiology/Types

- Slowly progressive muscle weakness
- Rapid onset with fever, widespread vasculitic rash, and profound weakness
- Rare tumor-associated
- Amyotrophic dermatomyositis = subclinical muscle involvement

Epidemiology

- Commonly ages 5 to 15; peak onset 5 to 10 years
- 5.5 cases/million people

Pathogenesis

- Unknown
- Possible complement-mediated vascular inflammatory process or tumor necrosis factor alpha abnormality

Risk Factors

- HLA types DR3, DR5, and DR7

Clinical Features

- Proximal, symmetric muscle weakness
- Commonly follows skin disease
- Possible systemic disease affecting esophagus, lungs, or heart
- Characteristic heliotrope rash and Gottron's papules (erythematous symmetric lesions over the metacarpophalangeal and interphalangeal joints)
- Poikiloderma on exposed skin (i.e., the shawl sign) or extensor arm surfaces
- Pruritic rash → insomnia, alopecia
- Nail fold changes
- Calcinosis (calcium deposits throughout the muscle which may come out through the skin) in 40%; children and adolescents >> adults

Natural History

- In 40% only skin disease at onset
- Weakness progressive over weeks or months
- Calcinosis usually 1 to 3 years after onset
- Children often not diagnosed until cutaneous disease clearly seen

Diagnosis

Differential diagnosis

- Scleroderma
- Progressive systemic sclerosis
- Polymyositis
- Inclusion body myositis
- Hypothyroidism
- Steroid myopathy
- Sarcoidosis
- CREST syndrome
- Systemic lupus erythematosus
- Rosacea
- Tinea corporis
- Other myopathies

History

- Presenting complaint often increasing fatigue
- Child not able to keep up or asks to be carried
- Difficulty going up and down stairs
- Characteristic rashes
- Proximal muscle weakness, stiffness, or soreness
- Arthralgia, arthritis, dyspnea, dysphagia, dysphonia, arrhythmia, and uncommonly, previous malignancy

Exam

- Characteristic rashes
- Vasculitic nail lesions
- Proximal muscle weakness
- Extensor > flexor forearm affected
- Decreased to normal reflexes
- Muscle atrophy
- Calcifications
- Joint swelling in small joints of hand

Testing

- ↑CK, aldolase or SGOT, LDH
- Electromyography: fibrillations, positive sharp waves, complex repetitive discharges, short duration, low-amplitude polyphasic motor unit potentials

- Muscle biopsy: perivascular and interfascicular infiltrates with fiber degeneration and regeneration
- Magnetic resonance imaging: used to establish presence of muscle abnormalities in those without weakness, to select biopsy site, or differentiate steroid myopathy from inflammatory myopathy
- Myositis-specific antibodies

Pitfalls

- Nail fold capillary dilatation and Gottron's papules almost always signal dermatomyositis but may occur in scleroderma or progressive systemic sclerosis
- Swallow evaluation necessary at presentation and flare-ups to avoid aspiration
- Fulminant dermatomyositis requires inpatient care

Red Flags

- Multiorgan vasculitic complications possible
- Watch out for mental status changes, skin rashes, abdominal pain, and chest infections
- Untreated bowel vasculitis can lead to thrombosis, infarction, and perforation

Treatment

Medical

- High-protection sunscreen and protective clothing needed; avoid sun
- Topical corticosteroids for skin rashes as needed
- Oral/IV prednisone is the treatment of choice
- Steroids often started IV at diagnosis then changed to oral and titrated down as symptoms better controlled
- Methotrexate (MTX) often added to shorten steroid course or other immunosupressants if severe

- Biologics and intravenous immune globulin under study
- Hydroxychloroquine good for heliotrope rash
- Diltiazem helpful for calcinosis

Exercises

- PROM to prevent contractures
- Hold AROM and isometrics until muscle enzyme levels declining
- Maintain active lifestyle
- Strengthening exercises long term
- Adaptive equipment as needed

Modalities

- Icing, both acute and chronic

Surgical

- As needed to remove painful or infected calcium deposits
- Gastrostomy tube for dysphagia

Consults

- Rheumatology
- Dermatology
- Psychology or psychiatry as needed for support and adjustment
- Cardiology, pulmonology, nutrition, and surgical oncology

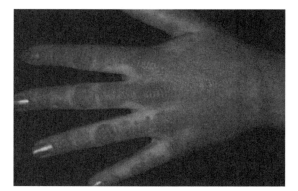

Lesions on the dorsal side of the hand demonstrate the photodistribution of dermatomyositis. Note the sparing of the interdigital web spaces. With permission from eMedicine.com, 2010.

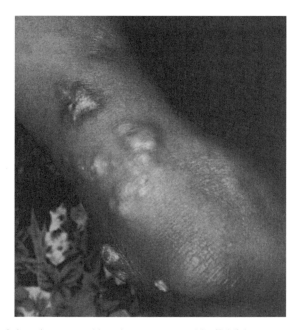

Calcinosis caused by dermatomyositis (DM) in childhood. With permission from eMedicine.com, 2010.

Complications of treatment
- Steroid-induced myopathy and atrophy
- MTX-induced hepatotoxicity and leukocytosis

Prognosis
- With treatment, symptoms usually resolve
- Some children have a chronic relapsing, remitting course; a few others are refractory to therapy
- Children with severe disease often develop contractures
- Calcinosis more likely in those with delayed diagnosis or less aggressive therapy

Helpful Hints
- Rash plus proximal weakness is likely dermatomyositis; check for key cutaneous and vasculitic findings
- Refer early to rheumatologist if suspected as better prognosis with earlier treatment

Suggested Readings

Callen JP, Wortmann RL. Dermatomyositis. *Clin Dermatol.* 2006;24(5):363–373.

Iorizzo LJ 3rd, Jorizzo JL. The treatment and prognosis of dermatomyositis: an updated review. *J Am Acad Dermatol.* 2008;59(1):99–112.

Connective Tissue Disease: Juvenile Rheumatologic Arthritis

Charles E. Sisung MD

Description

Juvenile rheumatoid arthritis (JRA), also called juvenile idiopathic arthritis (JIA), is a group of diseases of unknown etiology which manifest as chronic joint inflammation.

Etiology/Types

- The cause, though unknown, is felt to be environmentally triggered in a genetically primed host
- JRA subtypes are as given below:
  - Pauciarticular
  - Polyarticular
  - Systemic onset

Epidemiology

- Prevalence in the United States is 10 cases per 100,000 children but variable by study location (prevalence range 11–83/100,000)
- Pauci/polyarticular disease more common in girls
- Systemic onset equal in both sexes
- Occurs more frequently in certain populations, particularly in Native Americans
- Age variables are as given below:
  - pauciarticular: early childhood
  - systemic onset: early childhood through adolescence

Pathogenesis

- Unknown trigger
- Chronic synovial inflammation with B lymphocytes
- Macrophage and T lymphocyte invasion and cytokine release with further synovial proliferation
- Pannus (thickened synovium) leads to joint destruction

Risk Factors

- Genetic predisposition
- Family history of other autoimmune disease, including thyroiditis and diabetes

Clinical Features

- Evidence of joint inflammation as noted by the following factors:
  - swelling or effusion
  - limitation in range of motion (ROM)
  - tenderness or pain with ROM
  - warmth
- Present for at least 6 weeks
- Onset before age 16 years
- Onset type within the first 6 months:
  - pauciarticular: four or fewer joints
  - polyarticular: five or more joints
  - systemic onset: fever, rash, arthritis/arthralgias

Natural History

- Variable by onset type
- Onset insidious or abrupt
- Morning stiffness/limping
- Arthralgias
- Constitutional symptoms:
  - fever
  - weight loss
  - fatigue
- Decline in activity level
- Weakness/secondary muscle atrophy
- Loss of joint movement with persistent disease

Diagnosis

Differential diagnosis

- Trauma or orthopedic injury
- Infections with preceding illness
- Travel/exposure in Lyme disease
- Diarrhea/gastrointestinal symptoms in inflammatory bowel disease
- Weight loss/anorexia/fatigue in acute lymphocytic anemia

History

- Decreased activity level, especially in the morning
- Fatigue
- Fever
- Rash
- Joint swelling, warmth

Exam

- Joint fullness, tenderness
- Limitations in ROM

- Fever
- Rash
- Adenopathy
- Hepatosplenomegaly

Testing
- Lab: antinuclear antibody (ANA) positive in 25%, complete blood count, differential, platelet count erythrocyte sedimentation rate, and rheumatoid factor (RF) is rarely positive
- Other studies including urinalysis, total protein, albumin helpful, especially in systemic onset and polyarticular disease with more constitutional symptoms
- Radiography of affected joints
- Rarely arthrocentesis and synovial biopsy

Pitfalls
- Unusual presentation of monoarticular arthritis is a sign of possible infectious etiology or early hip arthritis in possible spondyloarthropathy

Red Flags
- Nonarticular complaints:
  - visual changes—iridocyditis
  - chest pain/shortness of breath—pericarditis
- ANA+ greater risk of eye disease
- High titer ANA:
  - disease evolution to another rheumatologic disease, including systemic lupus erythematosus

Treatment

Medical
- Lab studies support the diagnosis, and help with prognosis and disease management
- Nonsteroidal anti-inflammatory medication
- Corticosteroids
- Disease-modifying antirheumatic drugs such as methotrexate
- Biologic drugs, including etanercept (blocks tumor necrotic factor, thereby minimizing inflammation)

Exercises
- General strengthening, endurance, and fitness
- Maintain ROM and flexibility

Modalities
- Heat
- Cold
- Orthoses

Injection
- Selective pain control, treatment for focal joint disability with corticosteroids

Surgical
- Joint replacement

Consults
- Orthopedic surgery
- Rheumatology
- Orthotist
- Opthalmology
- Cardiology

Complications
- Visual loss
- Joint destruction with persistent disease

Prognosis
- Seldom life threatening, with mortality less than 1%
- From pericarditis or infection/immune suppression
- Persistent and/or additive arthritis associated with poor functional outcome
- Early wrist and later hip disease, especially symmetrical, associated with poor functional outcome
- RF+ a marker of persistent/life long, aggressive disease
- Presence of ANA+ status associated with eye disease risk

Helpful Hints
- Recognize persistent disease and markers of poor prognosis: total joint count and RF+, then treat aggressively

Suggested Readings
Foster HE, Marshall N, Myers A, et al. Outcome in adults with juvenile idiopathic arthritis: a quality of life study. *Arthritis Rheum.* 2003;48(3):767–775.

Wallace CA, Huang B, Bandeira M, et al. Patterns of clinical remission in select categories of juvenile idiopathic arthritis. *Arthritis Rheum.* 2005;52(11):3554–3562.

Connective Tissue Disease: Juvenile Rheumatologic Arthritis—Pauciarticular

Charles E. Sisung MD

Description

Juvenile rheumatoid arthritis (JRA) is a group of diseases of unknown etiology which manifest as chronic joint inflammation. Pauciarticular JRA has four or fewer joints involved within the first 6 months of disease onset.

Etiology

- The cause, though unknown, is felt to be environmentally triggered in a genetically primed host

Epidemiology

- 40% to 50% of cases of JRA
- Girls more than boys
- Often younger age: 3 to 6 years

Pathogenesis

- Unknown trigger
- Chronic synovial inflammation with B lymphocytes
- Macrophage and T lymphocyte invasion and cytokine release with further synovial proliferation
- Pannus leads to joint destruction

Risk Factors

- Genetic predisposition
- Family history of other autoimmune disease, for example, thyroiditis; diabetes

Clinical Features

- Typically involves larger joints, for example, knees, ankles, and wrists
- Monoarticular arthritis possible (rarely hip, unless spondyloarthropathy)
- Affected knee often associated with quadriceps muscle wasting, limping, and flexion contracture

Natural History

- Persistent swelling leads to progressive muscle wasting, weakness around the joint, and muscle contracture

Diagnosis

Differential diagnosis

- Consider lyme arthritis, infectious arthritis (including tuberculosis), postinfectious arthritis, foreign body, tumor with monoarthritis which is persistent and resistant to treatment
- Consider spondyloarthropathy, especially in the older child (>8 years) with asymmetric hip involvement, limited range of motion (ROM), tenderness with ROM, and decreased back/lumbar spine ROM with hamstring tightness

History

- Onset may be subtle/insidious
- Morning stiffness presents with decreased play activity in the toddler
- Prominent limping with stiffness, weakness, and contractures
- Joint fullness, warmth may be noted intermittently by the family

Exam

- Joint fullness and tenderness
- Limitations in ROM
- Strength of limbs

Testing

- Complete blood count/erythrocyte sedimentation rate usually normal
- Antinuclear antibody (ANA+), a marker for uveitis risk especially in younger girls
- Radiographs: most common finding is soft tissue swelling

Pitfalls

- Early onset hip disease, especially in an older child, is most likely spondyloarthropathy

Red Flags

- Positive ANA, especially in young girls, is a strong marker for possible uveitis. Though only 10% to 15% of children have or develop uveitis, 90% will be from this risk group

Treatment

Medical

- Nonsteroidal anti-inflammatory drugs and other pain medications
- Remittive agent if persistent additive disease and evidence of erosions on radiography

Exercise

- ROM and gentle strengthening
- General endurance and fitness
- Cautious management of knee contracture to prevent tibia subluxation

Modalities

- Heat
- Cold
- Serial casting to rest a joint and improve ROM
- Orthoses

Injections

- Steroid joint injection for more painful joint not responding to other medications

Surgical

- Joint replacement (knee most common) in adulthood

Consults

- Opthalmology
- Rheumatology

Complications

- Medication effects

Prognosis

- Excellent remission rate

Helpful Hints

- ANA+ is a marker for eye disease which is "silent" and needs to be routinely screened for by opthalmology

Suggested Readings

Arabshahi B, Dewitt DM, Cahill AM, et al. Utility of corticosteroid injection for temporomandiular arthritis in children with juvenile idiopathic arthritis. *Arthritis Rheum.* 2005;52(11):3563–3569.

Ilovwite NT. Current treatment of juvenile rheumatoid arthritis. *Pediatrics.* 2001;109(1): 109–115.

Connective Tissue Disease: Juvenile Rheumatologic Arthritis—Polyarticular

Charles E. Sisung MD

Description

Juvenile rheumatoid arthritis (JRA) is a group of diseases of unknown etiology which manifest as chronic joint inflammation. In polyarticular JRA there is joint inflammation in five or more joints within the first 6 months of disease onset. This type is most similar to adult rheumatoid arthritis (RA).

Etiology

- Unknown
- Felt to be environmentally triggered in a genetically primed host

Epidemiology

- 30% to 40% of cases of JRA
- Girls more than boys
- Can occur throughout childhood to early adolescence
- The later the onset, the more similar to adult RA

Pathogenesis

- Unknown trigger
- Chronic synovial inflammation with B lymphocytes
- Macrophage and T lymphocyte invasion and cytokine release with further synovial proliferation
- Thickened synovium leads to joint destruction

Risk Factors

- Genetic predisposition
- Family history of other autoimmune disease, including thyroiditis and diabetes

Clinical Features

- Often symmetrical arthritis involving the small joints of the hands, feet, jaw, and cervical spine
- Mild-to-moderate constitutional symptoms, that is, weight loss, fatigue, associated adenopathy, and organ inflammation
- Evidence of joint inflammation as noted by the following factors:
  - swelling or effusion
  - limitation in range of motion (ROM)
  - tenderness or pain with ROM
  - warmth
- Present for at least 6 weeks

Natural History

- With progressive disease, rapid progression of weakness and contractures possible
- Pain can be very severe, especially with hands/wrists, feet, and neck involvement
- Decline in activity level
- Weakness/secondary atrophy
- Loss of joint movement with persistent disease

Diagnosis

Differential diagnosis

- Malignancy (due to constitutional symptoms, ill appearance, concern for infection)
- Multiple organ system (systemic) disease with children often looking chronically ill

History

- Onset usually less subtle than systemic JRA with associated prominent morning stiffness
- Progressive joint complaints of swelling and warmth
- Fatigue
- Decreased activity level, especially in morning

Exam

- Often limited neck ROM
- Weakness in hands with symmetric joint swelling
- May see rheumatoid nodules at areas of pressure points, including elbows

Testing

- Complete blood count: may have elevated white blood counts, platelets, and anemia
- RF+ or may become positive in about 10% of patients
- Antinuclear antibody (ANA+): greater risk of eye inflammation

- Radiography of affected joints: periarticular soft tissue swelling, osteoporosis—juxta-articular, periostitis, overgrown or ballooned epiphyses, advanced skeletal maturation, late joint space loss, late erosive disease, and joint ankylosis
- Elevated erythrocyte sedimentation rate

Pitfalls

- Need to treat aggressively to prevent/decrease long-term disability from joint destruction

Red Flags

- ANA+: screen for eye disease routinely
- Monitor for functional decline: for example, missed school days, decreased ambulation endurance, self-care assistance, in conjunction with pain complaints to monitor treatment response
- Children may "feel better" due to curtailed activity and more sedentary lifestyle to reduce pain. Therapy program needs to maintain general fitness level

Treatment

Medical

- Disease-modifying antirheumatic drugs early, especially with RF+ or progressive joint disease
- Biologic agents such as etanercept
- Nonsteroidal anti-inflammatory drug and other pain medications to maintain movement/function
- Low dose short term steroids for constitutional symptoms

Exercise

- General physical fitness
- ROM and gentle strengthening
- Focus on neck, shoulder, pelvis flexibility, and general endurance
- Individualized Education Plan and school modifications as needed

Modalities

- Heat
- Cold

- Orthoses

Injections

- Steroid joint injections for more painful, limiting joints

Surgical

- Plan joint replacements as necessary to maintain activity level in late adolescence, young adulthood

Consults

- Rheumatology
- Opthamology

Complications

- Persistent joint disease and progressive contractures with pain and functional decline affecting mobility and self care
- Early joint fusion, especially arm/hand, limiting self-care independence

Prognosis

- Markers of bad disease 2 years postdiagnosis: persistent synovitis; additive joint count despite medical management
- Often early, profound disability due to joint involvement
- Ninety percent better within 2 years
- Up to 10% may have persistent disease and severe functional decline

Helpful Hints

- Remember to follow activity level/performance to monitor response to treatment, and to time joint replacements

Suggested Readings

Foster HE, Marshall N, Myers A, et al. Outcome in adults with juvenile idiopathic arthritis: a quality of life study. *Arthritis Rheum.* 2003;48(3):767–775.

Ravelli A, Martini A. Early predictors of outcome in juvenile idiopathic arthritis. *Clin Exp Rheumatol.* 2003;21(5 suppl 31):589–593.

Connective Tissue Disease: Juvenile Rheumatologic Arthritis—Systemic

Charles E. Sisung MD

Description

Juvenile rheumatoid arthritis (JRA) is a group of diseases of unknown etiology which manifest as chronic joint inflammation. There is joint pain ± swelling with associated spiking fever and evanescent rash.

Etiology

- Unknown
- Felt to be environmentally triggered in a genetically primed host

Epidemiology

- 10–20% of cases of JRA
- Equal distribution boys and girls

Pathogenesis

- Unknown trigger
- Chronic synovial inflammation with B lymphocytes
- Macrophage and T-lymphocyte invasion and cytokine release with further synovial proliferation
- Thickened synovium leads to joint destruction

Risk Factors

- Genetic predisposition
- Family history of other autoimmune disease, including thyroiditis and diabetes

Clinical Features

- Daily (usually afternoon) or twice daily fever (99–104°F) spike with return to baseline
- Fleeting rash, typically linear, often during fever, on trunk/extremities; 10% puritic
- Arthralgias often worse during the fever; joint swelling is atypical early
- Generalized myalgia
- Possible panserositis; for example, pericarditis, pleuritis
- Other constitutional symptoms including weight loss, nausea, and fatigue
- Adenopathy
- Hepatosplenomegaly
- Evidence of joint inflammation as noted by:
  - swelling or effusion
  - limitation in range of motion (ROM)
  - tenderness or pain with ROM
  - warmth
- Present for at least 6 weeks

Natural History

- Fever and other systemic features (organomegaly, adenopathy, etc.) usually dissipate with time
- Arthritis can become a long term problem and become polyarticular with joint destruction

Diagnosis

Differential diagnosis

- Multiple organ system (systemic) disease with children often looking chronically ill
- Cancer, for example, acute lymphocytic leukemia
- Infection

History

- Onset may be subtle/insidious
- Rash more prevalent with fever, during warm bath
- Daily fevers with normal baseline between spikes
- Progressive joint complaints of swelling, warmth

Exam

- Joint fullness, tenderness
- Limitations in ROM
- Fever
- Rash
- Adenopathy
- Hepatosplenomegaly

Testing

- Complete blood count—may have elevated white blood counts, platelets, erythrocyte sedimentation rate; anemia

- Rheumatoid factor/antinuclear antibody (ANA) negative
- Radiography of affected joints

Pitfalls
- With slow/insidious onset may have symptoms for several weeks before arthralgias/arthritis worsen

Red Flags
- With erratic fever (persistent or not returning to baseline) consider another diagnosis, for example, infection, cancer
- With positive serologies (ANA) likely another rheumatic disease, for example, systemic lupus erythematosis

Treatment

Medical
- Nonsteroidal anti-inflammatory drug
- Tylenol
- Steroids for more persistent systemic features with persistent arthritis +/- polyarticular disease
- Disease-modifying antirheumatic drugs: methotrexate, hydroxychloroquine, sulfasolazine
- Biologic agents: etanercept, infliximab

Exercises
- ROM and gentle strengthening

Modalities
- Cold
- Orthotics

Surgical
- Joint replacement

Consults
- Orthopedics
- Cardiology—pericarditis

Complications
- Persistent polyarticular disease/joint destruction/fusion

Prognosis
- Ninety percent better within 2 year
- Up to 10% may have persistent disease

Helpful Hints
- Short-term low-dose steroids help control systemic complaints and result in better therapy tolerance

Suggested Readings
Adams A, Lehman TJ. Update on the pathogenesis and treatment of systemic onset juvenile rheumatoid arthritis. *Curr Opin Rheumatol.* 2005;17(5):612–616.

Spiegel LS, Schneider R, Lang BA, et al. Early predictors of poor functional outcome in systemic-onset juvenile rheumatoid arthritis: a multi center cohort study. *Arthritis Rheum.* 2000;43(11):2402–2409.

Connective Tissue Disease: Kawasaki's Disease

Rajashree Srinivasan MD

Description

An acute febrile vasculitis of childhood, described by Dr Tomisaku Kawasaki of Japan in 1967. Asians are at high risk. It is the leading cause of acquired heart disease in children in Japan and the United States, replacing acute rheumatic fever. It is also known as mucocutaneous lymph node syndrome or infantile polyarteritis nodosa.

Etiology

- Hypothesis is that an aberrant immune response causes Kawasaki disease in genetically predisposed individuals
- Ubiquitous microbe, not identified

Epidemiology

- Three thousand cases diagnosed annually in the United States
- Occurs worldwide with increased incidence in Asians
- Seen mostly in children—80% less than 5 years, though occasionally adolescents and adults are affected
- Boys more than girls 1.5: 1

Pathogenesis

- Severe vasculitis of all blood vessels, predominantly affecting medium-sized arteries, with coronary artery predilection
- Edema of endothelial and smooth muscle cells seen
- Intense inflammatory infiltration of vascular wall
- Elevated levels of immunoglobulins

Risk Factors

- Genetic
- Environmental—epidemics in Japan; New York
- Viral infection—thought to be due to presence of cytoplasmic inclusion bodies in ciliated bronchial epithelium
- Immunologic—rare in infants <3 months suggesting passive maternal antibody; almost absent in adults suggesting widespread immunity

Clinical Features

- High fever (up to 104° F)—remittent, unresponsive to antibiotics. Lasts for 1 to 2 weeks
- Bilateral bulbar conjunctival injection, without exudate
- Erythema of oral and pharyngeal mucosa with "strawberry" tongue and dry, cracked lips
- Erythema and swelling of hands and feet
- Rash: maculopapular, erythema multiforme, or scarlatiniform, with accentuation in groin area
- Nonsuppurative cervical lymphadenopathy (node size of 1.5 cm or more).

Natural History

- Untreated symptoms are usually self limited by 4 to 8 weeks
- Risk of coronary artery disease, usually aneurysms
- Fatal in 1%

Diagnosis

Differential diagnosis

- Adenovirus infection
- Scarlet fever
- Epstein-Barr virus infection
- Fifth disease
- Rocky Mountain spotted fever
- Measles
- Polyartertis nodosa
- Toxic epidermal necrolysis
- Staphylococcal scalded skin syndrome
- Toxic shock syndrome

History

- High unremitting fever for 3 to 5 days with mucocutaneous manifestations

Exam

- Fever
- Rash, including strawberry tongue
- Conjunctivitis
- Lymphadenopathy
- Edema of hands and feet

Testing

- Lab—normocytic anemia, thrombocytosis, elevated erythrocyte sedimentation rate (ESR), elevated C-reaction protein, inflammatory hepatic changes
- Urine—sterile pyuria
- Echocardiography—may show pancarditis, pericardial effusion, coronary artery thrombosis, or coronary aneurysms
- Electrocardiography—showing conduction abnormalities and ischemic changes
- Repeat echocardiograms at 6 to 8 weeks, then 6 to 12 months, then consider depending on the American Heart Association risk stratification; for I–II: no coronary artery obstruction, in 5 years; for III–V: aneurysm or obstruction, biannual.
- Stress tests and serial imaging if evidence of coronary abnormalities
- Cardiac catheterization with angiography to delineate morphology once inflammation is resolved

Pitfalls

- Difficult to diagnose early
- Delay in diagnosis can lead to coronary artery involvement
- Relapse possible after initial treatment

Red Flags

- Arrhythmia

Treatment

Medical

- Intravenous immune globulin (IVIG) within the first 10 days of illness to decrease risk of coronary aneurysm
- High-dose aspirin until defervescence, or until day 14 with normal platelet and ESR
- Plasmapheresis if unresponsive to aspirin and IVIG
- Low dose aspirin after defervescence
- Annual immunization for influenza
- Antiplatelet agent to treat thrombocytosis
- Anticoagulation may be needed if coronary disease is present
- Use of corticosteroids controversial

Exercises

- General strengthening, closely monitored due to coronary artery anomalies
- Usually no restrictions after first 6 to 8 weeks

Modalities

- N/A

Injections

- N/A

Surgical

- Rare, cardiac

Consults

- Cardiology

Complications of treatment

- Blood clots

Prognosis

- Usually resolves by 4 to 8 weeks, untreated

Helpful Hints

- Early and extended treatment important

Suggested Readings

Burns JC. The riddle of Kawasaki disease. *N Engl J Med.* 2007;356:659–661.

Pinna GC, Kafetzis DA, Tselkas OI, Skovaki CL. Kawasaki disease: an overview. *Curr Opin Infect Dis.* 2008;21:263–270.

Connective Tissue Disease: Lyme Disease

Rajashree Srinivasan MD

Description

Infectious disease caused by a spirochete, *Borrelia burgdorferi*, borne by a tick.

Etiology

- Most common vector-borne disease in the United States
- Caused by the spirochete, *B burgdorferi*, which is transmitted by the bite of infected tick species *Ixodes scapularis* and *Ixodes pacificus*
- Babesiosis can occur as a coinfection, caused by *Babesia microti*. The other coinfection can be *Anaplasma phagocytophilum* (*Ehrlichia phagocytophilia*) causing human granulocytic anaplasmosis or human granulocytic ehrlichiosis

Epidemiology

- Lyme disease reported in more than 50 countries
- In the United States, most cases reported in New England, eastern parts of Middle Atlantic States, and upper Midwest, a small endemic focus along Pacific coast
- In Europe seen more in Scandinavian countries, Central Europe—Germany, Austria, and Switzerland
- Highest among children 5 to 10 years of age

Pathogenesis

- Skin infected as primary target. Inflammation produces erythema migrans, a characteristic rash
- Early disseminated disease is due to the spread of spirochetes, through the blood stream to tissues through the body
- Symptoms of early and late disease are due to inflammation mediated by interleukin-1 and other lymphokines in response to the organism's presence
- Inflammatory lesions containing both T and B cell lymphocytes, macrophages, plasma cells and some mast cells characterize inflammatory lesions in Lyme disease
- Lyme disease is a zoonosis caused by *B burgdorferi*, through the bite of an infected tick of Ixodes species, to humans. Ixodes ticks have a 2 year 3 stage life cycle

- Larvae hatch in early summer, uninfected with *B burgdorferi*
- Tick can become infected at any stage by feeding on a host, like white footed mouse—a natural reservoir for *B burgdorferi*
- Larvae emerge during winter to nymph form in spring, the stage that transmits infection
- Nymphs molt to adults in fall
- Females lay eggs the following spring before they die
- Risk of transmission of *B burgdorferi* is related to duration of feeding of the tick

Risk Factors

- Expansion of suburban neighborhood leads to deforestation, decreasing the primary reservoirs for Lyme disease
- Increased transmission due to increased human contact

Clinical Features

- Skin, joints, nervous system, and heart are involved typically
- Divided into early and late stages
  - **Early** localized disease—first manifestation is the annular rash—erythema migrans
  - Occurs 7 to 14 days after the bite
  - Initial lesion is at the site of the bite
  - Rash may be uniformly erythematous or like a target lesion with a central clearing
  - Rash can occur anywhere on the body. Can be associated with fever, myalgia, malaise, and headache. Rash remains for 1 to 2 weeks
  - Early disseminated disease—secondary erythema lesions develop in 20% of cases, caused by hematogenous spread of organisms to multiple skin sites. Secondary lesions are smaller than primary lesions and are accompanied by fever, myalgia, headache, malaise, conjunctivitis, and lymphadenopathy
  - Other presentations include aseptic meningitis, carditis with heart block, papilledema, uveitis, or

focal neurological findings, including cranial nerve involvement
- **Late** disease—arthritis, starting weeks to months after initial infection, is the presentation of late disease
- Arthritis involves large joints, like the knee, presenting as tender and swollen. Resolution is seen in 1 to 2 weeks
- Late manifestations involving central nervous system—called, tertiary neuroborreliosis, seen in adults, present with encephalitis, polyneuritis, and memory problems
- Congenital lyme disease may be seen in endemic areas though extremely rare

Natural History
- Untreated patients can develop chronic and severe symptoms affecting various organ systems
- Paraplegia or chronic polyneuropathy can occur

Diagnosis

Differential diagnosis
- GBS
- Encephalitis
- Polyneuritis

History
- History of being in a tick-infested area

Exam
- Circular, outwardly expanding rash called erythema migrans. Inner-most part is red and indurated, outer edge is red, the portion between the two areas is clear, appears like a "bulls eye"
- Neurology evaluation for nerve involvement
- Joints tender and swollen

Testing
- IgM antibodies are elevated at 6 to 8 weeks

- ELISA against antibodies to *B burgdorferi*
- Western blot
- Culture takes 4 weeks, though is diagnostic
- Increased white cell count, elevated erythrocte sedimentation rate, mild pleocytosis, and elevated cerebrospinal fluid protein

Pitfalls
- Due to absorption from the skin, insect repellents can cause toxicity in children
- Vaccine—introduced in 1998 and withdrawn in 2002

Red Flags
- Delay in diagnosis

Treatment
- Removal of tick and treatment with antibiotic
- Wear appropriate protective clothing when in tick infested areas, check skin. Skin repellants provide only transient protection
- Empiric treatment—for patients with erythema migrans, and in endemic areas, if prolonged, unexplained constitutional symptoms in absence of erythema migrans and who test positive for Lyme, doxycycline is the drug of choice. Not recommended in children less than 8 years of age due to discoloration of teeth, so other drugs can be used: Cefuroxime, Ceftriaxone

Prognosis
- Excellent in children and in those treated at the beginning of the late phase

Suggested Readings
Foy AJ, Studdiford JS. Lyme Disease. *Clinics Fam Pract.* 2005;7:191–208.
Patricia D, Robert BN. Erythema migrans. *Infect Dis Clin North Am.* 2008;22:235–260.

Connective Tissue Disease: Rheumatic Fever

Rajashree Srinivasan MD

Description

Rheumatic fever is a multisystem inflammatory disease seen in genetically predisposed individuals 2 to 3 weeks after a Group A Streptococcal infection. It is thought to be due to antibody cross reactivity in the heart, skin, joints, and brain.

Etiology

- Group A Beta Hemolytic Streptococcal infection such as sore throat or scarlet fever

Epidemiology

- Seen in children 5 to 15 years of age
- Common throughout the world
- In the United States, prevalence is less than 0.05/1000 population. Higher incidence in Maori and native Hawaiians
- Male to female ratio is equal
- Incidence—0.1% to 3% in patients with untreated streptococcal pharyngitis
- Increased incidence in crowding, poverty, and young age
- There may be familial disposition

Pathogenesis

- Occurs after untreated Group A hemolytic streptococcal infection
- Thought to be due to antibody cross reactivity, a type II hypersensitivity reaction
- M protein present in Group A *Streptococcus pyogenes* cell wall is very antigenic. Antibodies formed against the M protein cross react with myosin in cardiac muscle, heart muscle glycogen, and smooth muscle arteries
- Inflammation produced causes immune reactions

Risk Factors

- Genetic
- Environmenta—crowding and poverty
- Streptococcal infection

Clinical Features

- Fever
- Signs of migratory polyarthritis involving large joints with cephalic spread
- Signs of carditis, congestive heart failure, pericarditis, and new heart murmur
- Erythema marginatum—serpiginous evanescent rash. Never starts on face, worse with heat
- Abdominal pain and epistaxis
- Sydenham's chorea (St. Vitus' dance) can occur as an isolated manifestation after group A respiratory tract streptococcal infection, or precede, or accompany other manifestations

Natural History

- Acute rheumatic fever—pericarditis resolves without sequelae
- Involvement of endocardium leads to thickenings called MacCallum plaques
- Chronic rheumatic heart disease causes leaflet thickening, commissural fusion, and shortened and thickened chorda tendinae; aortic and mitral valve stenosis seen
- Recurrence is less common if low dose antibiotics are used

Diagnosis

Differential diagnosis

- Rheumatoid arthritis
- Juvenile rheumatoid arthritis (Still's disease)
- Bacterial endocarditis
- Systemic lupus erythematosus
- Serum sickness
- Viral infection

History

Jones Major Criteria

- Cardiac involvement may include pancarditis, mitral valve stenosis and regurgitation, aortic stenosis and regurgitation
- Migratory polyarthritis is seen in large joints. Arthritis persists for 12 to 24 hours and can last a week or so
- Erythema marginatum is seen in 5% to 13 % of patients with rheumatic fever. Defined as pink-red nonpruritic macules or papules

- Subcutaneous nodules are seen on the extensor surface of joints
- Sydenham's chorea is characterized by rapid involuntary movements of all extremities, sometimes involving tongue
- Prior history of rheumatic fever or inactive heart disease

Exam
- Fever
- Migratory polyarthritis
- Carditis, congestive heart failure, pericarditis, and new heart murmur
- Erythema marginatum
- Sydenham's chorea

Testing
- Increased antistreptolysin O titers, AntiDNase B (streptozyme), streptococcal antibodies may be helpful
- Chest x-ray for cardiomegaly
- Echocardiogram
- Aschoff bodies-made up of swollen eosinophilic collagen from cardiac tissue, surrounded by lymphocytes and macrophages are seen on light microscopy
- Lab—increased C-reactive protein and erythrocyte sedimentation rate, also leukocytosis
- Electrocardiography—Prolonged PR interval
- Evidence of strep infection—Increased ASO titer, DNAse, may have negative strep cultures

Pitfalls
- Delay in diagnosing Streptococcal infection leads to Rheumatic fever

Red Flags
- New heart murmur

Treatment

Medical
- Acute phase—Aspirin to treat arthralgia

- Penicillin to treat carriers
- Prednisone for carditis and heart failure
- Chronic phase—benzathine penicillin monthly to prevent recurrence in patients at risk: multiple previous attacks, children, adolescents, teachers, military recruits, individuals living in crowded dormitories, economically disadvantaged
- Duration varies: usually for 5 years, or until 21 years, or until age 40 years, or lifelong

Exercises
- Bed rest for severe carditis, then gradual supervised increase in activity

Surgical
- Rarely for cardiac valve sequelae

Consults
- Cardiology
- Rheumatology
- Infectious disease

Prognosis
- Variable
- Risk of recurrence greatest in the first 3 years, so take antibiotics to minimize

Helpful Hints
- Index of suspicion should be low to diagnose and treat rheumatic fever as its effects can be minimized with prompt care
- Low dose antibiotics to prevent recurrence

Suggested Readings
Cilliers AM. Rheumatic fever and its management. *BMJ*. 2006;333:1153–1156.

Tubridy-Clark M, Carapetis JR. Subclinical carditis in rheumatic fever: a systematic review. *Int J Cardiol*. 2007;119:54–58.

Connective Tissue Disease: Septic Arthritis

Rajashree Srinivasan MD

Description

Septic arthritis is an infection in a joint which results in arthritis occurring due to occult bacteremia. It is also known as suppurative arthritis. Hips, knees, and sacroliliac joints (SIJ) are most commonly involved.

Etiology/Types

- In the pediatric population, the most common joints involved are hips > knees > SIJ
- For children: most commonly due to Staphylococci, Streptococci, gram-negative anaerobes, and community acquired methicillin-resistant Staphylococcus aureus
- Prosthetic joint infections are due to Staphylococcus aureus, mixed flora, and gram-negative organisms
- Brucellosis—exposure to unpasteurized diary products

Epidemiology

- 2 to 10/100,000 in the United States
- Most cases occur by 5 years of age
- Hip, knee, and SIJ are commonly involved

Pathogenesis

- Majority of infection is of hematogenous origin
- Usually a result of occult bacteremia
- Lack of a protective basement membrane predisposes the highly vascular synovium to bacterial seeding
- Microscopic breaks in skin or mucous membranes allow bacteria access to bloodstream
- Infections with gram-negative organisms come up from the gastrointestinal and urinary tracts
- Penetrating trauma
- Joint damage is due to bacterial invasion, host inflammation, and tissue ischemia
- Enzymes and toxins released from bacteria are harmful to cartilage
- Avascularity of cartilage and its dependency on oxygen diffusion from synovium leads to increased joint pressure due exudate accumulation with tamponade of synovial blood flow causing cartilage hypoxia

Risk Factors

- Preexisting joint disease, recent trauma, prior joint surgery, and connective tissue disease, including SLE
- Rheumatoid arthritis patients at high risk due to joint damage, immunosuppressive medication, and skin breakdown. Periarticular disease can cause sinus tracts, bursitis, and rupture of synovial cysts
- Conditions causing loss of skin integrity
- Conditions with compromised immunity
- Anti-inflammatory treatment with tumor necrosis factor blockers
- Infection of bones and joints can occur after penetrating injuries or procedures
- Risk-taking behavior, seen more commonly in boys predisposes to trauma
- Impaired host defenses predispose

Clinical Features

- Classic presentation—fever; rigors; warm, swollen, and painful joint
- Serum leukocytosis
- Knee joint most involved with bacterial septic arthritis
- FABERE test—flexion, abduction, external rotation, and extension stresses the sacroiliac joint
- Pubic symphysis infection presents with fever, suprapubic and hip pain, waddling, antalgic gait
- Other joints that can be involved are shoulder, elbows, and sternoclavicular joints

Natural History

- Variable, but with proper antibiotics, can do well

Diagnosis

Differential diagnosis

- Trauma, cellulitis, pyomyositis, sickle cell disease, hemophilia, Henoch Schonlein purpura, collagen vascular disease, and rheumatic fever
- For hip: toxic synovitis, Legg-Calve-Perthes disease, slipped capital femoral epiphysis, psoas abscess, proximal femoral, pelvic, or vertebral osteomyelitis

■ For knee: distal femoral or proximal osteomyelitis, pauciarticular rheumatoid arthritis, referred pain from hip

History
■ Fever
■ Lack of movement
■ Joint pain

Exam
■ Septic, swollen joints
■ Decreased or refusal to weight bearing
■ Antalgic gait
■ Decreased range of motion

Testing
■ Blood cultures
■ X-rays, computed tomography, magnetic resonance imaging and radionuclide studies
■ Aspiration of joint fluid sent for gram stain and culture; synovial leukocytosis may be seen
■ Lab: C-reactive protein >20 mg/L, erythrocyte sedimentation rate >40, and white blood cell >12,000

Pitfalls
■ Perception of joint pain can be blunted in patients on corticosteroids, leading to delay in diagnosis
■ Needs long-term treatment

Red Flags
■ High index of suspicion in patients with sickle cell and anyone with compromised immune status

Treatment

Medical
■ Joint drainage decompresses the joint
■ Empirical broad spectrum antibiotics
■ Duration of therapy varies between 4 and 6 weeks, depending on the joints involved

Exercises
■ Nonweight bearing postoperatively
■ Passive range of motion as infection improves
■ Progress to isometric strengthening, then active range of motion

Modalities
■ Splint in position of function
■ Avoid topical heat

Injection
■ Needle aspiration

Surgery
■ Drainage and lavage of joint if not quickly improving
■ Central line for long-term antibiotics

Consults
■ Infectious disease
■ Surgery

Complications
■ Osteoarthritis and joint degeneration
■ Sepsis

Prognosis
■ Outcome is good with drainage of exudate and antibiotic therapy

Helpful Hints
■ Monitor C-reactive protein during treatment

Suggested Readings
Donatto KC. Orthopedic management of septic arthritis. *Rheum Dis Clin North Am.* 1998;24:276–286.
John JR. Septic arthritis. *Infec Dis Clin North Am.* 2005;19:799–817.

Connective Tissue Disease: Systemic Lupus Erythematosus

Maureen R. Nelson MD

Description

Systemic lupus erythematosus (SLE) is an autoimmune disease that is quite variable and can affect multiple body systems. Almost everyone with SLE has arthritis. The word lupus means wolf, and some say the classic malar rash on the face looks either like a wolf facial pattern or like having been bitten by a wolf.

Etiology/Types

- Twenty percent of cases begin in childhood
- Most children have migratory arthritis

Epidemiology

- Cause is not known
- Thought to occur after infection with organism that resembles body protein which is later targeted
- May occur after medications
- Can occur at any age, but is more frequent after 5 years, and is most common between ages 10 and 50
- Girls are affected more than boys by about 5:1
- Asians, blacks, and Hispanics are much more commonly affected than whites

Pathogenesis

- Inappropriate immune response with immune complex deposition leading to inflammatory response

Risk Factors

- Infection
- At least 38 medications have been implicated, with procainamide, hydralazine, and quinidine mentioned as highest risks

Clinical Features

- Joint pain, most commonly in fingers, hands, wrists, and knees
- Arthritis
- Pericarditis, myocarditis, and endocarditis
- Fatigue and malaise
- Pulmonary disease
- Fever
- Skin rash, particularly the butterfly (malar) rash over the cheeks and nasal bridge and especially after sun exposure in 30% to 50%
- Seizures

Natural History

- Variable
- Commonly migratory arthritis
- Joint deformity over time
- May get glomerulonephritis due to immune complex deposition; rarely may lead to renal failure

Diagnosis

Differential diagnosis

- Scleroderma
- Conversion disorder
- Arthritis
- Teenage adjustment problems

History

- Variable joint pain
- Fatigue and malaise
- Respiratory disease
- Anorexia
- Photosensitivity

Exam

- Joint abnormalities
- Malar butterfly rash
- Lymphadenopathy
- Pleural rub
- Oral or nasopharyngeal ulcer

Testing

- Antibody tests, including antinuclear antibody panel, antidouble strand DNA, antiphospholipid antibodies, anti-Smith antibodies
- Radiographs of involved joints to check for arthritis or medication effects
- Chest x-ray to evaluate both heart and lungs
- Urinalysis to check for proteinuria or hematuria
- Erythrocyte sedimentation rate

- Complete blood count—anemia in up to 50%, with thrombocytopenia, and leukopenia from SLE or medications
- Kidney biopsy if hematuria or proteinuria, since renal failure may develop from lupus nephritis
- Pulmonary function studies may show restrictive pattern

Pitfalls
- Difficult to evaluate effectiveness of treatment due to relapsing, variable disease course

Red Flags
- Lupus nephritis can lead to renal failure; urinalysis is followed; if problematic: 24-hour urine collection
- Cardiac complications
- Hemolytic anemia
- Seizures

Treatment

Medical
- Nonsteroidal anti-inflammatory medications
- Corticosteroids
- Hydroxychloroquine (plaquenil)
- Immunosuppressive medications including methotrexate, azathioprine, cyclophosphamide, and cyclosporine
- Plasmapheresis

Exercises
- General strengthening and stretching

Modalities
- Whirlpool

Injection
- Corticosteroid injection into joints

Surgical
- For associated disease, including renal

Consults
- Rheumatology
- Nutrition
- Nephrology

Complications
- Proximal weakness may be due to illness, myositis, or steroid use
- Avascular necrosis of the femoral head due to steroid use
- Stomach ulcer due to medications
- Cataracts due to steroids, other medications, SLE
- Osteopenia due to the disease, medications used, and difficulty exercising due to lupus
- Infection since SLE and medications to treat it affect the immune system

Prognosis
- Good, with 5-year survival 100%, 10-year survival >85%
- Poorer with low socioeconomic status, more extensive disease activity, and central nervous system and renal involvement

Helpful Hints
- Be aware of psychological impact of disease and treatment on teenagers

Suggested Readings
Bader-Meunier B, Armengaud JB, Haddad E, et al. Initial presentation of childhood onset systemic lupus erythematosus: a French multicenter study. *J Pediatr.* 2005;146:648–653.

Hiraki LT, Benseler SM, Tyrrell PN, et al. Clinical and laboratory characteristics and long-term outcome of pediatric systemic lupus erythermatosus: a longitudinal study. *J Pediatr.* 2008;152:550–556.

Conversion Reaction

Ellen S. Kaitz MD

Description

Conversion disorder is a condition in which symptoms and deficits in voluntary motor and/or sensory function suggest a neurologic or physical condition, but are without organic or physiologic explanation. It is one type of somatoform disorder.

Etiology/Types
- Psychiatric

Epidemiology
- Most common in 10 to 15 year old
- Rare in children <6 years
- If <10 years old, male = female
- In adolescents, 2 to 3:1 female to male

Pathogenesis
- Psychodynamic theory: symptom is a symbol of underlying psychologic conflict
- Learning theory: symptom is a maladaptive learned response to stress

Risk Factors
- Rigid obsessional personality trait
- Anxiety or depression
- Prior sexual abuse
- Personality disorder

Clinical Features
- Motor: paralysis, gait disturbance, incoordination, tremor, loss of speech, and astasia/abasia (the inability to stand or walk normally, with dramatic lurching, and falling only when someone is there to catch)
- Sensory: parasthesia, intractable pain, tunnel vision, hearing loss, and abdominal pain
- Other: pseudoseizures, headache, unremitting fatigue, and hiccups

Natural History
- Highly variable
- Many successfully treated by pediatrician with reassurance
- Spontaneous resolution of symptoms with removal of stressors
- Persistent symptoms and functional disability

Diagnosis

Differential diagnosis
- Malingering: conscious deception
- Other psychiatric disorder
- Personality disorder
- Multiple sclerosis or other neurologic disorder
- Complex regional pain syndrome
- Epilepsy
- Brain or spinal cord lesion

History
- Onset of symptoms often occurs around identifiable life stressor
- High-achieving student and/or athlete
- Limited prior coping strategies, poor interpersonal communication (males), family conflicts (females)
- Medical model of similar symptoms—patient knows someone with organic disease with similar presentation

Exam
- Variable, depending on manifestation
- Ratchet-like ("give way") weakness
- Inconsistent or changing symptoms
- Severe balance disturbance without falls
- Narrow-based gait with exaggerated forward flexion or dramatic sway
- Symptom magnification during observation

Testing
- Electroencephalography if pseudoseizure
- Electromyography and magnetic resonance imaging to rule out organic disease
- Once diagnosis is clinically evident, further testing should be avoided

Pitfalls
- Longer duration of symptoms often more resistant to treatment
- Presence of organic disease does not preclude coexisting conversion disorder

Red Flags
- Hostility toward medical query or investigation (suggests malingering)
- Abnormal reflexes

Treatment

Medical
- Behavioral: positive reinforcement (common) and negative reinforcement (uncommon)
- Modality based
- Psychiatric: psychotherapy, hypnosis

Exercises
- Graded program of progressively more complex motor tasks

Modalities
- Biofeedback
- Functional electrical stimulation

Injection
- Not indicated

Surgical
- Not indicated

Consults
- Neurology
- Psychiatry/psychology

Complications of treatment
- Psychologic distress
- Recurrence or persistence of symptoms
- Symptom substitution

Prognosis
- Early intervention is associated with high rates of symptom resolution and return to baseline functioning
- Limited studies in children suggest psychiatric and behavioral/rehabilitative models of treatment that have similar outcomes

Helpful Hints
- Avoid confronting the patient
- Avoid labeling, trivializing, or reinforcing symptoms
- Create expectation of recovery with child and family
- Resistant patients may respond to double-bind scenario: tell them that full recovery is proof of an organic etiology and that failure to recover is evidence of a psychiatric etiology
- Provide a structured environment with specific goals and expectations
- Individualized rewards for achievement of goals may improve compliance and speed of improvement

Suggested Readings

Gooch JL, Wolcott R, Speed J. Behavioral management of conversion disorder in children. *Arch Phys Med Rehabil.* 1997;78(3):264–268.

Pehlivantürk B, Unal F. Conversion disorder in children and adolescents: a 4-year follow-up. *J Psychosom Res.* 2002;52(4):187–191.

Cystic Fibrosis

Stephen Kirkby MD ■ Mark Splaingard MD

Description

Cystic fibrosis (CF) is the most common fatal genetic disorder affecting Caucasians. It is a multisystem disease caused by a defect in the cystic fibrosis transmembrane conductance regulator (CFTR) protein.

Etiology

- Genetic

Epidemiology

- Autosomal recessive inheritance
- Approximately 1:3000 Caucasians affected
- Average life expectancy is approximately 38 years

Pathogenesis

- The CFTR protein is a cell membrane ion channel
- Defective CFTR results in abnormal chloride secretion and leads to production of thick mucus
- Over 1500 known CF mutations; delta F508 is most common
- Altered chloride transport depletes airway surface liquid layer and results in thick mucus and altered mucociliary transport
- Chronic airway bacterial colonization and recurrent pulmonary infections (*Pseudomonas aeruginosa* and *Staphylococcus aureus* are common pathogens)
- Chronic airway inflammation leads to the development of bronchiectasis
- In the gastrointestinal tract, thick mucus leads to poor absorption of nutrients and results in malnutrition
- In the pancreas, thick mucus leads to pancreatic insufficiency and diabetes mellitus
- CF-related liver disease is common

Clinical Features

- Chronic cough
- Sputum production
- Shortness of breath and exercise limitation
- Wheezing
- Hemoptysis
- Pneumothorax
- Sinus congestion
- Malnutrition
- Loose, greasy stools
- Constipation—may be severe
- Pancreatic insufficiency
- Hyperglycemia/Diabetes mellitus
- Infertility
- Portal hypertension
- Osteopenia/Osteoporosis

Natural History

- Progressive obstructive lung disease
- Chronic respiratory failure is most common cause of death
- Diabetes mellitus frequently develops in adults

Diagnosis

Differential diagnosis

- Asthma
- Immunodeficiency
- Other causes of malnutrition

History

- Chronic cough
- Recurrent sinopulmonary infections
- Malnutrition, failure to thrive
- Decline in pulmonary function

Exam

- Hyperinflation of thorax
- Crackles
- Digital clubbing
- Malnutrition

Testing

- Sweat chloride
- Genetic analysis of CFTR gene
- Chest x-ray
- Chest computed tomography scan may demonstrate bronchiectasis
- Pulmonary function testing demonstrating airflow obstruction
- Sputum culture

Red Flags

- Acute chest pain may be associated with pneumothorax
- Hemoptysis can occur acutely and may be life-threatening

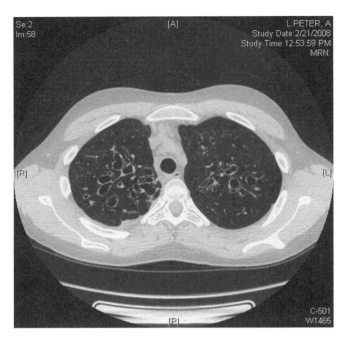

Chest CT scan demonstrating bronchiectasis in a patient with advanced CF lung disease.

Treatment

Medical

- Antibiotic therapy during periods of pulmonary exacerbations
- Oral azithromycin and inhaled tobramycin used chronically in patients colonized with *Pseudomonas aeruginosa*
- Chest physiotherapy enhances airway clearance
- Aerosolized dornase alpha decreases mucus viscosity
- Aerosolized hypertonic saline hydrates the airways
- Inhaled bronchodilators
- Digestive enzyme supplementation
- Caloric supplementation
- Insulin for diabetes

Exercises

- Regular physical exercise is encouraged
- Chest physiotherapy

Surgical

- Bilateral lung transplantation is an option for patients with end-stage pulmonary disease
- Sinus surgery

Consults

- Pulmonology
- Gastroenterology
- Nutrition

Complications

- Exacerbation of pulmonary disease
- Pneumothorax
- Hemoptysis
- Sinus disease
- Liver cirrhosis/portal hypertension
- Severe constipation
- Diabetes mellitus

Prognosis

- Patients can be expected to survive well into adulthood with aggressive management including treatment of pulmonary infections, regular chest physiotherapy, nutritional support, and close attention to nonpulmonary manifestations

Helpful Hints

- CF is a multisystem disease and requires an experienced multidisciplinary team for optimal long-term management
- An increase in pulmonary symptoms indicates an exacerbation; further evaluation by a pulmonologist is indicated
- Many patients harbor multidrug resistant bacteria and contact isolation is often indicated
- Abdominal pain in a CF patient is frequently caused by severe constipation

Suggested Readings

Davis PB. Cystic fibrosis since 1938. *Am J Respir Crit Care Med.* 2006;173:475–482.

Flume PA, O'Sullivan BP, Robinson KA, et al. Cystic fibrosis pulmonary guidelines: chronic medications for maintenance of lung health. *Am J Respir Crit Care Med.* 2007;176:957–969.

Developmental Delay

Marcie Ward MD

Description

Developmental delay is a lag in one or more domains of development; the delay may include gross motor, fine motor, speech and language, or social-emotional developmental delays.

Etiology/Types

- Global developmental delay
  - Delays in all domains
- Mixed developmental delay
  - Some motor delay plus another domain
- Pervasive developmental disorder
  - Deviance in development

Epidemiology

- Estimated incidence ranges from 16% to 18%

Pathogenesis

- Often due to CNS pathology
- Can be due to neuromuscular pathology
- Sometimes a result of severe environmental factors

Risk Factors

- Poor socioeconomic status
- Prenatal factors/maternal factors:
  - Previous pregnancy complications
  - Maternal medical comorbidities/infections
  - Prenatal complications
- Early (<30 weeks' gestation) or complicated birth
- Neonatal factors
  - Abnormal sucking/feeding/crying
  - Additional medical support needed at birth
  - Low birth weight
- Family history of developmental delay

Clinical Features

- Late or unrealized attainment of milestones

Natural History

- Delayed or arrested development
- Often identified by the school system when enrolled

Diagnosis

Differential diagnosis

- Speech and language delay
  - Hearing loss/poor language environment
  - Intellectual disability
  - Autism
  - Dysarthria
  - Specific learning disability
  - Developmental language disorder
  - Landau-Kleffner syndrome
- Gross motor delay alone
  - Cerebral palsy
  - Ataxia
  - Spina bifida
  - Spinal muscular atrophy
  - Myopathy
  - Benign congenital hypotonia
  - Developmental coordination disorder
- Fine motor delay alone
  - Hemiplegic cerebral palsy
  - Brachial plexus palsy
  - Fractured clavicle
  - Developmental coordination disorder
  - Disorder of written expression
- Motor delay plus speech and language delay
  - Intellectual disability
  - Visual impairment
  - Cerebral palsy
- Personal-social delay
  - Intellectual disability
  - Autism
  - Abuse/neglect/deprivation
  - Dysfunctional parenting

History

- Obstetric history
- Prenatal/perinatal course
- Developmental history
- Medical history
  - Significant illnesses
  - Chronic medical conditions
- Social history
  - Parental marital/custodial status

– Adoption or foster care history
– Current rehabilitation services
– Family history of developmental delay

Exam

- Microcephaly, macrocephaly, or normocephaly
- Obligatory/persistent primitive/brisk/Babinski/ abnormal postural reflexes
- Absent deep tendon reflexes
- Muscle tone evaluation
- Range of motion
- Symmetry of movement
- Evaluation of gait

Testing

- Administer standardized parent questionnaire
- Standardized clinical developmental screening tool
- MRI of brain and/or spine to evaluate for any structural abnormalities
- Genetic testing for chromosomal disorders
- Metabolic testing to identify any inborn errors of metabolism

Pitfalls

- Failure to identify delays impedes the child's connection with appropriate habilitative services

Red flags

- Loss of any previously acquired skill necessitates referral to evaluate for a progressive rather than static disease

Treatment

Medical

- Treat abnormally high tone with oral medications
- Follow nutrition to assure safe and adequate intake

Exercise

- Physical therapy for gross motor skills
- Occupational therapy for fine motor skills, adaptive social-emotional skills, and sensory integration
- Speech therapy for communication skills

Modalities

- Provide equipment to facilitate habilitation of skills
- Augmentative communication devices
- Functional neuromuscular stimulation

Injection

- Botulinum toxin and phenol neurolysis

Surgical

- Rare

Consults

- Neurology
- Ophthalmology
- Audiology/otolaryngology
- Developmental pediatrics
- Genetics
- Psychology/social work

Complications of treatment

- Oral medications: somnolence
- Injectable medications: weakness

Prognosis

- Variable
- Language delays may represent cognitive impairment if not explained by hearing loss or a specific disorder of speech production

Helpful Hints

- The American Academy of Pediatrics recommends that surveillance and screening take place in the primary care provider's office to capture as many children at risk for developmental delay as possible
- Standardized parental report questionnaires have a high degree of reliability for identifying developmental delays
- The sooner a delay is recognized, the sooner habilitative services can be implemented to assist the child in catching up to his or her peers developmentally

Suggested Readings

American Academy of Pediatrics. Identifying infants and young children with developmental disorders in the medical home: an algorithm for developmental surveillance and screening. *Pediatrics*. 2006;118:405–420.

PEDIATRICS Vol. 118 No. 1 July 2006, pp. 405–420 (doi:10.1542/ peds.2006–1231)

Tervo RC. Identifying patterns of developmental delays can help diagnose neurodevelopmental disorders. *Clin Pediatr*. 2006;45(6):509–517.

Down Syndrome

Joseph E. Hornyak MD PhD

Description
Down syndrome (DS) is the most commonly seen pattern of human malformation and known cause of intellectual disability.

Etiology/Types
- 95% complete trisomy 21
- 2.5% mosaic trisomy 21
- 2.5% Robertsonian translocation, 21 → 14

Epidemiology
- Incidence roughly 1 in 700 live births
- Common cause of miscarriage
- Higher risk with increasing maternal age, though most born to younger mothers

Pathogenesis
- On average, 50% increase in expression from genes on chromosome 21
- Overexpression results in abnormal fetal development as well as metabolic abnormalities
- No clear correlation of any gene to a specific phenotypic feature
- Overexpression of DS "critical region" necessary for syndrome features
- Likely most overexpression is not pathogenic
- Overexpression of microRNA's on chromosome 21 may play a pathogenic role in gene expression

Risk Factors
- Increasing maternal age: 0.1% in a 20-year-old woman, 1% in a 40-year-old woman, and >3.5% in a 45-year-old woman
- With higher pregnancy rates, most mothers of children with DS are actually younger
- Translocation carrier of DS critical region
- Recurrence rate approximately 1% (higher in translocation carriers) after one affected child in family

Clinical Features
- Global developmental delays
- Cognitive impairments
- Hypotonia
- Joint hypermobility/ligamentous laxity
- Flattened nasal bridge
- Prominent epicanthal folds
- Brushfield spots, small spots on the periphery of the iris
- Slanted palpebral fissures
- Brachycephaly
- Low set ears
- Unipalmar crease
- Short, broad digits
- Enlarged space between first and second toes
- 50% incidence of congenital heart defects
- Impaired growth
- Hypothyroidism, both congenital and acquired
- Hypogonadism—males are generally thought to be infertile, while it is estimated that 30% to 50% of females are fertile
- Congenital cataracts
- Hip dysplasia
- Atlantoaxial instability

Natural History
- Prenatal or neonatal diagnosis
- Increased mortality with cardiac defects
- Mortality greatly improved with improved cardiac care
- Improved tone with age
- Cognitive delays become more prominent with increasing age
- IQ range reported as 25 to 50
- Mean age of walking is 24 months
- High risk for overweight and obesity
- Improved performance noted with early intervention programs and special education
- Increased risk of early-onset dementia
- Shortened life expectancy, average now surpassing 50 years

Diagnosis

Differential diagnosis
- Wide variety of chromosomal disorders

History
- Developmental progress
- Nutrition

- Behaviors
- Upper motor neuron syndrome signs

Exam
- DS growth charts
- Cardiac auscultation
- Comprehensive neurologic exam
- Scoliosis exam
- Hip subluxation or dislocation
- Foot position
- Visual screening

Testing
- Karyotype
- Echocardiogram prior to hospital discharge
- Screening labs per DS healthcare guidelines
- Flexion-extension cervical spine x-rays once at age 3 to 5 years, also as indicated by history and exam to evaluate for cervical spine instability, particularly atlantoaxial instability
- Thyroid testing at birth, 6 and 12 months, then annually
- Screening antibodies for celiac disease at 3 to 5 years of age
- Audiologic testing at birth, then every 1 to 2 years as needed

Pitfalls
- Atlanto-occipital instability

Red Flags
- Spasticity with cervical cord compression from cervical spine instability may present as "normal" tone and muscle stretch reflexes ("normal" is hypotonic). Other upper motor neuron signs (eg, +Babinski) should be present as in typical population
- Undetected hypothyroidism may worsen developmental delays
- Sleep apnea may worsen behaviors and development

Treatment

Medical
- No treatments currently available for underlying pathophysiology

- Appropriate screening and referrals as necessary per DS Healthcare Guidelines
- Numerous "treatments" (eg, vitamins, stem cells) marketed, but have not been shown to be effective, may be harmful

Exercise
- Supported infant treadmill training
- Developmental goal-directed activities

Consults
- Ophthamology for cataracts
- Cardiology for congenital anomalies
- Early intervention for mobility, speech, and activities of daily living
- Audiology
- Special education services
- Family support groups
- Social security administration for supplemental security income benefits

Prognosis
- Variable outcome. Some high-functioning adults are able to live with minimal support in the community, while others require complete support
- In general, mosaicism results in a better functional outcome

Helpful Hints
- Orthoses have not been shown to hasten ambulation
- Neurologic exam is best screen for atlantoaxial instability issues
- Educate families early about mainstreaming and special education services

Suggested Readings
Down Syndrome Healthcare Guidelines, Revised. *Down Syndrome Quarterly.*1999;4(3).

Kuhn DE, Nuovo GJ, Terry AV Jr, et al. Chromosome 21-derived microRNAs provide an etiological basis for aberrant protein expression in human Down syndrome brains. *J Biol Chem.* 2010;285(2):1529–1543.

Pueschel SM. Should children with Down syndrome be screened for atlantoaxial instability? *Arch Pediatr Adolesc Med.* 1998;152(2):123–125.

Dysarthria

Stephanie Ried MD

Description

Dyarthrias are motor speech disorders that result from neurologic/neuromuscular impairments associated with weakness, abnormal tone, or incoordination of the musculature used to produce speech.

Etiology/Types

- Due to underlying neurologic disorder, congenital or acquired, including cerebrovascular accident, brain injury, cerebral palsy, myasthenia gravis, seizure disorder, high spinal cord injury, progressive neurologic disorder, and tumor
- Type of dysarthria depends on underlying etiology and site of lesion:
  - Spastic (bilateral upper motor neuron lesion)
  - Hypokinetic (extrapyramidal lesion)
  - Hyperkinetic (extrapyramidal lesion)
  - Ataxic (cerebellar lesion)
  - Flaccid (unilateral or bilateral lower motor neuron lesion)
  - Mixed (multiple lesion sites)

Epidemiology

- Prevalence unclear due to multiplicity of disorders in which it occurs and inclusion within statistics of pediatric "phonological" disorders that are present in approximately 5% of US children entering the first grade

Pathogenesis

- Although the underlying cause of the dysarthria may vary, in children it occurs in a context of brain maturation, rapid physical growth, and cognitive and psychosocial development
- Oral musculature and quality of oral movements change during development
- There is a syndrome with mutism followed by dysarthria that may occur after resection of a cerebellar tumor, so consequently the syndrome has been termed mutism and subsequent dysarthria (MSD)

Risk Factors

- Congenital or acquired neurologic disorders
- Neuromuscular disorders

Clinical Features

Effects generally broader rather than focal. Speech production systems that may be affected:
- Respiration
- Phonation
- Articulation
- Resonance
- Prosody
- Specifics dependent on underlying disorder and lesion site

Natural History

- If significant and untreated, dysarthria may disrupt or distort oral communication to the extent that it interferes with family relations, peer socialization, academic success, vocational potential, self-esteem, and overall quality of life

Diagnosis

Differential diagnosis

- Articulation disorders
- Velopharyngeal disorders
- Voice disorders

History

- Developmental delay and/or oral motor/feeding problems may presage motor speech problem
- May occur with progression of neurologic disorder or with acquired impairment/illness

Exam

- Slurred speech
- Imprecise articulation
- Weak respiratory support
- Low volume
- Incoordination of respiratory stream
- Harsh, strained, or breathy vocal quality
- Involuntary movements of the oral facial muscles
- Spasticity or flaccidity of the oral facial muscles
- Hypernasality
- Hypokinetic speech

Testing

- Hearing testing
- Oral agility assessment

- Perceptual methods of assessment may be supplemented with:
  - Acoustic analyses
  - Aerodynamic recordings
  - Imaging techniques
  - Movement transduction
  - Electropalatography

Pitfalls
- Progression of symptoms warrant thorough evaluation

Red Flags
- Vigilance for concomitant dysphagia is warranted

Treatment

Medical
- Perceptually based therapy—traditional drill exercises without instrumentation
- Treatment and supportive care for underlying condition

Exercises
- Exercises of the lips and/or tongue to increase the rate, strength, range, or coordination of the musculature supporting articulation
- Drill breathing exercises to increase respiratory/breath support for speech
- Voicing drills to increase loudness of phonation

Modalities
- Instrumentally based biofeedback approaches

- If severe, may benefit from use of alternative/augmentative communication intervention
- Biofeedback strategies may be useful

Injections
- N/A

Surgical
- N/A

Consults
- Neurology
- Neurosurgery

Complications of treatment
- N/A

Prognosis
- Prognosis is dependent upon underlying etiology

Helpful Hints
- One of the most common expressive language problems in children with traumatic brain injury
- Early evaluation and intervention is critical

Suggested Readings

Driver L, Ayyangar R, Van Tubbergen M. Language development in disorders of communication and oral motor function. In Alexander MA, Matthews DJ, eds. *Pediatric Rehabilitation. Principles and Practices.* 4th ed. New York, NY: Demos Medical; 2010.

Kent RD. Research on speech motor control and its disorders: a review and perspective. *J Commun Disord.* 2000(33):391–428.

Dysphagia

Stephanie Ried MD

Description

Dysphagia is an abnormality of swallowing (deglutition) function due to disruption in any aspect in transit of a liquid or solid bolus from its entrance into the oral cavity through the esophagus.

Etiology/Types

- Neurologic disorders, congenital or acquired
- Neuromuscular disorders
- Intracranial masses
- Bulbar dysfunction
- Craniovertebral abnormalities
- Cerebrovascular disorders
- Prematurity/immaturity
- Anatomic abnormalities of the digestive and/or respiratory tracts, congenital or acquired
- Genetic conditions/syndromes
- Degenerative diseases
- Inborn errors of metabolism
- Connective tissue disorders
- Myopathies
- Craniofacial anomalies
- Conditions affecting the coordination of suck/swallow/breathing
- Pervasive developmental delay
- Behavioral feeding disorders

Epidemiology

- Estimated 25% to 45% of normally developing children and 33% to 80% in those with developmental disorders have some type of feeding disorder
- 37% to 40% of infants/children with feeding/swallowing problems were born prematurely
- Incidence of dysphagia is unknown but described as increasing
- Increase in incidence of dysphagia is likely related to improved survival of premature infants and increasing life expectancy of children with developmental disorders and neuromuscular conditions, as well as better diagnostic tools

Pathogenesis

- Premature infants below 36 weeks' gestation lack coordination of the suck-swallow-breathe sequence

- Critical periods exist for development of normal feeding behaviors
- Chewing and swallowing skills approximate adults by 3 years of age
- Feeding success requires sufficient experience in addition to maturation
- Inappropriate head and neck alignment can impair transit of oral bolus and increase risk of aspiration
- Interruption in development of normal feeding skills due to illness may be prolonged and compounded by emergence of maladaptive behaviors, food aversions/refusals, and medical complications

Risk Factors

- Prematurity below 36 weeks' gestation
- Neurologic depression or insult
- Anatomic defects of digestive or respiratory tracts
- Craniofacial abnormalities
- Gastroesophageal reflux (GER)
- Respiratory disease
- Complex medical conditions, for example, cardiac disease
- Bulbar or muscle tone abnormalities

Clinical Features

- Changes in respiratory rate, decreased level of alertness, or drop in oxygen saturation with feeding
- Coughing, gagging, or choking during feeding
- Frequent respiratory infections, particularly right upper lobe pneumonia
- Wet, gurgling respirations associated with feeding
- Poor weight gain
- Irritability associated with feeding
- Food refusal or rigid feeding behaviors

Natural History

- Respiratory and nutritional sequelae with significant impact on overall growth and upon growth and development of specific organs
- Recurrent pneumonias and development of aspiration-induced chronic lung disease
- Impairment of normal caregiver-child interactions/bonding

Diagnosis

Differential diagnosis
- GER
- Achalasia
- Esophageal perforation

History
- Failure to thrive
- Prolonged feeding time
- Food aversions
- Recurrent respiratory infections

Exam
- Dependent on age and comorbidities
- Poor nutrition/underweight
- Irritable/altered level of alertness
- "Wet" voice
- Oral motor abnormalities, bulbar dysfunction
- Increased respiratory rate
- Neurologic findings

Testing
- Videofluoroscopy swallow study/modified barium swallow
- Fiber-optic endoscopic evaluation of swallowing

Pitfalls
- Caretaker compliance is critical

Red Flags
- Clinically significant rumination (effortless regurgitation into mouth immediately after eating)
- Recurrent hospitalizations for pneumonia

Treatment
- Diet modification/National Dysphagia Diet
- Altered route of enteral feeds—indicated when risk of aspiration is not ameliorated with dietary maneuvers or nutritional needs not attainable by oral feeding
- Nasogastric/nasojejunal tube—indicated when expected duration of non-oral feeding is less than 6 weeks
- Gastrostomy/jejunostomy tube—anticipated duration of non-oral feeding more than 6 weeks

Medical
- Management of GER

Exercises
- Therapy with a speech-language pathologist or occupational therapist may include exercises for oral musculature and desensitization strategies
- Posture/positioning interventions

Modalities
- Biofeedback may be useful in older children
- Electrical stimulation may improve swallow in some children via synchronous muscle stimulation

Surgical
- Feeding tube placement as noted earlier
- Fundoplication in severe GER

Consults
- Pulmonology
- Neurology
- Neurosurgery
- Gastroenterology

Complications
- Potential life-threatening respiratory compromise if complicated by aspiration
- Severe malnutrition

Prognosis
- Dictated by underlying etiologies/conditions

Helpful Hints
- Neurologic conditions are most common etiologies associated with dysphagia

Suggested Readings

Eicher, PS. Feeding. In: Batshaw ML, ed. *Children with Disabilities*. Baltimore, MD: Brooks; 2002: 549–599.

Lefton-Greif MA. Pediatric dysphagia. *Phys Med Rehabil Clin N Am*. 2008;19(4):837–851.

Endocrine Abnormalities

Susan Biffl MPT MD ■ Pamela E. Wilson MD

Description

The endocrine system functions to regulate hormones to control enzymatic and metabolic processes, energy production, maintain homeostasis of the internal environment, and regulate growth, pubertal development, and reproduction.

Etiology/Types

- Inherited
- Idiopathic
- Acquired—traumatic, exposures, and illnesses
- Hypopituitary dysfunction:
  - Multiple axis dysfunction
  - Hypo/hyperthyroid
  - Growth hormone deficiency (GHD)
  - Precocious puberty
  - Adrenal insufficiency
  - Diabetes insipidus (DI)
  - Diabetes mellitus type I (DM I) and II (DM II)

Pathogenesis

- Hypopituitary dysfunction—direct trauma, vascular insult, metabolic, or toxic insult to pituitary, hypothalamus or target organ, central nervous system (CNS) malformation, or other genetic process
- Hypothyroid: iodine deficiency, congenital, autoimmune, infiltrative, and toxic exposure
- Hyperthyroid: autoimmune, inflammatory
- Adrenal insufficiency—congenital, infection, trauma, vascular insufficiency, and end-organ resistance
- GH insensitivity
- Precocious puberty:
  - Gonadotropin dependent—CNS abnormality, idiopathic, and genetic
  - Gonadotropin independent—female-ovarian cysts, tumors, male-tumors, and both
  - Genetic and adrenal abnormality
  - Exogenous ingestion
- DM I/II: genetic factors, autoimmune process, and peripheral insulin resistance

Associated Syndromes/Conditions/Risk Factors

- DM I: autoimmune disorders, including systemic lupus erythematosus (SLE), juvenile rheumatoid arthritis (JRA), Friedrich's ataxia, cystic fibrosis, drug-induced
- DMII: obesity, immobility, and polycystic ovarian syndrome
- Hypopituitary dysfunction: traumatic brain injury, anoxic brain injury, CNS malformation (eg, septo-optic dysplasia, midline brain defects), infiltrative disorders, CNS mass and after chemotherapy and radiation, CNS infection or vascular insufficiency, multiorgan system failure, anorexia nervosa, and iatrogenic suppression
- Hyper/hypothyroid: autoimmune disease (SLE, JRA, DMI, thrombocytopenic purpura, and pernicious anemia), infiltrative process, oncologic process, thyroid hormone resistance, factitious, myasthenia gravis, Turner's syndrome, William's syndrome, and Trisomy 21

Clinical Features

- DM I: hyperglycemia, polyuria, polydipsia, polyphagia, weight loss, lethargy, fatigue, diabetic ketoacidosis (DKA), asymptomatic
- DM II: overweight, postpubertal presentation, acanthosis nigricans, polydipsia, polyuria, lethargy, fatigue, asymptomatic, less likely DKA
- ACTH/cortisol deficiency: death due to vascular collapse, postural hypotension with tachycardia, fatigue, anorexia, weight loss, eosinophilia, weakness, fatigue, myalgia, arthralgia, hypoglycemia, ± headache and visual field defects, may be asymptomatic
- Primary adrenal insufficiency: weakness, fatigue, myalgia, arthralgia, hypoglycemia, hyperpigmentation, hyponatremia, hyperkalemia, hypotensive shock
- Hypothyroid: fatigue, lethargy, cold intolerance, decreased appetite, constipation, dry skin, bradycardia, cognitive impairment (most dramatic in the first 3 years of life), growth delay, decreased deep tendon reflexes (DTRs), delayed puberty
- Hyperthyroid-goiter, opthalmopathy, proptosis, stare and lid lag, delayed pubertal development, increased cardiac output, mitral valve prolapse, accelerated linear growth, weight loss, malabsorption, hyperphagia, hyperdefecation, osteoporosis, increased

DTRs, warm smooth damp skin, sleep disturbance and distractability, Hashimoto's encephalopathy

- GHD: decreased growth and growth failure, hyperlipidemia, increased body fat, decreased lean muscle mass, decreased bone mineral density (BMD), anhedonia, delayed puberty, doll-like face
- Gonadotropin deficiency—female: oligo/amenorrhea, infertility, fatigue; male: decreased energy and muscle mass, decreased BMD
- Precocious puberty: secondary sexual development <8 year old for girls; <9 year old for boys (see Tanner stages in Ratings Scales chapter)

Natural History

- Ranges from abrupt onset of severe symptoms to insidious onset of symptoms, dependent upon etiology

Diagnosis

Tests

- Thyroid axis: TSH, fT4, tT4,T3, serum antithyroid antibody (TRS-Ab), thyroid-stimulating immunoglobulin, and radioactive iodine uptake
- Adrenal axis-cortisol level, random, morning or stimulated
- GHD: IGF-1, random level or stimulated test, and bone age
- Gonadal axis: LH/FSH estradiol female; testosterone male, pubertal staging, bone age
- Diabetes: plasma glucose, random or glucose tolerance test, HgA1C, pancreatic autoantibodies

Pitfalls

- Failure to consider endocrine abnormalities in patients with risk factors or symptoms

Red Flags

- Hypotension

- Hypertension
- Electrolyte abnormalities
- Shock
- Pathologic fracture
- Unexplained weight loss or gain

Treatment

- Hyperthyroid: antithyroid drug or thyroidectomy
- Hypothyroid: thyroid hormone replacement with synthetic T4
- ACTH deficiency: hydrocortisone or other glucocorticoid, may unmask DI
- Leutenizing hormone (LH)/follicle stimulating hormone (FSH) deficiency/hypogonadism: gender, age, and desire for fertility specific, may include testosterone, gonadotropins, GnRH, estrogen/progesterone
- GHD: recombinant human GH
- Precocious puberty: GnRH agonist, treat underlying pathology

Consults

- Endocrinology

Prognosis

- Dependent upon etiology, associated conditions, and provision of appropriate therapy

Helpful Hints

- Consider routine screening in high-risk patients even if asymptomatic

Suggested Readings

Acerini CL, Tasker RC. Traumatic brain injury induced hypopituitary dysfunction: a paediatric perspective. *Pituitary.* 2007;10(4):373–380.

Hay W, Hayward A, Levin M, Sondheimer J. *Current Diagnosis and Treatment in Pediatrics.* New York: McGraw Hill;2009.

Fetal Alcohol Syndrome

Desirée Rogé MD

Description

Fetal alcohol syndrome (FAS) is the leading preventable cause of birth defects and developmental disability. Features such as birth defects, behavioral and learning delays and disabilities may be present at birth or develop over time. These may persist into adulthood.

Etiology/Types

- Fetal alcohol spectrum disorders (FASD) represent a spectrum of structural anomalies, behavioral problems, and neurocognitive disabilities
- FASD encompasses different syndromes that result from in utero alcohol exposure:
  - FAS (Table)
  - Partial FAS
  - Alcohol-related birth defects
  - Alcohol-related neurodevelopmental disorder

Epidemiology

- FASD is the leading preventable cause of birth defects
- Incidence of FAS in the Western world is 1.9 affected infants in 1000 births
- Incidence of FASD in the Western world is 3.5 affected infants in 1000 births

Pathogenesis

- Teratogenic effects of alcohol during pregnancy
- Alcohol and its metabolites cross the placenta and affect DNA synthesis, cell division, and repair
- First-trimester exposure can cause craniofacial and structural organ (especially cardiac and brain) abnormalities
- Second-trimester exposure leads to a higher number of spontaneous abortions
- Third-trimester exposure has more severe effects on birth weight and length

Risk Factors

- In utero alcohol exposure
- No specific alcohol amount has been identified

Clinical Features

- Microcephaly with head circumference less than 10th percentile
- Short palpebral features
- Thin vermillion border of the upper lip
- Smooth philtrum
- Height or weight less than the 10th percentile
- Congenital anomalies and dysplasias such as:
  - Cardiac: septal defects
  - Skeletal: radioulnar synostosis, vertebral segmentation defects, large joint contractures, scoliosis, and pectus carinatum/excavatum
  - Renal: kidney/ureter abnormalities
  - Eyes: strabismus, ptosis, retinal vascular abnormalities, and optic nerve hypoplasia
  - Ears: conductive and/or sensorineural hearing loss
  - Minor abnormalities: hypoplastic nails, short digits, clinodactyly of fifth finger, and hockey-stick palmar creases
- Neurobehavioral problems
- Neurostructural abnormalities observed through neuroimaging

Natural History

Persistence into adulthood of primary and secondary disabilities.

- Primary disabilities:
  - Abnormal cognitive function: impaired memory, attention, concentration, math skills
  - Abstract reasoning deficits
  - Behavioral and conduct problems different from those identified in other forms of intellectual disability
  - Maladaptive social functioning
- Secondary disabilities:
  - Mental health problems
  - Chemical dependency
  - Inappropriate sexual behavior
  - Trouble with the law

Diagnosis

Differential diagnosis

- Velocardiofacial syndrome, microdeletion chromosome 22q11, cleft palate, cardiac anomalies, and learning problems
- William's syndrome, microdeletion chromosome 7q11, unusual face, attention-deficit hyperactivity disorder, reflux, and intellectual disability
- Cornelia de Lange syndrome, unusual face, short, developmental delay, and behavior issues
- Dubowitz syndrome, unusual face, short, microcephalic
- Fragile X syndrome (see chapter)

History

- Confirmed or suspected alcohol exposure during pregnancy
- Growth retardation
- Dysmorphic features
- Developmental delays
- Behavioral problems

Exam

- See Clinical Features
- Sensory—processing deficits
- Behavioral problems
- Cognitive deficits

Testing

- Clinical diagnosis based on the revised Institute of Medicine 1996 Criteria, or Center of Disease Control diagnostic guidelines
- Neuro-imaging to document structural brain abnormalities
- Multidisciplinary assessment to make diagnosis
- Routine screening for primary and secondary disabilities

Pitfalls

- Among pregnant women aged 15 to 44 years, 9.8% used alcohol and 4.1% reported binge drinking

Treatment

Medical

- No cure
- Multidisciplinary team for planned intervention
- Pharmacology treatment: stimulants

Therapies

- Early intervention
- Sensory integration therapy
- Behavioral therapy
- Social skills training
- Virtual reality training

Consults

- Genetics
- Behavioral and developmental pediatrician
- Neurology
- Psychiatry
- Cardiology

Prognosis

- Life span varies depending on the severity
- Early diagnosis and intervention may help decrease the incidence of secondary disabilities

Helpful Hints

- Lifetime cost of caring for a child with FAS is approximately $1.4 million
- Prevention, screening tools have been developed— T-ACE, TWEAK

Suggested Readings

American Academy of Pediatrics. Committee on substance abuse and Committee on Children with Disabilities. Fetal alcohol syndrome and alcohol-related developmental disorders. *Pediatrics.* 2000;106(2):358–361.

Hoyme HE, May PA, Kalberg WO, et al. A practical clinical approach to diagnosis of fetal alcohol related spectrum disorders: clarification of the 1996 Institute of Medicine Criteria. *Pediatrics.* 2005;115;39–47.

Floppy Baby

Marcie Ward MD

Description
Infant with low resistance to passive movement; marked head lag and floppiness of the trunk, arms and legs; delay in achieving gross motor milestones.

Etiology/Types
- Hypotonia with weakness (paralytic)
- Hypotonia without weakness (nonparalytic)

Epidemiology
- Incidence is unknown due to the multiple etiologies
- The most common paralytic hypotonia in infancy is spinal muscular atrophy (SMA) with an incidence of 5 to 7 per 100,000 live births
- The most common cause of nonparalytic hypotonia in infancy is nonspecific intellectual disability

Pathogenesis
- Malformation, injury or structural abnormality anywhere along the pathway from the precentral cortex to the muscle cell
- The insult may result from genetic causes, infectious causes, environmental causes, or unknown etiology

Risk Factors
- Intrauterine/perinatal drug or teratogen exposure
- Breech presentation
- Reduced fetal movements
- Polyhydramnios
- Maternal epilepsy
- Maternal diabetes
- Advanced maternal age
- Consanguinity
- Maternal intellectual disability
- Sibling with hypotonia
- Family history of neuromuscular disease
- Traumatic/difficult birth

Clinical Features
- Low muscle tone
- "Frog-leg position" and flaccid extension of the arms
- May require respiratory assistance at birth
- May exhibit feeding difficulty
- May exhibit seizures
- May demonstrate congenital abnormalities in other organ systems

Natural History
- Variable depending on etiology
- For those without weakness but with cognitive impairment, expectation is for normal motor development with persistent cognitive delays
- Without weakness or cognitive impairment, will likely catch up gross motor skills to peers
- With weakness, natural history depends on whether the process is static or progressive, and how severe

Diagnosis

Differential diagnosis
- With weakness:
  - SMA
  - Congenital or metabolic myopathies
  - Congenital myotonic or muscular dystrophies
  - Myasthenia gravis
  - Botulism
  - Acquired or hereditary peripheral neuropathies
  - Leukodystrophies and other progressive central nervous system disorders
  - Spinal cord injury
  - Chiari malformation
  - Use of benzodiazepines or lithium by the mother while pregnant
- Without weakness:
  - Nonspecific cognitive deficiency
  - Genetic disorders such as Down syndrome, Prader-Willi syndrome
  - Cerebral dysgenesis
  - Hypotonic cerebral palsy
  - Hypoxia
  - Perinatal drug exposure
  - Metabolic disorders
  - Connective tissue disorders
  - Nutrition and endocrine disorders
  - Benign congenital/essential hypotonia

History
- May report poor active movements
- Gross motor delays

- Perhaps difficulty swallowing/sucking

Exam
- Low muscle tone
- No resistance to passive movement
- Frog-legged posture (external hip rotation with hips abducted)
- Head lag
- Poor ventral suspension response

Testing
- Without weakness
  - Magnetic resonance imaging (MRI) of the brain
  - Karyotype
- With weakness
  - Electromyography (EMG)/nerve conduction study (NCS)
  - Genetic testing
  - Muscle biopsy
  - Creatine kinase level
  - Urine organic amino acids
  - Serum ammonia, lactate, and amino acids
  - Potassium and magnesium levels

Pitfalls
- Low tone is normal in the preterm infant
- Sepsis and congenital heart disease may initially present with hypotonia and must be ruled out

Red Flags
- Loss of a previously acquired skill suggests progressive disorder

Treatment

Medical
- Respiratory support/pulmonary toilet
- Nutritional support

Exercise
- As tolerated, but avoid fatigue
- Range of motion

Modalities
- Orthoses to support weak/lax joints and maintain good joint alignment
- Adaptive equipment

Surgical
- Tracheostomy for prolonged respiratory support/ toileting
- Gastrostomy tube placement for nutritional support
- Shunting of hydrocephalus

Consults
- Pediatric neurology
- Palliative care
- Pediatric surgery

Prognosis
- Variable depending on etiology

Helpful Hints
- Begin by determining if the hypotonia is without weakness (typically central etiology: usually exhibit brisk reflexes) or with weakness (typically a motor unit etiology: usually exhibit absent reflexes)
- If central etiology, consider MRI
- If motor unit etiology, begin with EMG/NCS unless family history suggests genetic testing would confirm the diagnosis

Suggested Readings
Bodensteiner JB. The evaluation of the hypotonic infant. *Semin Pediatr Neurol.* 2008;15:10–20.

Dubowitz V. *The floppy infant.* In: *Clinics in Developmental Medicine.* Vol 76. 2nd ed. London: William Heinemann Medical Books Ltd; 1980:133–138.

Fragile X Syndrome

Desirée Rogé MD

Description

Fragile X syndrome (FXS) is the most common form of inherited intellectual disability (ID) and the most common genetic cause of autism. It is characterized by a broad spectrum of morphologic, cognitive, behavioral, and psychologic features.

Etiology/Types

- X-linked dominant inheritance
- FXS is caused by decreased or absent levels of fragile X mental retardation protein (FMRP).
- FXS is caused by a full mutation: >200 CGG repeats on the fragile mental retardation gene (FMR1) located in chromosome Xq27
- Premutation 55–200 CGG repeats on the *FMR1* gene, leads to primary ovarian insufficiency, fragile X associated tremor ataxia syndrome (FXTAS), neuropathies, and milder cognitive and behavioral difficulties
- Severity of physical phenotype and intellectual impairment correlates with the magnitude of the FMRP deficit
- Prader-Willi phenotype of FXS: subgroup of males with hyperphagia and obesity with negative results for Prader-Willi molecular testing

Epidemiology

- FXS is the most common cause of inherited ID:
  - Males: 1/3600
  - Females: 1/ 4000 to 6000
- Incidence of the premutation: 1/130–250 females and 1/250–800 males
- 2% to 7% children with autism have a mutation in the *FMR1* gene
- Prevalence of autism in children with FXS ranges from 20% to 35%

Pathogenesis

- Genetic defect Xq27

Risk Factors

- Familial inheritance
- Spontaneous mutation risk factors are unknown

Clinical Features

- Male phenotypic features of full mutations vary by age:
  - Prepubertal boys: >50th percentile head circumference, late motor and speech milestones, abnormal behavior, and autism
  - Pubertal boys: long face, prominent forehead, large ears, prominent jaw, and large genitalia
- Facial features in females are rarely noted
- Connective tissue problems: ligamentous laxity, velvet-like skin
- Flat feet
- Heart murmurs
- Hypotonia
- Seizures: 15% of males, 5% of females
- Eighty percent of males have cognitive delays and ID
- Fifty percent of females with full mutation have ID and 35% have IQ < 85
- Behavioral difficulties: attention deficit hyperactivity disorder (ADHD), autistic related behavior, hand flapping, chewing/biting, sensory processing problems, tics, anxiety, coprolalia, psychosis, and schizophrenia

Natural History

- Infancy: normal or slightly delayed milestones
- Childhood: fine motor skill deficits, severe language and expressive speech problems, and cognitive and behavioral impairments are noted
- Normal life span

Diagnosis

Differential diagnosis

- Ehlers-Danlos syndrome
- Pervasive developmental disorders
- Autism
- ADHD
- Retts syndrome
- Prader Willi syndrome
- Sotos syndrome
- Lujan-Fryns syndrome

History

- Developmental delays
- Behavioral difficulties
- Family history

Exam

- Males show pubertal facial features: long face, prominent forehead, large ears, and prominent jaw, as well as large genitalia
- Connective tissue problems, including ligamentous laxity, and velvet-like skin
- Flat feet, scolosis, and pectus excavatum
- Recurrent ear infections
- High arched palate
- Decreased visual acuity
- Heart murmurs
- Hypotonia

Testing

- FMR1 DNA testing
- High-risk screening is recommended in children with autistic behavior and family history of IDs
- Screening is recommended for individuals with features of FXS, learning disabilities, females with primary ovarian insufficiency, and adults with FXTAS
- Neuro-imaging may reveal: enlarged hippocampal volumes, large cerebrum with small posterior cerebellar vermis, and larger hypothalamus
- Electroencephalogram

Red Flags

- Family history of ID
- Family history of females with primary ovarian insufficiency and adults with FXTAS

Treatment

Medical

- No cure

- Pharmacological management of behavior: stimulants, clonidine, guanfacine, SSRI's, and antipsychotics
- Early intervention: behavioral therapy, occupational therapy, speech therapy, sensory integration therapy
- Treatment of seizures

Consults

- Genetics
- Neurology
- Developmental-behavioral pediatrics
- Psychology/psychiatry

Prognosis

- Depends on the severity of the condition
- Normal life span
- High-functioning individuals may succeed in lower level jobs

Helpful Hints

- High-risk screening is recommended in children with autistic behavior and a family history of IDs
- Screening is recommended for individuals with features of FXS or learning disabilities, females with primary ovarian insufficiency, and adults with FXTAS

Suggested Readings

Chonchaiya W, Schneider A, Hagerman RJ. Fragile X: a family of disorders. *Adv Pediatr.* 2009;56(1):165–186.
Hagerman RJ, Berry-Kravis E, Kaufman WE, et al. Advances in the treatment of fragile X syndrome. *Pediatrics.* 2009;123(1)1:378–390.

Friedreich's Ataxia

Gregory T. Carter MD ■ Jay J. Han MD

Description

Friedreich's ataxia (FA) is a progressive neuromuscular disorder. Symptoms include weakness, ataxia, and loss of balance and coordination. A cardiomyopathy is common and may be severe. Cognition is not affected. Disease onset is typically at age 10 to 15 years old. Earlier onset is associated with a more severe clinical course.

Etiology/Types

- Autosomal recessive
- Caused by a repeating mutation in the frataxin gene located on chromosome 9
- Protein product frataxin regulates levels of iron inside mitochondria
- Most common mutation is a trinucleotide repeat expansion
- Normally the gene contains 5 to 30 GAA repeats but in FA, the gene can contain hundreds to thousands of GAA repeats
- Longer repeat expansions are associated with more severe disease

Epidemiology

- FA is the most common of a group of related disorders called hereditary spinocerebellar ataxias (HSCAs)
- In the United States, the carrier rate is 1 in 100
- FA affects 1 in 50,000 people

Pathogenesis

- The current prevailing theory holds that frataxin acts like a storage depot for iron, releasing it only when it is required by the cell
- In the absence of frataxin, free iron accumulates in mitochondria producing oxidative stress that ultimately leads to damage and impaired cellular respiration
- Widespread mitochondrial damage explains why FA is a multisystem disorder, affecting cells of the peripheral and central nervous system as well as the heart and endocrine systems
- In FA carriers, the frataxin gene may contain either a repeat expansion (95%) or a point mutation (5%). Rarely there is a permutation, a number of expanded repeats occurring just below the disease-causing range. Permutations may or may not further expand into the disease-causing range in a given ova or sperm.

This complicates the ability to definitively assess risk of transmission for carriers.

Risk Factors

- Family history
- Cajun (Acadian) ancestry in North America

Clinical Features

- Progressive ataxia
- Sensory impairment
- Loss of flexibility
- Scoliosis is common (63%). Curve patterns do not necessarily resemble idiopathic curves
- Cardiomyopathy (hypertrophic) is seen in approximately 2/3, with variable severity; severity is not concordant with electrocardiography abnormalities or severity of the ataxia
- Approximately 10% have diabetes, both type I and II
- An additional 20% have hypoglycemia

Natural History

- Significant ataxia, usually presenting in the legs
- Unsteady gait or impaired athletic performance
- Coordination and balance progressively decline, along with weakness and fatigue in skeletal muscles
- Most FA patients will become wheelchair users within 5 to 15 years after disease onset
- Concomitant axonal sensory neuropathy
- Progressive scoliosis
- Dysarthria, producing a typically "ballistic" speech pattern. Word production is slow with an irregular pattern
- Dysphagia may develop, increasing risk for aspiration
- The sensory neuropathy further impairs coordination through loss of proprioception
- Dysesthesias/parasthesias are not common
- FA also impairs motor planning and coordination of movement
- Cause of death in FA is usually related to cardiomyopathy or complications of diabetes; otherwise life span can be normal or near normal

Diagnosis

Differential diagnosis

- Other types of HSCAs—type 1 (HSCA1); additional dominant gene mutations cause HSCA2 and HSCA3

101

- Familial spastic paraparesis
- Cerebral palsy
- Brain or spinal cord tumors
- Stroke
- Central nervous system demyelinating diseases (i.e., multiple sclerosis)

History
- History of tripping, falling, with loss of coordination
- Cardiac symptoms
- Speech disturbances

Exam
- Loss of reflexes
- Decreased vibration and temperature sensation
- Impaired proprioception
- Widespread ataxia with impaired balance and gait
- Scoliosis

Testing
- Electrodiagnostic testing shows absent sensory nerve action potentials (or of reduced amplitude)
- Magnetic resonance imaging (MRI) to rule out brain or cerebellum tumors
- White blood cells for DNA to assess for frataxin mutations
- DNA may be used for prenatal screening and to determine carrier status
- Echocardiogram
- Scoliosis spine films

Pitfalls
- Patients mistakenly diagnosed with a type of HSCA, which can appear clinically very similar to FA
- Cardiac symptoms may be "silent" initially
- Scoliosis may not progress in a linear fashion and needs to be monitored regularly with radiographs

Red Flags
- Progression of scoliosis

Treatment

Medical
- Idebenone (a short-chain coenzyme Q10 analogue) dose at 5 to 20 mg/kg/day—may help with cardiac function and muscle performance
- Analgesics for muscle and joint pain
- Scoliosis screening and management with timely spinal fusion. This should be done before the primary curve becomes greater than 25°. Surgery done in curves greater than 40° has a diminished likelihood of successful correction. Scoliosis does not respond to bracing.
- Cardiomyopathy management includes after load reduction with angiotensin-converting-enzyme

inhibitors, and positive ionotropic agents like digoxin
- Tachyarrhythmias should respond to β-blockers
- All FA patients with significant cardiomyopathy should be evaluated by a cardiologist

Exercise
- Rehabilitation goals include increased walking distance; decreased falls; improved gait stability; more normal gait speed, step length, and cadence; and increased independence in activities of daily living
- Physical therapy for gait training, muscle balance, core stabilization programs; wheelchair evaluation and training; instruction on use of assistive devices—canes, walkers, etc.
- Occupational therapy for assistive device evaluation and for home program of sensory integration and neuromuscular coordination exercises
- Speech-language pathology for linguistic and oropharyngeal exercises; augmentative communication devices

Surgical
- Spinal fusion for progressive scoliosis
- Surgical correction of joint contractures if needed

Consults
- Neurosurgery or orthopedic spine surgery
- Cardiology

Complications of treatment
- Progressive pain and dysfunction
- Pseudarthrosis

Prognosis
- Variable
- Poor if severe cardiomyopathy is present

Helpful Hints
- DNA testing, although expensive, is highly reliable and should be done in the proband and anyone at risk for either being affected or being a carrier
- All patients and their families should have formal genetic counseling
- FA is covered by the Muscular Dystrophy Association (MDA). Patients with FA can receive treatment through MDA clinics. Information is available at http://www.mda.org/

Suggested Reading
Fogel BL, Perlman S. Clinical features and molecular genetics of autosomal recessive cerebellar ataxias. *Lancet Neurol.* 2007;6(3):245–257.

Pandolfo M. Friedreich ataxia. *Arch Neurol.* 2008;65(10):1296–1303.

Growing Pains

Joshua Jacob Alexander MD FAAP FAAPMR

Description
Occasional nighttime leg pain without an apparent cause. Named in 1823 when it was (incorrectly) assumed the pain was related to periods of rapid linear growth at night.

Etiology/Types
- Unclear

Epidemiology
- Most commonly occurs between the ages of 4 and 12
- Prevalence is 37% in children of ages 4 to 6 years

Pathogenesis
- Unknown
- Possibly related to decreased pain threshold, decreased bone strength

Risk Factors
- Increased activity levels (running, climbing, and jumping) earlier that day
- Family history of growing pains

Clinical Features
- Aching or throbbing in the muscles of the leg, most often in the anterior thigh, popliteal fossa, or calves
- Usually involves both legs
- Often occurs in the late afternoon and early evening
- Pain can last from minutes to hours
- Pain disappears by morning
- Does not limit daytime activities

Natural History
- Frequency of attacks can vary widely, from almost daily to once every few months
- Self-resolve over time
- Typically end by the teen years

Diagnosis

Differential diagnosis
- Osteoid osteoma
- Trauma
- Tumor
- Infection
- Restless leg syndrome
- Rheumatoid arthritis
- Somatization
- Fibromyalgia

History
- Young child
- Intermittent, bilateral leg pain, occurring in late afternoon and at night
- Pain in muscles, not joints
- Pain gone upon waking in the morning
- Does not affect daytime activity
- No swelling, redness, fever, limping, rash, anorexia, weight loss, weakness, or fatigue

Exam
- Normal exam
- No fever, weight loss, tenderness to palpation, rashes, swelling, fatigue, or limp

Testing
- Not warranted unless history or physical exam raises suspicion for another condition

Pitfalls
- Missing an infection, injury, rheumatologic or other pathologic condition by assuming that leg pain "is just growing pains" when history and/or physical examination includes any red flags

Red Flags
- Unilateral leg pain
- Symptoms still present in the morning
- Associated with an injury
- Pain worse, not better, with massage
- Joint pain
- Morning stiffness
- Easy bruising or bleeding
- Night sweats
- Accompanied by swelling, redness, fever, limping, rash, anorexia, weight loss, weakness, or fatigue
- Reduced range of motion
- Reduced physical activity during the day

Treatment

Medical
- Acetaminophen
- Ibuprofen

Exercises
- Gentle massage
- Stretching of affected muscles

Modalities
- Warm bath before bedtime
- Heating pad (with supervision)

Consults
- None needed if history and physical exam consistent with growing pains

Complications of treatment
- Do not use aspirin as pain reliever as this may increase risk of Reye's syndrome

Prognosis
- Excellent
- Spontaneously resolves by teen years

Helpful Hints
- An ultimately benign condition, growing pains can be diagnosed by a thorough history and physical examination that rules out other, more serious causes of nighttime leg pain
- Once diagnosis is made, reassurance should be given to parent and child with parental encouragement to provide symptomatic relief at night for this self-limiting condition

Suggested Readings
Goodyear-Smith F, Arroll B. Growing pains. *BMJ*. 2006;333(7566):456–457.
Lowe RM, Hashkes PJ. Growing pains: a noninflammatory pain syndrome of early childhood. *Nat Clin Pract Rheumatol*. 2008;4(10):542–549.

Guillain-Barré Syndrome

Douglas G. Kinnett MD

Description

Guillain-Barré syndrome (GBS) is an acute or a subacute inflammatory process of the peripheral nervous system resulting in demyelination of the axons involved. This syndrome is also known as:

- Acute inflammatory demyelinating polyradiculopathy (AIDP)
- Acute idiopathic polyneuritis
- Landry's syndrome
- Postinfectious polyneuritis

Etiology/Types

- Acute inflammatory demyelinating polyradiculopathy (AIDP)
- Acute axonal motor neuropathy (AMAN)
- Miller Fisher syndrome (cranial nerves/ataxia)
- Acute sensory neuropathy (motor intact)
- Rare forms involving isolated regions as face/arms or autonomic nervous system
- Chronic form of GBS (ongoing or relapsing)

Epidemiology

- Incidence (children and adults) is 1 per 100,000
- Seasonal outbreaks can be seen (AMAN form related to *Campylobacter jejuni* infection)
- Average age of children with GBS is 4 to 8 years but ranges throughout childhood

Pathogenesis

- The inflammatory response is believed to occur as a result of the immune system being triggered by a viral or bacterial infection with subsequent attack on the peripheral nerves
- Segmental involvement of the myelin is classically seen, however, the axon can be involved as well, which can result in other variants of this syndrome
- Abnormal T-cell response initiated by the preceding infection
- Initial demyelination occurs at nodes of Ranvier, followed by segmental myelin loss
- Axon injury can occur in the absence of significant demyelination or inflammation
- Initially affects the most proximal part of the axon, then the most distal, then the entire axon

- Initially with nerve recovery, myelin can be thinner and with more internodes than prior to injury

Risk Factors

- Known association from infection with *Campylobacter jejuni*, cytomegalovirus, Epstein-Barr virus, varicella-zoster virus, mycoplasma pneumoniae, and human immunodeficiency virus
- No genetic or race predisposition
- Slight predominance of males over females

Clinical Features

- Ascending weakness from lower extremities
- Paresthesias and numbness in some cases
- Pain (aching/throbbing) in many cases
- Ataxia and autonomic symptoms in some cases
- Respiratory involvement with ascending weakness

Natural History

- Symptoms can appear 2 to 4 weeks after illness
- Half of the children have respiratory weakness but only 10% to 20% require mechanical ventilation
- Mild autonomic symptoms more common in children
- <5% mortality in children; 5% to 10% with disability

Diagnosis

Differential diagnosis

- Acute form of GBS:
  - Myasthenia gravis and botulism (infants)
  - Toxic neuropathies (heavy metals)
  - Infections (Lyme disease, HIV)
  - Spinal cord lesions (including transverse myelitis, tumors, vascular malformations)
- Chronic form of GBS:
  - Hereditary motor/sensory neuropathies (HMSN)
  - Critical illness polyneuropathy
  - Metabolic neuropathies
  - Myopathies (dermatomyositis)

History

- History of prodromal illness
- Ascending weakness in legs (ataxic gait initially)
- Pain in extremities and back

- Autonomic symptoms (blood pressure changes, sweating, tachycardia, bowel/bladder disturbance)
- Sensory changes (vibration/position sense)

Exam
- Foot drop initially followed by leg weakness that can progress to the point of inability to ambulate
- Areflexia
- Decreased position sense/vibration, rarely touch is affected
- Can have sweating, tachycardia, and orthostatic hypotension (or hypertension) due to autonomic involvement
- Decreased vital capacity
- Check for involvement of cranial nerves (variant)

Testing
- Lumbar puncture with protein elevation >45 mg/dL (within 3 weeks of symptom onset, no active infection)
- Magnetic resonance imaging of lumbosacral spine with gadolinium will show enhancement of nerve roots in 80% to 90% of cases
- Electrodiagnostic studies (EMG/NCS) show:
  - Reduced conduction velocities (<60% to 80% normal)
  - Conduction block or temporal dispersion
  - Prolonged latencies (>125% to 150% normal)
  - Prolonged or absent F wave
- Serum anti-ganglioside antibodies in some cases

Pitfalls
- Not recognizing respiratory compromise
- Not recognizing conduction block on NCS

Red Flags
- Fever
- Generalized weakness not ascending
- Isolated leg paralysis and bladder/bowel dysfunction
- Symptoms without improvement for >1 month

Treatment

Medical
- Intravenous immunoglobulin (IVIG)
- Plasmapheresis
- Supportive care (gastric prophylaxis, antihypertensives, and pain management)

Exercises
- Initially in the very weak patient—range of motion and positioning to prevent contractures
- Submaximal strengthening program followed by endurance training as recovery progresses
- Long-term recovery is usually good in children but arm strength may need to be addressed

Modalities
- Bracing, if losing range of motion

Surgical
- If prolonged mechanical ventilation needed, then tracheotomy and feeding tubes may be placed

Consults
- Neurology
- Pulmonology
- Pain medicine
- Psychology
- Surgery
- Cardiology

Complications of treatment
- Side effects of IVIG (serious reactions are thrombotic events, pulmonary edema, and meningitis)
- Side effects of plasmapheresis (serious reactions are hypotension, hemorrhage, septicemia, and arrhythmias)

Prognosis
- Generally favorable in children, deaths are uncommon, full recovery in 90% of patients in 3 to 12 months

Helpful Hints
- Closely monitor cardiac and pulmonary status early to prevent respiratory failure
- Pain treatment should not be overlooked in the pediatric population with GBS
- Systematic periodic re-evaluation of strength and endurance as an outpatient should be done to help families with return to activities such as sports

Suggested Readings
Bolton CF. polyneuropathies. In: Jones HR, Bolton CF, Harper Jr CM. eds. *Pediatric Clinical Electromyography.* New York, NY: Lippincott-Raven; 1996:315–332.

Tseng BS, Markowitz JA. Guillian-Barre Syndrome in Childhood. eMedicine Web site (updated Sept 2008) http://emedicine.medscape.com

Hearing Loss

Stephanie Ried MD

Description

Hearing loss includes a variety of disorders and degrees of loss, both congenital and acquired. The degree and type of hearing loss is determined by the nature and location of the dysfunction in the auditory pathway.

Etiology/Types

- Hearing loss may be conductive, sensorineural, mixed, or central
  - Conductive hearing loss (CHL)—results from interference with the mechanical transmission of sound through the external and middle ear
  - Sensorineural hearing loss (SNHL)—dysfunction involves the cochlea or vestibulocochlear nerve
  - Mixed hearing loss is a combination of CHL and SNHL
  - Central hearing loss—dysfunction is in the brainstem or higher processing centers of the brain
- Congenital etiologies
  - CHL due to structural abnormalities, for example, cleft palate
  - SNHL may be caused by:
    ○ Genetic disorders
    ○ In utero infections (eg, TORCH)
    ○ Anatomic abnormalities involving the cochlea or temporal bone
    ○ Maternal exposure to ototoxic agents
    ○ Hyperbilirubinemia at levels requiring exchange transfusion
- Hearing loss due to genetic disorders may present at birth or in later childhood and may be progressive
- Mixed, progressive hearing loss may be seen in CHARGE association (coloboma of the eye, heart defects, atresia of the choanae, retardation of growth or development, genital and urinary abnormalities, ear abnormalities, and deafness)
- Numerous complex syndromes are associated with hearing loss
- Connexin 26 (Cx26) protein gene encoding mutations are the most common nonsyndromic genetic cause of hearing loss
- Acquired hearing loss can occur at any age
- Acquired CHL causes:

- Infection
- Otitis media with effusion–most common
- Foreign body/ear canal obstruction
- Trauma
- Cholesteatoma
- Acquired SNHL causes:
  - Infections—viral or bacterial illnesses
  - Brain or acoustic trauma
  - Neurodegenerative or demyelinating disorders
  - Ototoxic agents
  - Radiation therapy

Epidemiology

- 2 to 3/1000 children in the United States are born with a detectable hearing loss
- Approximately 10% to 15% of children fail school hearing screening
- Prevalence of hearing loss in children younger than 18 years of age has been estimated at 1.3%
- Only 50% of children with hearing loss are identified by use of risk indicators as listed below
- Genetic causes account for 80% of congenital SNHL and 30% to 50% of all childhood SNHL

Pathogenesis

- Dependent upon underlying etiology
- Onset may vary in genetic disorders
- Mild loss (26–40 dB)—may miss up to 50% of speech, and so present as a poor listener or behavior problems
- Moderate loss (41–55 dB)—may miss 50% to 100% speech, which may result in poor speech quality, or decreased vocabulary
- Severe (70–90 dB)—speech and language delay if loss is prelingual, or declining speech abilities and atonal if loss is postlingual
- Profound (90+ dB)—sound vibrations are felt not heard, so visual cues are primary for communication, and socially, usually prefers hearing loss peers

Risk Factors

- Infections—TORCH, measles, mumps, rubella, meningitis, and chronic ear infections
- Low Apgar scores, prematurity
- Neonatal hyperbilirubinemia

- Family history
- Disorder/syndrome associated with hearing loss
- Parent concern regarding speech/language delay, cognitive, behavior/attention problems
- Ear/craniofacial abnormalities
- Ototoxic medications (eg, aminoglycosides, alkylating agents)

Clinical Features

- Sleeping child not awakened by loud noise
- Failure to respond to verbal instructions and significant improvement with addition of visual cues
- Speech and language delay
- Behavior problems and/or attention deficits
- Difficulty in sibilant consonant production ("s" and "sh") with high-frequency hearing loss

Natural History

- Comprehension of speech development is dependent upon hearing
- Hearing loss early in development can have impact on linguistic and cognitive development and cause problems in social-emotional arena
- Affects both receptive and expressive language development, the extent to which depends upon type and severity of the hearing loss, and age at onset
- Hearing loss acquired after language is established has less impact

Diagnosis

- In the United States, universal newborn hearing screening is mandated before 1 month of age via evoked otoacoustic emission, auditory brainstem response, or both
- Infants who fail newborn hearing screening require full audiological evaluation by 3 months of age
- Hearing screening typically done at entrance into preschool or kindergarten
- Primary care providers must be vigilant for assessing risk factors for hearing loss at each contact
- Education staff should be aware of behaviors that may indicate hearing problems

Differential diagnosis

- Cognitive impairment
- Pervasive developmental disorder
- Attention deficit disorder

History

- Speech and language delay
- High visual vigilance
- Loud TV/music volumes

Exam

- Difficulty following verbal commands
- Reliance on visual information
- Dysmorphic features
- Craniofacial abnormalities
- Abnormal ear exam

Testing

- Thorough audiological assessment
- ENT evaluation
- Speech and language evaluation
- Visual and developmental evaluations

Pitfalls

- Caretaker/family education critical

Red Flags

- Regression in speech and language skills, decreased attention/auditory responsiveness

Treatment

Medical

- Treat underlying conditions; appropriate referrals

Exercises

- Family education and involvement in facilitating child's speech and language development and establishing functional communication is critical
- Auditory training
- Sign language instruction
- Speech and language therapy
- Appropriate individual education plan and school program
- Anticipatory guidance for hearing conservation

Modalities

- Appropriate amplification—hearing aids, assistive listening devices
- Cochlear implants—for children who are deaf and do not benefit from amplification; they convert sound into electrical impulses that stimulate the vestibulocochlear nerve

Surgical

- Myringotomy and placement of pressure-equalization tubes for chronic middle ear effusion
- Surgical removal of cholesteatoma
- Cochlear implantation

Consults
- Otolaryngology
- Plastic surgery
- Speech-language pathology

Complications
- Surgical complications

Prognosis
- In infants with isolated hearing loss, prognosis for speech, language and cognitive development is significantly improved when the loss is identified by 6 months of age and appropriate hearing aids/intervention initiated, and, in these cases, can be communicating within normal limits by 3 years of age

Helpful Hints
- Hearing assessment is warranted in any child with speech and language delay or a history of recurrent otitis media
- Young children diagnosed with hearing loss should undergo both visual and development assessments to determine if other deficits exist that may further effect on development

Suggested Readings

Gifford KA, Holmes MG, Bernstein HH. Hearing loss in children. *Pediatr Rev.* 2009;30:207–216.

Moeller MP. Early intervention and language development in children who are deaf and hard of hearing. *Pediatrics.* 2000;106(36):E43.

Section II: Pediatric Diseases and Complications

Hemophilia

Maurice Sholas MD PhD

Description

A heritable disorder of blood coagulation caused by the absence of key proteins required for the clotting cascade, leading to variable deficits, depending on the location of the bleeding.

Etiology/Types

- Two main types of hemophilia, A and B
- A and B are both X-linked recessive diseases
- Hemophilia A is the most common type and it is due to a deficiency of factor VIII
- Hemophilia B (Christmas disease) is due to a deficiency of factor IX
- Severe disease: less than 1% factor activity
- Moderate: 1% to 5% factor activity
- Mild: greater than 5% factor activity
- Minor factor IX deficiency is transmitted in an autosomal recessive pattern from disorders on chromosome 4
- Hemophilia C is due to a very rare factor XI deficiency and can occur in either gender

Epidemiology

- Factor VIII deficiency: 1 in 5000 males in the United States
- Factor IX deficiency: 1 in 25,000 males in the United States
- Minor factor IX deficiency: 1 in 100,000 males
- The most severe form of hemophilia C has a prevalence 10 times less than hemophilia A with the exception of Ashkenazi and Iraqi Jews, who have a rate of heterozygosity of 8%

Pathogenesis

- The clotting cascade is a complex series of chemical reactions that result in a cross-linked fibrin clot
- Both hemophilia A and B cause alterations in the intrinsic pathway
- Intrinsic pathway obstruction ultimately prevents the final common pathway of blood clotting
- The lack of a normal clotting mechanism leads to spontaneous bleeding and exaggerated bleeding response to trauma

Risk Factors

- Genetic inheritance
- Nearly exclusively affects males

Clinical Features

- Progressive back pain
- Progressive weakness
- Loss of flexibility/range of motion
- Intermittent joint swelling
- Excessive bleeding

Natural History

- Bleeding may occur anywhere, most commonly in joints (80%), muscles, and gastrointestinal (GI) tract; ankles most common in childhood; knees, elbows, and ankles in teens
- May bleed multiple sites at once
- Untreated hemophilia A is usually diagnosed in the first year due to excessive bleeding following circumcision (50%) or minor trauma
- In hemophilia A, spontaneous bleeding occurs 2 to 5 times per month into the joints, kidneys, GI tract, brain, and deep muscles
- Untreated hemophilia B is diagnosed in the first year or two of life due to spontaneous bleeding and excessive ooze following trauma
- In hemophilia B, spontaneous subcutaneous hematomas are common. These patients can have bleeding into the joints, GI tract, brain, and nose as well
- In hemophilia C, there is a delayed presentation as the condition is milder, can affect females, and does not typically cause joint bleeding

Diagnosis

Differential diagnosis

- von Willebrand disease
- Mild combined factor V and factor VIII deficiencies
- Factor XI deficiency
- Factor XII deficiency
- Prothrombin, factor V, factor X, and factor VII deficiencies
- Fibrinogen disorders

- Factor XIII deficiency
- Platelet function disorders
- Iatrogenic bleeding disorders
- Vitamin K deficiency

History
- Excessive bleeding and bruising following circumcision
- Large subgaleal hematoma following minor trauma
- Excessive blood loss following tooth extraction
- Hemarthrosis without antecedent trauma
- Unexplained intracranial hemorrhages
- Deep muscle hematomas
- Gross hematuria

Exam
- Bruising
- Joint swelling
- Progressive joint stiffness
- Neurologic findings consistent with brain or spinal cord compromise

Testing
- Coagulation screening tests
- Coagulation factor assays
- Molecular/genetic testing
- Carrier testing

Pitfalls
- Missed diagnosis of nonaccidental trauma
- Missed use of medications that impair clotting
- Missed nutritional deficiencies

Red Flags
- Excessive bleeding in male child
- Gross hematuria in male child
- Excessive blood loss following tooth extraction
- Compartment syndrome

Treatment

Medical
- Contraindication: Aspirin and nonsteroidal anti-inflammatory drugs
- DDAVP (vasopressin), which increases circulating factor VII levels
- Replacement of clotting factor

Exercises
- Support maximal range of motion for weight-bearing joints

Modalities
- Ice
- Compression of the affected area

Injection
- Avoid intra-articular injections
- Give intramuscular injections (vaccinations) subcutaneously

Surgical
- Will need extra factor supplementation beyond maintenance for all procedures

Consults
- Hematology/oncology

Complications
- Joint destruction
- Development of inhibitor antibodies so supplements stop working in 25% with type A and 3% with type B
- End-organ damage
- Anemia
- Central nervous system compromise

Prognosis
- High probability of debilitating events without treatment

Helpful Hints
- Hemophilia B is commonly misdiagnosed as non-accidental trauma
- Many individuals who received blood products to reconstitute factor VIII concentrate from 1979 to 1985 contracted HIV and died of AIDS, but not since the mid-1980s

Suggested Readings
Browser C, Thompson AR. Hemophilia A: classic hemophilia, factor VIII deficiency. *GeneReviews*. National Institutes of Health/University of Washington. 2008;1–24.

Browser C, Thompson AR. Hemophilia B: classic hemophilia, factor IX deficiency. *GeneReviews*. National Institutes of Health/University of Washington. 2008;1–20.

Hereditary Motor Sensory Neuropathy/ Charcot Marie Tooth Disease

Olga Morozova MD

Description
Charcot-Marie-Tooth disease hereditary motor sensory neuropathy (CMT HMSN) is a group of disorders with a chronic motor and sensory polyneuropathy in the upper and lower limbs resulting in progressive symmetric distal muscle weakness and atrophy, sensory loss, and depressed tendon reflexes

Etiology/Types
- Autosomal dominant (CMT 1, CMT 2)
- Autosomal recessive (CMT 4)
- X-linked (CMTX)

Epidemiology
- The most common genetic cause of neuropathy
- 1 person per 2500 population

Pathogenesis
- Demyelination, as a result of abnormal myelin, can lead to axonal death and Wallerian degeneration
- Slowing of conduction velocity in sensory and motor nerves with weakness and numbness

Risk Factors
- Familial inheritance

Clinical Features
- Distal muscle weakness and wasting
- Diminished or absent tendon reflexes
- Decreased vibration and proprioception, preserved pain and temperature sensation
- High-arched feet (pes cavus)
- Thoracic scoliosis
- Sensorineuronal hearing loss (CMTX)
- Intellectual disability (CMTX)
- Sensory gait ataxia

Natural History
- Onset is in the first to third decades
- Slowly progressing weakness
- Normal lifespan

Diagnosis
Differential diagnosis
- Autosomal dominant, autosomal recessive, or X-linked recessive disorders with neuropathy
- Hereditary ataxias with neuropathy
- Hereditary motor neuropathies or hereditary sensory neuropathies
- CMT syndrome with spasticity
- Distal myopathies
- Mitochondrial disorders associated with peripheral neuropathy
- Acquired peripheral neuropathy

History
- Slowly progressive symmetrical distal weakness and muscle atrophy
- Difficulty walking, frequent tripping and falls
- Progressive foot drop; steppage gait
- Clumsy or uncoordinated
- Musculoskeletal or neuropathic pain
- Decreased fine motor skills

Exam
- Distal weakness and muscle wasting
- Vibration and proprioception loss
- Depressed or absent tendon reflexes
- Characteristic stork leg, inverted champagne bottle
- Foot deformities: high arches, hammertoes, and hindfoot varus
- Enlarged and palpable peripheral nerves (CMT1)

Testing
- Electrodiagnosis: slow conduction velocity
- Sural nerve biopsy may be helpful
- Molecular genetic testing

Pitfalls
- Negative molecular genetic testing does not rule out a diagnosis of CMT

Red Flags
- Avoid medications that can cause nerve damage: vincristine, cisplatin, isoniazid, and nitrofurantoin

Treatment

Medical
- No treatment is available to correct the underlying abnormal myelin or slow myelin or axonal degeneration
- Acetaminophen or nonsteroidal anti-inflammatory drugs for musculoskeletal pain
- Tricyclic antidepressants or antiepileptic drugs for neuropathic pain
- Modafinil can be used to treat fatigue

Exercise
- Stretching to prevent contractures
- Submaximal strengthening program
- Aerobic exercise

Modalities
- Cautious use of cold/heat for musculoskeletal pain. Monitor skin (decreased sensation)
- Proper fitted shoes: high top, extra depth, or custom made
- Orthoses: inserts for arch support, inframalleolar or supramalleolar orthoses for arch support and control hindfoot varus, ankle foot orthoses (AFO) with dorsiflexion assist for foot drop

Injection
- Trigger point injections

Surgical
- Orthopedic surgery for severe foot deformity and scoliosis

Consults
- Neurology
- Orthopedic surgery
- Genetic counseling

Complications
- Progressive contractures
- Skin breakdown, burns, and nonhealing foot ulcers due to sensory loss

Prognosis
- Disability due to progressive weakness and deformities
- Normal life span

Helpful Hints
- Shoes with good ankle support
- AFO for distal muscle weakness and safe and efficient ambulation
- Adaptive equipment

Suggested Readings
Bird TD. Charcot-Marie-Tooth Hereditary Neuropathy Overview. Available at www. GeneTests.org
McDonald CM. Peripheral neuropathies of childhood. *Phys Med Rehabil Clin N Am.* 2001; 12(2):473–490.

Section II: Pediatric Diseases and Complications

Heterotopic Ossification

Paul Bryan Kornberg MD FAAPMR MSRT

Description

Heterotopic ossification (HO) is defined as the formation of trabecular bone in a location in the body where it normally does not exist.

Etiology/Types

- Myositis ossificans—typically associated with trauma and restricted to a single or contiguous sites. Terminology misleading because nonmuscular tissue may be involved and inflammation is rare.
- Neurogenic—without trauma, after burns or neurologic injury (traumatic brain injury [TBI], spinal cord injury [SCI])
- Precipitating factor is repetitive trauma in up to 70% of cases, noted after severe burns, TBI, and SCI
- Myositis ossificans progressiva (MOP)—rare, severely disabling, autosomal dominant with variable expressivity

Epidemiology

- Adult population—studies of total hip arthroplasty reveal incidence of 43% with only 2% to 10% of patients demonstrating restricted range of motion (ROM), with or without pain
- Pediatric spinal cord injury incidence—3.3% to 9.9%
- HO incidence in pediatric traumatic brain injury—4% to 15%

Pathogenesis

- Osteoblastic cells form via pluripotent mesenchymal cells
- Metaplasia of local cell lines, such as fibroblasts
- Transplantation of osteoprogenitor cells as a consequence of instrumenting medullary canal
- Role of growth factors and angiogenesis factors
- Unclear role of central nervous system (CNS) and neuropeptides
- Transformation of mesenchymal to bone-forming cells in response to a variety of stimuli such as immobilization, microtrauma, spasticity, disturbance of protein/electrolyte balance, alteration of vasomotor outflow, circulatory stasis, and tissue hypoxia

Risk Factors

- Repetitive trauma
- TBI/SCI
- Immobilization
- Spasticity
- Burns/wounds
- Hip dislocation
- Instrumentation of medullary canal
- Inflammatory myopathies
- Parathyroid disorders/vitamin D excess

Clinical Features

- Swelling
- Warmth
- Pain
- Low-grade fever
- Decreased ROM

Natural History

- Onset in pediatric population may be later than in adults; 1 to 20 months after onset; rarely years
- Initially may see swelling/warmth followed by development of firm mass and pain
- Pain may diminish with time
- Hip joint most commonly affected, other common sites are elbow and shoulder
- Usually resorbs spontaneously in children
- For MOP, severely disabling recurrent episodes of painful swelling and tumors start in infancy and progress with hand and feet malformations

Diagnosis

Differential diagnosis

- Infection/cellulitis
- Fracture
- Soft-tissue injury
- Deep venous thrombosis

History

- Trauma
- CNS injury
- Spasticity/hypertonia
- Warmth
- Swelling
- Pain
- Change in ROM

Exam
- Neurologic deficits
- Spasticity/hypertonia
- Swelling
- Warmth
- Limited ROM

Testing
- Complete blood count, erythrocyte sedimentation rate/C-reactive protein, alkaline phosphatase (alk phos)
- Three-phase bone scan—abnormal 3 to 4 weeks prior to plain x-rays
- X-ray, though may be normal in early stages
- Computed tomography (CT) helps define the localization of HO to assist with planning of surgical resection

Pitfalls
- Early x-rays may be normal
- Alkaline phosphatase ± normal
- Surgical resection too early can lead to recurrence

Red Flags
- Changes in neurologic exam (may be due to nerve compression)
- High fever
- Vascular compromise (may be due to vascular compression)

Treatment

Medical
- Nonsteroidal anti-inflammatory drugs
- Bracing
- In adult population, etidronate; NOT in growing children
- For prophylaxis in high-risk adult patients, radiation therapy

Exercises
- ROM and positioning
- Functional strength training

Modalities
- Cold
- Compression
- TENS

Surgical
- Excision—bone needs to be mature, usually wait at least 1 year. Normal alkaline phosphatase and CT can help with surgical planning

Consults
- Orthopedic surgery
- Vascular surgery

Complications
- Limited ROM impacting comfort/positioning/function/hygiene
- Vascular involvement
- Nerve compression

Prognosis
- Good, if identified early and treatment initiated

Helpful Hints
- High index of suspicion
- Monitor for loss of ROM as presentation may be insidious

Suggested Readings
Garland DE, Shimoyama ST, Lugo C, Barras D, Gilgoff I. Spinal cord insults and heterotopic ossification in the pediatric population. *Clinical Orthop Relat Res.* 1989;245:303–310.

Kluger G, Kochs A, Holthausen. Heterotopic ossification in childhood and adolescence. *J Child Neurol.* 2000;15:406–413.

Hip: Developmental Hip Dysplasia

Elizabeth Moberg-Wolff MD

Description

Developmental hip dysplasia (DDH) is an anatomic abnormality of the hip that occurs in 0.15% of infants. It may be congenital or develop during infancy, but its presence contributes substantially to development of adult degenerative arthritis.

Etiology/Types

- A multifactorial polygenetic etiology is suspected
- Ninety percent of DDH have normal anatomy with normal bony components
- Ten percent of cases involve teratologic deformities of the acetabulum or femur

Epidemiology

- Female: male 4:1
- Unilateral, left hip most common, thought due to intrauterine positioning limiting left hip movement

Pathogenesis

- Shallow and misdirected acetabulum
- Proximal femoral anteversion and coxa valga
- Iliopsoas tendon may be tight and depress the joint capsule
- Hypertrophy of ligamentum teres or transverse ligament may impede reduction of femoral head

Risk Factors

- Breech intrauterine positioning
- Female
- High birthweight
- Cultural use of swaddling (hips extended)
- Presence of club foot or torticollis
- Positive family history
- Primiparity

Clinical Features

- Positive Ortoloni sign (hip adducted then abducted and lifted, with clunk of hip reduction)
- Positive Barlow sign (instability when hip is adducted, then clunk of dislocation at the posterior acetabulum)
- Shortened femur on affected side on Galeazi's test
- Trendelenberg gait when ambulatory

Natural History

- May resolve spontaneously with proper positioning at a young age
- Avascular necrosis can occur in untreated or incompletely treated DDH
- Delay in diagnosis or management, relates to a high risk of young adult degenerative arthritis of the hip, lumbar lordosis, knee pain, and degenerative changes of the spine

Diagnosis

Differential diagnosis

- Muscle contracture
- Muscle disease

History

- Family history
- Torticollis
- Club foot
- First child, breech birth, and high birthweight

Exam

- Click or clunk felt as hips are flexed and abducted
- Asymmetric thigh crease
- Difference in knee height in supine

Testing

- An anteroposterior radiograph of the hip is reliable by 2 to 3 months of age; acetabular index (AI) is calculated
- AI is a measurement of the slope of the ossified part of the acetabular roof—the angle between the Hilgenreiner line and a line drawn from the triradiate epiphysis to the lateral edge of the acetabulum
- AI>30° is abnormal
- Ultrasound of the hip can be used to confirm suspicious exams in younger infants and to follow progress of treatment.
- Computed tomography scan
- Arthrogram

Pitfalls

- Overinterpretation of imaging studies
- Misdiagnosis by not repeating exams

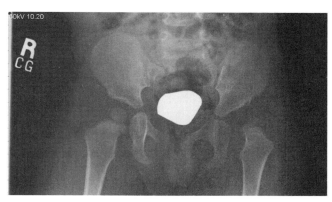

Abnormal acetabular index and humeral head on the left hip.

Red Flags
- Pain with movement
- Fracture
- Associated neurologic dysfunction

Treatment

Medical
- Triple diapering in abduction
- Pavlik harness positioning with weekly follow-up
- If hip reduced by 3 to 4 weeks—night splint and monitor until stable radiographically
- If not stable—proceed to surgery
- If not stable and infant is 6 months old—proceed to surgery

Surgical
- Closed or open reduction with spica cast immobilization
- Percutaneous adductor tenotomy
- Psoas tenotomy
- Femoral osteotomy
- Pericapsular osteotomy

Consults
- Orthopedic surgery

Complications of treatment
- Avascular necrosis
- Pressure sores
- Limp
- Knee flexion contracture
- Infection

Prognosis
- Best if treated before 6 months

Helpful Hints
- Repeated exams are important
- Bilateral hip dislocations are more difficult to identify and can be missed

Suggested Readings
Am Academy of Pediatrics. Clinical practice guideline: early detection of developmental dysplasia of the hip. Committee on Quality Improvement, Subcommittee on Developmental Dysplasia of the Hip. *Pediatrics*. 2000;105:896–905.
Staheli L. *Practice of Pediatric Orthopedics*. 2nd ed. Philadelphia, PA: Lippincott Williams & Wilkins; 2006.

Hip: Legg-Calve-Perthes Disease

Edward A. Hurvitz MD

Description
Legg-Calve-Perthes disease is an avascular necrosis of the hip in children.

Etiology/Types
- Temporary loss of blood flow to the femoral head

Epidemiology
- Children aged 4 to 10
- Male:female 5:1
- International incidence 1 in 1200
- Bilateral in 10% to 12%

Pathogenesis
- Death and necrosis of femoral head
- Related to pattern of vascular supply running alongside the femoral neck—can be sensitive to changes in the growth plate and other problems
- Changes with age, which allows for healing by molding with the femoral head positioned in the acetabulum
- Inflammation and irritation

Risk Factors
- Malnutrition
- Hypercoaguable states
- Low birthweight
- Older parents
- Delayed bone age
- Does not appear to be genetic

Clinical Features
- Child walks with a limp
- Pain in groin, also in thigh and knee
- Muscle spasm around hip

Natural History
- Can have complete recovery, especially in younger children
- May lead to early arthritis and eventual joint replacement

Diagnosis

Differential diagnosis
- Transient synovitis
- Hip trauma
- Joint infection
- Slipped capital femoral epiphysis (generally seen in older children)

History
- Limp, usually over a few weeks
- Pain in groin, starts mild over weeks or months
- Pain in other parts of leg—knee, thigh
- Often the child does not complain of pain until asked

Exam
- Pain increases with stressing range of motion (ROM) of the hip
- ROM of hip decreased
- Antalgic limp

Testing
- Serial x-rays demonstrate necrosis and regrowth of femoral head (as noted in the right hip in figure)
- Magnetic resonance imaging scan may be helpful to see early signs in the other hip
- Arthrogram may be useful to assess cartilage

Pitfalls
- Missing diagnosis with knee pain presentation

Red Flags
- Continuing pain and symptoms, or lack of improvement of x-rays, surgical treatment may be indicated

Treatment

Medical
- Containment—position the hip to help the femoral head recover to as close to normal as possible. The goal is to keep the hip in the acetabulum as much as possible, while still allowing motion, which is needed for cartilage health. The hip should be kept in abduction as much as possible during recovery.
- Anti-inflammatory medication
- Traction, including home traction

Exercises
- ROM
- Strengthen hip adductors, abductors, and rotators
- Ambulation training without weightbearing—crutches, wheelchair use—moving back to weightbearing with healing
- Therapy can begin immediately after diagnosis

Modalities

- Hip abduction orthosis, such as a Scottish Rite Orthosis, or similar, can be worn during ambulation
- Sometimes Petrie casts are used: hold the legs in abduction with a bar worked into the cast at the knees

Injection

- Botulinum toxin may be useful to reduce adductor spasm and to improve positioning in braces and therapy compliance

Surgical

- Tendon lengthenings of contracted muscles
- Femoral or pelvic osteotomy for realignment. Plates and screws are used to hold alignment

Consults

- Orthopedic surgery
- Physical therapy

Complications

- Inadequate treatment and/or healing leads to immobility of the hip joint and decreased mobility

Prognosis

- Most children return to normal activities in 18 months to 2 years
- Girls usually have more extensive involvement, and can have worse prognosis
- Problems may develop years later, leading to arthritis and joint replacement

Helpful Hints

- Younger children may need a less aggressive program, whereas older children bear more watching

Suggested Readings

Herring JA. *Tachdjian's Pediatric Orthopedics*. Philadelphia, PA: Saunders; 2007.

Herring JA, Kim HT, Browne R. Leg-Calve-Perthes disease: part I and II. *J Bone Joint Surg Am.* 2004;86-A:2103–2134.

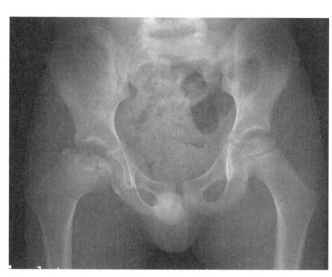

Necrosis and remodeling of right femoral head.

Hip: Slipped Capital Femoral Epiphysis

Elizabeth Moberg-Wolff MD

Description

Slipped capital femoral epiphysis (SCFE) is the most common adolescent hip disorder, defined as displacement of the femoral epiphysis on the metaphysis.

Etiology/Types

- A multifactorial etiology is typical with acute (<3 weeks), chronic, and acute-on-chronic slips possible
- Slips are classified in several ways: stable or nonstable, and mild (<1/3), moderate (1/2–2/3), or severe (>2/3) depending on percent of displacement

Epidemiology

- 1 in 50,000 teens
- Males more common
- Black and Hispanic ethnicity have higher risk
- Peak age 13 years (male), 11 years (female)
- Bilateral approximately 25% of the time
- Regional differences are seen (risk higher in Northeast and Western United States)

Pathogenesis

- The hip carries four times its body weight (due to muscle contraction); adolescent growth plates are weaker and more prone to injury
- The acetabulum is normal but the physis slips inferiorly and posteriorly
- Most slips are gradual, but can occur acutely
- Cessation of growth with physeal closure halts progression
- Severe slips in older children increase risk of osteoarthritis, avascular necrosis, and chondrolysis

Risk Factors

- Male gender
- Renal osteodytrophy
- Radiation
- Down syndrome
- Obesity
- Hypothyroidism
- Hypopituitarism
- Metabolic disorders (rickets)

Clinical Features

- Acute or chronic groin, thigh, or knee pain
- Left side more often affected than right
- Out toed gait
- Abductor lurch: pelvis drops in single leg stance, then the trunk shifts toward side with hip abductor weakness to compensate, usually in children with hip dysplasia
- Limb atrophy
- Refusal to move leg or weight bear

Natural History

- Avascular necrosis can occur in untreated or incompletely treated SCFE
- Delays in diagnosis or management relates to a high risk of young adult degenerative arthritis of the hip, further resulting in knee pain and secondary degenerative changes of the spine

Diagnosis

Differential diagnosis

- Knee injury
- Chondrolysis
- Legg-Calve-Perthes disease
- Muscle strain
- Fracture
- Infection

History

- Sudden pain without preceding trauma
- Chronic pain over several weeks leading to limp
- Inability to extend or internally rotate leg
- Adolescent growth spurt concurrent
- Premenstrual, if female
- Knee pain complaints
- Groin or thigh pain complaints
- Refusal to weight bear

Exam

- Loss of internal rotation of the hip
- Pain with extension and internal rotation
- Externally rotated and flexed leg
- Lack of swelling, instability, and tenderness at the knee
- Limping gait

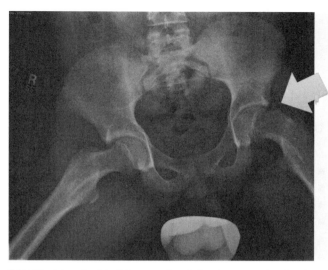

Displacement of left femoral epiphysis on metaphysis, at arrow.

Testing
- Anteroposterior and lateral radiograph of the hip; may miss slip early, and may need computed tomography or magnetic resonance imaging (MRI) to diagnose
- Ultrasound to view step off
- Bone scan, if "preslips" suspected
- MRI, if avascular necrosis suspected

Pitfalls
- Causing further slip by allowing weight bearing or forcing internal rotation on exam

Red Flags
- Acute pain and history of injury
- Fracture
- Associated neurologic dysfunction

Treatment

Medical
- Crutch walking/partial weight bearing if stable slip
- Traction or immobilization if unstable and compressed joint

Surgical
- Open reduction and fixation with single central screw. Non-weight-bearing until callous seen
- Osteotomy

Consults
- Orthopedic surgery

Complications of treatment
- Avascular necrosis—increases with severity of slip
- Chondrolysis, with prolonged immobilization and multiple hardware
- Knee flexion contracture

Prognosis
- Early diagnosis and treatment is essential as risk of arthritis increases with the severity of the slip
- Those with avascular necrosis or chondrolysis have more rapid arthritic deterioration and may require hip fusion or replacement at an early age

Helpful Hints
- Unstable, acute slips need immediate surgical treatment
- Delays in diagnosis are common

Suggested Readings
Hotchkiss BL, Engels JA, Forness M. Hip disorders in the adolescent. *Adolesc Med State Art Rev.* 2007;18(1):165–181,x-i.
Staheli L. *Practice of Pediatric Orthopedics.*2nd ed. Philadelphia, PA: Lippincott Williams & Wilkins; 2006.

Section II: Pediatric Diseases and Complications

Hip: Transient Synovitis of the Hip

Elizabeth Moberg-Wolff MD

Description

Transient synovitis (TS) of the hip is an idiopathic, benign inflammation of the joint, often seen in children who have recently had an upper respiratory infection. It is also known as irritable hip, toxic synovitis, or observation hip, and its symptoms typically subside within several days.

Etiology/Types

- Unknown

Epidemiology

- Children younger than 10 years of age; 3 to 8 years classic
- Boys more than girls at 2:1
- Unilateral in 95%
- Contralateral ultrasound findings in 25%

Pathogenesis

- May be an immune-mediated response to viral infection in some patients

Risk Factors

- Upper respiratory infection

Clinical Features

- Unilateral knee, hip, or thigh pain
- Acute or insidious onset
- Duration of days to weeks
- Refusal to weight bear due to pain with ambulation and abduction of the hip
- Mild fever or normal temperature
- Improvement in symptoms when leg positioned in flexion and external rotation

Natural History

- Pain develops acutely or gradually, often following a viral illness
- Symptoms improve within 10 days typically
- Long-term outcomes are benign
- Recurrent TS may occur but is not associated with long-term orthopedic conditions

Diagnosis

Differential diagnosis

- Septic arthritis
- Slipped capital femoral epiphysis
- Legg-Calve-Perthes
- Lyme disease
- Sickle cell crisis
- Avascular necrosis
- Rheumatoid disease
- Muscle pull
- Leukemia
- Malignancy
- Fracture

History

- Absence of current signs of systemic illness (fever, joint inflammation)
- Child comfortable at rest, worsens with weightbearing
- Pain improves with positioning in flexion, abduction, and external rotation

Exam

- Adduction and internal rotation of leg will elicit pain
- Generally nontender to palpation
- No spasms or muscular rigidity

Testing

- Radiographs of hip (should be normal)
- Ultrasound may show effusion
- C-reactive protein (<20 mg/L)
- ESR (<20 mm/hour)
- WBC (<12,000 cells/mm3)
- Body temperature (should be normal)
- Aspiration of joint if concern about sepsis

Pitfalls

- Septic joint misdiagnosed as TS

Red Flags

- Failure to resolve in a few days
- Fracture associated
- Radiographic changes

Treatment

Medical

- Rest—reduce weightbearing
- Position for comfort
- Nonsteroidal anti-inflammatory medication

Consults

- Orthopedic surgery
- Infectious disease

Prognosis

- Excellent for full recovery

Helpful Hints

- Repeated exams, including checking for fever, are important, with suspicion of sepsis crucial

- Presence of fever, with elevated WBC, C-reactive protein, and ESR should lead to high suspicion of sepsis

Suggested Readings

Caird MS, Flynn JM, Leung YL, et al. Factors distinguishing septic arthritis from transient synovitis of the hip in children. A prospective study. *J Bone Joint Surg Am.* 2006;88(6):1251–1257.

Hardinge K. Etiology of transient synovitis of the hip in childhood. *J Bone Joint Surg Br.* 1970;52-B(1):100.

Uziel Y, Butbul-Aviel Y, Barash J, et al. Recurrent transient synovitis of the hip in childhood. Long-term outcome among 39 patients. *J Rheumatol.* 2006;33(4):810–811.

HIV/AIDS

Michelle A. Miller MD

Description

Human immunodeficiency virus (HIV) is a retrovirus from the Lentivirinae family. It targets the CD4 T lymphocytes thereby weakening the immune system.

Etiology/Types

- HIV-1
- Vertical transmission from infected mother to child in perinatal period is most common means of infection in children
- No race, gender, or socioeconomic status risk factors

Epidemiology

- Pandemic with especially high numbers in sub-Saharan Africa
- Estimated 2.3 million children younger than 15 years living with HIV in 2006
- 410,00 to 600,000 new pediatric cases reported in 2006

Pathogenesis

- Infection via blood to blood contact, through breast milk, or vaginal secretions
- HIV enters CD4 cells and creates a DNA replica of the viral RNA
- CD4 cells are destroyed in the process
- CD4 cells are a subset of T cells, that activate other white blood cells for an immune response
- Viral load increases within the blood and then seeds lymph nodes, other organs, and tissues
- Body develops antibodies to fight infection which may lead to an autoimmune reaction

Risk Factors

- HIV infected mother
- Limited or no access to antiretroviral therapy

Clinical Features

- Failure to thrive
- Delays in motor and language developmental milestones
- Opportunistic infections, especially pulmonary

Natural History

- Stage 1—HIV serology positive, but zero to one symptoms of infections
- Stage II—mildly symptomatic with two or more of the following: infection of lymph nodes, recurrent or persistent upper respiratory infection, skin infection, hepatomegaly, splenomegaly, or parotitis
- Stage III—moderately symptomatic with anemia, persistent fever, diarrhea, fatigue, pneumonia, persistent thrush, hepatitis, persistent chicken pox, herpes stomatitis, shingles, and/or cardiomyopathy
- Stage IV (AIDS)—severely symptomatic with opportunistic infections, cancers, or wasting syndrome, often leading to death

Diagnosis

Differential diagnoses

- Inflammatory demyelinating polyneuropathy
- Leukodystrophies
- Metabolic myopathies
- Other viral or bacterial encephalopathy
- Paraneoplastic syndrome
- Spinal muscular atrophy
- Viral meningitis

HIV-associated diagnoses

- HIV-associated encephalopathy
- Meningitis
- Distal sensory polyneuropathy
- Autonomic neuropathy
- Inflammatory demyelinating polyneuropathy
- HIV-associated neuromuscular weakness syndrome (HANWS)
- Mononeuropathy multiplex
- Progressive polyradiculopathy
- Myopathy

History

- HIV serology positive or HIV positive mother
- Delay in achieving or loss of motor and/or cognitive milestones
- Poor suck or difficulty feeding
- Progressive weakness
- Sensory loss

- Declines in spelling, reading, and reading comprehension

Exam
- Linear growth failure
- Oral thrush
- Proximal weakness
- Poor head and trunk control
- Decreased sensation to light touch and pinprick
- Flaccid paraparesis with decreased rectal tone
- Spastic diplegia or hemiplegia
- Expressive language and articulation deficits

Testing
- Positive serology for HIV and lower CD4 count
- Electromyography findings consistent with acute inflammatory demyelinating polyneuropathy (AIDP)/ chronic inflammatory demyelinating polyneuropathy (CIDP), myopathy, sensory neuropathy, or radiculopathy
- Brain magnetic resonance imaging with atrophy, calcification of the basal ganglia, encephalitis, toxoplasmosis, diffuse leukoencephalopathy, or tumor
- Videofluoroscopic swallow evaluation may demonstrate abnormalities in oral, pharyngeal, and esophageal phases
- Significant delays in mental and motor domains of the Bayley scales of infant development

Pitfalls
- Often have more than one disease process

Red Flags
- CD4 count less than 500

Treatment

Medical
- Highly active antiretroviral therapy (HAART) treatment in mother decreases vertical transmission and slows disease process
- Standard immunizations except varicella
- Pneumococcal vaccine at age two and annual influenza vaccine
- Antibiotics, antivirals, and antifungals
- Antiepileptics or tricyclic antidepressants for neuropathic pain

- Intravenous immune globulin or corticosteroids for myopathy, AIDP/CIDP, HANWS, or mononeuropathy

Exercises
- Moderate aerobic or resistive conditioning but monitor pulmonary status

Modalities
- Massage therapy
- Ice or cold foods to desensitize mouth and oropharynx

Equipment
- Bracing
- Walker or wheelchair for mobility
- Augmentative and alternative communication systems

Consults
- Infectious diseases or HIV team
- Neurology
- Psychology

Complications of treatment
- HAART may be neurotoxic leading to further impairment
- Exhaustive physical conditioning can be immunosuppressive

Prognosis
- Highly variable with multiple confounding factors including environment, access to medical care, and socioeconomic status
- HAART has significantly improved life expectancy, but has not had a reliable, positive impact on cognitive function

Helpful Hints
- Set realistic goals for therapy and re-evaluate neuromuscular and cognitive function often

Suggested Readings
Van Rie A, Mupuala A, Dow A. Impact of the HIV/AIDS epidemic on the neurodevelopment of preschool-aged children in Kinshasa, Democratic Republic of the Congo. *Pediatrics.* 2008;122(1):e123–e128.

Willen, E. Neurocognitive outcomes in pediatric HIV. *Men Retar Dev Disabil Res Rev.* 2006;12:223–228.

Section II: Pediatric Diseases and Complications

Intellectual Disability

Benjamin Katholi MD ■ Deborah Gaebler-Spira MD

Description

Intellectual disability (ID) is characterized by limitation in intellectual functioning and adaptive behavior (conceptual, social, and practical adaptive skills) originating before age 18.

Etiology/Types

- More than 1000 identifiable causes
- Common causes —Fragile X, Down syndrome, and fetal alcohol syndrome
- More prenatal than perinatal or postnatal causes, often coexists with cerebral palsy and autism
- Acquired due to traumatic brain infection, tumor, and brain irradiation
- Most ID is mild to moderate

Epidemiology

- 3/100 people in the United States have ID
- 1/10 children needing special education have ID

Pathogenesis

- Mainly cortical structure dysfunction (hippocampus and medial temporal cortex)
- 3% to 7% due to inborn errors of metabolism complicated by multiorgan disease. Alcohol exposure in utero accounts for 8% of mild ID
- Factors include genetic abnormalities, problems during pregnancy/birth, infancy, childhood, or adolescence (i.e., head injury, infection, and stroke)
- Most individuals with mild ID and other learning disorders have no other neurologic problems. They are more likely to be born into families of low socioeconomic status, low IQ, little education

Risk Factors

- Prenatal—central nervous system dysgenesis, chromosomal disorders, complex malformations, toxin exposures, and congenital infections.
- Perinatal—prematurity, intrauterine growth restriction, and neonatal infection
- Postnatal—infection, lead, metabolic disorders, trauma, severe deprivation, and social disadvantage

Clinical Features

- Expressive and receptive language delays
- IQ below 75 (mild 50–75, moderate 35–50, severe 20–35, profound ≤ 19) combined with difficulty in conceptual, social, and practical adaptive skills

Natural History

- Mild ID may not be diagnosed until elementary school; moderate ID may be noted in preschool years; severe and profound ID may be noted in the first year of life.
- Diagnosis delayed until appropriate age for complete testing for ID

Diagnosis

Differential diagnosis

- Developmental delays
- Specific learning disabilities
- Autism/Autism spectrum disorder

History

- Behavioral and emotional disturbances
- Language delay, social developmental delay
- Delays in adaptive and problem-solving skills
- Cognitive delays: problems with short-term memory, concept formation, understanding social rules or problem solving, using logic, understanding cause-and-effect relationships
- 10% to 40% comorbid mental health disorder (attention deficit disorder, anxiety, and depression)
- Infantile hypotonia of central origin may precede cognitive impairment

Exam

- Head circumference
- Dysmorphic features
- Neurological exam, assessment of muscle tone
- Ophthalmological exam
- Observations of communicative, perceptual, and social behavioral skills
- Growth parameters

Testing

- Developmental questionnaires, followed by formal testing possibly including Stanford-Binet, Wechsler-IV, Vineland Adaptive Behavior Scales II
- Adjunctive testing may include the following: karyotype, FISH for subtelomeric abnormalities to

check for very small rearrangements, Fragile X testing, molecular genetic testing, magnetic resonance imaging, metabolic testing; all to evaluate for treatable causes
- Audiological and opthalmological consultation
- Psychological and specialized testing, especially in communicative, behavioral, adaptive skills

Pitfalls
- Misdiagnosis delays proper treatment or therapies
- Too early a diagnosis may not allow for normal developmental variation
- Non-English speaking patients from different cultural background or low socioeconomic status may perform poorly on formal testing

Red Flags
- Progressive decline concerning for other etiology
- Underlying acute medical condition explaining symptoms

Treatment

Medical
- Most causes of ID are untreatable
- Growth, developmental, and behavioral surveillance
- Management of possible sensory/motor deficits
- Monitoring for sleep disorders
- Management of behavioral, psychiatric, and neurologic comorbidities (i.e., seizures)
- If ID etiology is clear, medical management should include specialty services, monitoring based on associated comorbidities with specific diagnosis
- Anticipatory guidance following child's developmental age, functional strengths rather than chronological age

Therapeutic/Educational
- Physical therapy, occupational therapy, speech-language pathology, with behavioral, social skills training

- Early childhood services followed by special education services, community living, vocational support/supported employment services
- Family care with support and counseling unless family cannot provide care. Transition services for adult care

Consults
- Pediatric neurology or developmental pediatrician
- Genetics and genetic counseling

Prevention/Prognosis
- Parental counseling: teratogen avoidance, prepregnancy vaccinations, prematurity prevention, recurrence risk (up to 25% with unknown etiology)
- Life expectancy possibly shortened due to coexisting medical conditions (i.e., recurrent seizures, gross motor function classification system IV or V cerebral palsy, congenital heart disease)
- Patients with mild to moderate ID can support themselves, live independently, and be successful at jobs requiring basic intellectual skills

Helpful Hints
- Language development is best predictor of future intellectual function
- ID should be defined for parents to initiate necessary planning
- ID may be present in conjunction with other disabilities (i.e., cerebral palsy and autism)

Suggested Readings

Curry CJ, Stevenson RE, Aughton D, et al. Evaluation of mental retardation: recommendations of a Consensus Conference: American College of Medical Genetics. *Am J Med Genet.*1997; 72(4):468–477.

Luckasson R, Schalock RL, Spitalnik DM, et al. *Mental Retardation: Definition, Classification, and Systems Of Support.* 10th ed. Washington, DC: American Association on Mental Retardation; 2002.

Section II: Pediatric Diseases and Complications

Klippel-Feil Syndrome

Robert J. Rinaldi MD

Description

Klippel-Feil Syndrome is a heterogeneous collection of clinical findings all unified by the presence of congenital synostosis of some or all cervical vertebrae.

Etiology/Types

- Exact etiology and underlying genetic components are unknown
- Likely due to disruption in genes regulating segmentation and resegmentation of somites
- Possible roles for *BMP-13, FGFR3, Notch, and PAX* genes
- Numerous classification systems proposed

Epidemiology

- Proposed incidence of 1:40,000 to 42,000 births
- Slight female predominance (3:2)
- Large phenotypic heterogeneity
- Most cases sporadic, though autosomal dominant and autosomal recessive inheritance patterns are described

Pathogenesis

- Disruptions in the regulation of somite segmentation and resegmentation
- Difficult to define due to large patient heterogeneity and broad spectrum of anomalies associated with sporadic cases

Risk Factors

- Sporadic mutation risk factors are unknown
- Some are genetic

Clinical Features

- Characteristic triad including short neck, low hairline, and limited cervical mobility in 50%
- Fusion of one or multiple cervical levels
- Broad spectrum of associated findings, including the following:
  - Congenital scoliosis (50%)
  - Torticollis and facial asymmetry (20%–50%)
  - Hearing deficits (30%)
  - Sprengel anomaly (20%–30%)
  - Rib abnormalities (30%)
  - Renal anomalies, major and minor (30%)
  - Synkinesia (30%)
  - Cardiovascular anomalies (15%)
  - Congenital limb deficiencies
  - Craniosynostosis
  - Craniofacial abnormalities
  - Spinal dysraphism
  - Cognitive impairment
  - Genitourinary anomalies

Natural History

- May be asymptomatic in minor cases
- Risk of cervical disc degeneration, vertebral subluxation, and spinal stenosis with increasing age
- Degenerative changes may lead to radicular findings or myelopathies
- Cervical instability and hypermobility may develop at interspaces between fused vertebrae
- Increased risk of sustaining spinal cord injury with minor and major trauma
- Scoliosis may be progressive over time

Diagnosis

Differential diagnosis

- Congenital anomalies of C1
- Cervical fusions due to juvenile rheumatoid arthritis

History

- Limitations in cervical range of motion
- Progressive cervical pain
- Neurologic changes due to cervical radiculopathy or myelopathy
- Progressive congenital scoliosis

Exam

- Short neck
- Low hairline
- Limited cervical range of motion
- Scoliosis
- Upper motor neuron and/or lower motor neuron findings in those with neurologic compromise
- Associated congenital anomalies as per clinical features

Testing

- X-ray of the cervical spine including anteroposterior and lateral views, with flexion-extension views if instability is suspected

- X-rays of entire spine to rule out associated spinal anomalies
- Flexion and extension magnetic resonance imaging to assess for instability, cervical stenosis, and other associated central nervous system abnormalities
- Audiologic testing
- Kidney ultrasound
- Echocardiography

Pitfalls
- Missed diagnosis on plain films of younger children
- Missed diagnosis of associated findings

Red Flags
- Cervical spinal cord injury following minor trauma
- Progressive cervical radiculopathy or myelopathy

Treatment

Medical
- Management of associated clinical findings
- Bracing of scoliosis

Injection
- Epidural steroid injection for radicular symptoms

Surgical
- Occipitocervical fusion for atlanto-occipital instability
- Discectomy/fusion for degenerative disc disease
- Posterior decompression and fusion for cervical stenosis

Consults
- Neurosurgery or orthopedic surgery
- Nephrology
- Cardiology
- Audiology

Complications
- Progressive neurologic compromise
- Progressive scoliosis
- Acute spinal cord injury

Prognosis
- Variable: dependent upon severity, associated clinical findings, and medical management

Helpful Hints
- Full physical evaluation must be done to assess for associated conditions

Suggested Readings
Klimo P, Rao G, Brockmeyer D. Congenital anomalies of the cervical spine. *Neurosurg Clin N Am.* 2007;18(3):463–478.
Tracy MH, Dormans JP, Kusumi K. Klippel-Feil syndrome: clinical features and current understanding of etiology. *Clin Orthop Relat Res.* 2004;(424):183–190.

Section II: Pediatric Diseases and Complications

Metachromatic Leukodystrophy

Teresa Such-Neibar DO

Description

Metachromatic leukodystrophy (MLD) is one of a group of autosomal recessive genetic disorders with abnormalities of the myelin sheath. MLD is one of several lysosomal storage diseases and is caused by a deficiency of the enzyme arylsulfatase A.

Etiology/Types

- Late infantile—The most common MLD. Affected children have difficulty walking after the first year of life
- Juvenile—Children with the juvenile form of MLD (between 3 and 10 years of age) usually begin with impaired school performance, mental deterioration, and dementia and then develop symptoms similar to the infantile form but with slower progression

Epidemiology

- It is estimated the carrier defect occurs in the general population at 1 in every 100 people
- The affected birth rate is 1:40,000

Pathogenesis

- Cause impairment in the growth or development of the myelin sheath
- Defect in the arylsulfatase A enzyme that helps produce the myelin sheath
- Results in the toxic buildup of lipids in cells in the nervous system, liver, and kidneys. This toxic buildup destroys the myelin sheath.

Risk Factors

- Family history

Clinical Features

- Late infantile MLD
  - Period of months of apparently normal growth and development
  - Deterioration of skills such as walking and speech
  - Symptoms often appear to progress rapidly over a period of several months to years, with alternating periods of stabilization and decline
  - Eventually, the child is unable to speak or feed independently
  - Seizures may occur and will eventually disappear
  - Contractures are common and apparently painful
  - The child is still able to smile and respond to parents at this stage, but eventually may become blind and largely unresponsive
  - Swallowing eventually becomes difficult and a feeding tube becomes necessary
  - With modern treatment and care, the child may survive for 5 to 10 years
  - Other symptoms include loss of cognitive ability, hypertonia, motor regression, and eventual absence of voluntary functions
- Juvenile onset
  - Diagnosis 3 to 10 years of age
  - Noted deterioration of motor and cognitive abilities

Natural History

- Late infantile MLD—death occurs usually 5 to 10 years after diagnosis with supportive care
- Juvenile onset—more individuals are living into adulthood with supportive medical care

Diagnosis

Differential diagnosis

- Cerebral palsy
- Batton's disease
- Attention deficit hyperactivity disorder

History

- Loss of motor and speech milestones

Exam

- Blindness
- Loss of cognitive ability
- Hypertonia
- Spasticity
- Motor regression and eventual absence of voluntary functions

Testing

- Usually a blood test is done first to check for enzyme levels

- A urine test to confirm the presence of sulfatides
- Cerebrospinal fluid for elevated protein
- Electromyography for slowed nerve conduction
- Prenatal diagnosis for MLD is available
- Brain magnetic resonance imaging to look for white matter disturbances characteristic of MLD

Pitfalls
- Misdiagnosis

Red Flags
- Loss of motor and speech milestones
- Hypotonia and hypertonia

Treatment

Medical
- No cure
- Monitor swallowing and refer for gastrostomy tube when supplemental feeding is necessary
- Bone marrow transplantation has been performed for patients with MLD with the aim to repopulate recipient hematopoietic and lymphoid compartments with cells with a functional hydrolase. Results have been limited due to the slow pace of replacement of resident tissue compared to the progressive nature of the disease
- Other treatment is symptomatic and supportive
- Oral antispasticity medications
- Antiseizure medications
- Antireflux medications
- End of life directives

Exercises
- Range of motion (ROM), braces

Modalities/Equipment
- Supportive equipment, for example, wheelchair, positioning devices, and lifts

Injection
- Intramuscular injections, including botulinum toxin and phenol, may be helpful to maintain ROM and decrease discomfort

Surgical
- Intrathecal baclofen pump may be useful to maintain ROM and decrease pain

Consults
- Orthopedic surgery
- Hematology/oncology (bone marrow transplant)
- Neurosurgery
- Gastroenterology

Prognosis
- Poor
- Most children with the infantile form die by age 5
- Progression in the juvenile forms is slower; may live a decade or more following diagnosis

Helpful Hints
- Begin supportive care early, and connect families with similar diagnosis
- Testing asymptomatic brothers and sisters of patients who have MLD

Suggested Readings

Biffi A, Lucchini G, Rovelli A, Sessa M. Metachromatic leukodystrophy: an overview of current and prospective treatments. *Bone Marrow Transplant.* 2008;42:S2–S6.

http://www.ninds.nih.gov/disorders/metachromatic_leukodystrophy/metachromatic_leukodystrophy.htm

http://www.ulf.org/types/MLD.html

http://www.mldfoundation.org

Louhiata P. Bone marrow transplantation in the prevention of intellectual disability due to inherited metabolic disease: ethical issues. *J Med Ethics.* 2009;35:415–418.

Section II: Pediatric Diseases and Complications

Morquio/Mucopolysaccharidose Type 4

Rajashree Srinivasan MD

Description

Neurometabolic genetic disorders which occur due to a defect in glycosaminoglycan (GAG) metabolism. They are characterized by skeletal changes, intellectual disability, and involvement of the viscera.

Etiology

- Autosomal recessive disorders due to absence of or malfunction of the lysosomal enzymes, which break down GAG
- Type I—Hurler syndrome, deficiency of alpha L-iduronidase, most severe type
- Type II—Hunter syndrome, deficiency of iduronate sulfate sulfatase, X-linked
- Type III—Sanfillipo syndrome, deficiency of Heparan sulfamidase or alpha N acetylglocosaminidase
- Type IV—Morquio syndrome, deficiency of N-acetylgalactosamine-6-sulfatase, autosomal recessive
- Type VII—Sly syndrome, deficiency of beta glucoronidase
- Autosomal recessive usually, except Hunter syndrome

Epidemiology

- 1 in 25,000 in the United States

Pathogenesis

- Lysosomal enzymes are needed to break down GAG, which are long chains of carbohydrates which help build bone, cartilage, skin, tendons, cornea, and connective tissue
- GAG is also found in the joint fluid
- People with mucopolysaccharidosis (MPS) do not produce enough of the 11 enzymes needed to break down GAG or produce defective enzymes. This leads to the collection of GAG in the connective tissue, cells, and blood, leading to cell damage.

Risk Factors

- Familial

Clinical Features

- Severe skeletal dysplasia and short stature (Types IV and VII)
- Macroglossia (Types I and II)
- Coarse facial features with prominent forehead
- Macrocephaly
- Micrognathia
- Motor dysfunction and developmental delay
- Spasticity (Type III)
- Retinal degeneration (Types I, II, III)
- Intellectual disability (all except for Type IV)
- Corneal clouding (Types I, II, VII)
- Mitral regurgitation (Types I, II)
- Aortic valve disease (Types I, IV, VI)
- Hepatosplenomegaly (Types I, II, VI, VII)
- Joint stiffness (most except Type IV)
- Spinal cord compression (Type IV)

Natural History

- No cure
- Death by second decade for some (not Type IV)
- Cardiac complications due to cardiac valve, myocardial, and ischemic factors lead to death by 15 years

Diagnosis

Differential diagnosis

- Hypothyroidism
- Mucolipidoses

History

- Period of normal growth then slowing
- Repeated respiratory infections
- Repeated otitis media infections

Exam

- Joint abnormalities
- Coarse facies
- Umbilical hernias
- Corneal clouding

Testing

- Urinalysis—for GAG
- Enzyme assay, cultured fibroblasts—for lysosomal enzymes
- Prenatal diagnosis on cultured amniotic fluid cells or chorionic villus biopsy

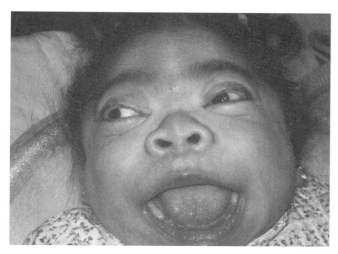

A child with a neurometabolic disorder.

Pitfalls
- Growth retardation
- Airway compromise

Red Flags
- Seemingly normal period of development followed by developmental delay leads to prolongation of diagnosis

Treatment

Medical
- Enzyme replacement trials using recombinant technique are in progress
- Supportive management, attention to respiratory and cardiovascular complications, hearing loss, carpal tunnel syndrome, spinal cord compression, and hydrocephalus
- Bone marrow transplant in MPS I—recommended in patients less than 24 months
- End of life directives

Exercise
- Strengthening

- Gait training

Modalities
- Wrist hand orthoses
- Ankle foot orthoses

Injection
- N/A

Surgery
- Orthopedic procedures needed—Femoral osteotomies, acetabular reconstruction, and posterior spinal fusion
- Corneal grafting
- Bone marrow transplant (Type I)

Consults
- Orthopedic surgery
- Opthalmology
- Pulmonology
- Cardiology
- Genetics
- Transplant surgery

Complications
- Cervical myelopathy
- Cardiac complications
- Obstructive sleep apnea

Prognosis
- Poor without aggressive intervention
- Many require ventilatory assistance

Helpful Hints
- Avoid contact sports

Suggested Readings
Cormier-Daire V. Spondylo-epi-metaphyseal dysplasia. *Best Pract Res Clin Rheumatol.* 2008;22:33–44.

Martins AM, Dualibi AP, Norato D, et al. Guidelines for the management of mucopolysaccharidoses type I. *J Pediatr.* 2009;155:S32–46.

Section II: Pediatric Diseases and Complications

Multiple Sclerosis

Glendaliz Bosques MD ■ David W. Pruitt MD

Description

Autoimmune progressive demyelinating disease of the central nervous system (CNS), which is prevalent in adults but uncommon in children.

Etiology/Types

- Relapsing-remitting (most common)
- Primary progressive
- Secondary progressive
- Progressive-relapsing

Epidemiology

- Approximately 10% of all multiple sclerosis (MS) patients are younger than 16 years of age
- Disease manifestation before age 5 is extremely rare, and should be considered an equivocal diagnosis
- Incidence is higher in females (2.8:1)
- Unknown prevalence

Pathogenesis

- Immunopathogenic hypothesis suggests the presence of antimyelin autoreactive T cells which get activated
- Activation of these autoreactive T cells may occur through molecular mimicry
- Activation of B cells may also be important in severe demyelination due to production of autoantibodies which attack the myelin coating of nerves

Risk Factors

- Environmental factors (viral exposure, country of origin, sun exposure, and temperate climate) may play a role
- Genetic and ethnic factors are suggested

Clinical Features

- Polyfocal or polysymptomatic neurologic deficits
- Isolated optic neuritis (higher risk of developing MS if bilateral)
- Isolated brain-stem dysfunction
- Isolated dysfunction of the long tracts
- Fatigue (severe enough to limit school performance or recreational activities)
- Encephalopathic signs (usually absent in adults) such as headaches, vomiting, seizures, and altered mental status
- Bladder dysfunction (urgency and frequency more frequent than obstructive symptoms)
- Heat sensitivity (Uhthoff's phenomenon) causes exacerbation or worsening of symptoms with increased body temperature

Natural History

- Involvement of CNS white matter leads to clinical neurological impairments. Remission usually follows. Other episodes involve different areas of the white matter
- Episodes are spread over time (at least two distinct neurologic episodes) and location (evidence of lesions seen by clinical findings, magnetic resonance imaging (MRI), computed tomography, or evoked potentials)
- Time to recover from clinical exacerbation is shorter in children (4.3 weeks vs up to 8 weeks in adults)
- Length of time between first and second neurologic episodes can extend up to 2 years

Diagnosis (Table 1)

Differential diagnosis

- CNS infection
- CNS malignancy
- Primary small-vessel vasculitis of the CNS
- Macrophage-activation syndrome
- Inherited white matter leukodystrophies
- Transverse myelitis

History

More than one clinical episode of the following occurs:
- Muscular weakness
- Sensory deficits
- Visual disturbances: blurry vision, partial blindness, and diplopia

- Coordination deficits
- Bulbar impairments
- Dysautonomia: vertigo, headaches, somnolence, tinnitus, and sphincter incompetence
- Depending on the subtype, the patient may recover or evolve into a progressive chronic course

Exam
- Muscle weakness
- Ataxia
- Dysmetria
- Upper motor neuron signs: hyperreflexia, spasticity, and presence of Babinski's or Hoffmann's reflexes
- Visual changes: pale optic disc, gaze paralysis, and nystagmus
- Altered mental state: confusion, euphoria, and emotional lability; Psychosis is unusual

Testing
- Cerebrospinal fluid analysis: oligoclonal bands and increased IgG
- Visual, brainstem, or somatosensory delayed evoked potentials
- MRI of the brain: >2 periventricular ovoid lesions
- McDonald criteria lists required testing for definitive MS diagnosis
- Neuropsychological assessment
- Bladder function: low threshold to check postvoid residual volumes or urodynamic testing—detrusor hyperreflexia (2/3 of patients) and/or detrusor-sphincter dyssynergia

Table 1. McDonald criteria for diagnosis of MS

Attacks	Clinical evidence	Requirements for diagnosis
2 or more	2 or more	None
2 or more	1 lesion	Dissemination in space by MRI (or CSF or await further attack)
1 attack	2 lesions	Dissemination in time by MRI (or second clinical attack)
1 attack	1 lesion	Dissemination in space and time by MRI (or CSF and second attack)
0 attack	Insidious neurological progression	Positive brain MRI Positive spinal cord MRI Positive CSF (2 of 3)

Pitfalls
- MRI lesions in children may be fewer and less dramatic than adults
- Oligoclonal bands may be seen in other disorders of the CNS

Red Flags
- Dysphagia
- Respiratory depression
- Profound encephalopathy
- Quadriplegia

Treatment
Medical
- Acute exacerbations: steroids
- Life-threatening demyelination and no response to steroids: plasma exchange
- Possible reduction in relapse rate with immunomodulatory therapies but no specific studies for dose or effectiveness in children
- Spasticity: spasmolytic medications
- Neuropathic pain: anticonvulsants or tricyclic antidepressants
- Musculoskeletal pain: nonsteroidal anti-inflammatory drugs and/or analgesics
- Fatigue: neurostimulants
- Bladder dysfunction: timed voids, anticholinergic or alpha blocking medications, intermittent catheterization program, and continent diversion surgery
- Fall risk: mobility aids and orthoses to enhance gait stability

Exercises
- General strengthening and stretching
- Gait training or ambulation component integrated into program
- Aquatic exercise program (pool temperature 80–84° F)

Modalities
- Cooling vests or other techniques to decrease body temperature
- Energy conservation

Injection
- Chemodenervation procedures

Surgical
- Intrathecal baclofen pump implantation

Section II: Pediatric Diseases and Complications

Consults

- Neurology
- Speech therapy: dysphagia and dysarthria
- Neuropsychology
- Urology

Complications

- Rapid cognitive decline
- Loss of mobility
- Bladder dysfunction

Prognosis

- Pediatric onset MS progression takes longer than in adults, but the disability occurs at a younger age
- Predictors of greater severity and worse outcome: female, no encephalopathy at onset, well-defined lesions on MRI, <1 year between first and second attacks, and secondary progressive disease

Helpful Hints

- Children with MS have similar memory problems as adults, but also have the ability to express themselves better. Therefore, cognitive impairments may be missed during a routine office visit.

Suggested Readings

Chabas D, Strober J, Waubant E. Pediatric multiple sclerosis. *Curr Neurol Neurosci Rep.*2008;8(5):434–441.

MacAllister WS, Boyd JR, Holland NJ, et al. The psychosocial consequences of pediatric multiple sclerosis. *Neurology.* 2007;68(16 Suppl 2):S66–69.

Muscular Dystrophy: Becker

Nanette C. Joyce DO

Description

Becker muscular dystrophy (BMD) is a dystrophinopathy more mild in phenotypic expression than Duchenne muscular dystrophy (DMD). It is characterized by a progressive limb-girdle pattern of weakness, calf hypertrophy, and loss of ambulation after age 15.

Etiology/Types

- X-linked recessive inheritance pattern
- Mutations are located in the dystrophin gene Xp21
- Sixty five percent of mutations are deletions, approximately 5% are duplications
- Clinical severity more dependent on in-frame versus out-of-frame mutation ("reading-frame rule"), rather than the location of the mutation along the gene
- In-frame mutations produce semifunctional dystrophin, resulting in the BMD phenotype
- Approximately 89% of BMD patients with a deletion mutation are in-frame

Epidemiology

- Incidence: 5 per 100,000
- Prevalence: 17 to 27 per 1 million
- Primarily affects males; though translocation at the Xp21 site may cause female presentation of the BMD phenotype

Pathogenesis

- Results from mutations in the dystrophin gene
- One of the largest genes identified in humans with 79 exons, coding a 14-kb transcript
- Dystophin, along with dystrophin-associated proteins, form a complex, connecting cytoskeletal actin to the basal lamina
- The complex stabilizes the sarcolemmal membrane during contraction/relaxation and if abnormal, leads to increased tears with subsequent necrosis

Risk Factors

- Familial inheritance
- Ten percent to 30% of cases due to spontaneous mutations

Clinical Features

- Progressive proximal muscle weakness affecting lower limbs before upper limbs
- Pseudohypertrophy of the calves
- Relative preservation of neck flexor muscle strength until later in the disease course
- Contractures are less frequent than in DMD; most commonly plantar flexion contracture
- Scoliosis rare in BMD, but may develop after transition to wheelchair
- Myalgias may be severe with possible episodes of myoglobinuria
- Cardiomyopathy may precede skeletal muscle weakness

Natural History

- Onset is later than DMD, typically occurring between the ages of 5 and 15 years, but may present as late as the third or fourth decade
- Pelvic girdle and thigh muscles are affected first
- Patients typically ambulate beyond the age of 15
- Most survive past the age of 30
- Life span is shortened, with death often occurring from respiratory or cardiac disease

Diagnosis

Differential diagnosis

- Fascioscapulohumeral dystrophy
- Limb-girdle muscular dystrophy
- Spinal muscular atrophy type III
- Emery-Dreifuss muscular dystrophy
- Congenital muscular dystrophy
- Duchenne muscular dystrophy

History

- Delayed gross motor milestones
- Falls more frequently than contemporaries
- Toe-walking
- Difficulty arising from the floor and climbing stairs

Exam

- Symmetric weakness worse in the hip girdle and quadriceps versus the upper limbs
- Preserved neck flexion strength

- Pseudohypertrophy of the calf muscles
- Gower's sign, using the arms to push up from a squatting position due to hip weakness
- Toe-walking with heel cord contractures
- Decreased or absent reflexes
- Intact sensation

Testing
- Serum creatine kinase may be 5 to 100 times the upper limit of normal
- DNA testing
- Muscle biopsy with immunohistochemical staining and Western blot to quantify dystrophin

Pitfalls
- Genetic testing may not identify causative mutation
- Genetic testing to determine carrier status of the mothers and sisters of the patient should be provided; daughters are obligate carriers

Red Flags
- Cardiac disease from cardiomyopathy may be presenting symptom
- Increased risk for malignant hyperthermia with anesthesia

Treatment

Medical
- No large randomized controlled trials, but small series suggest benefits of corticosteroids
- Prednisone 0.75 mg/kg/day or 5 mg/kg given both days on weekends
- Possible benefit from short courses of creatine monohydrate at 5 to10 mg/day
- Angiotensin converting enzyme inhibition or use of angiotensin receptor blockers for treatment of cardiomyopathy

Exercise
- Range of motion exercises to reduce contractures
- Aquatherapy to maintain cardiovascular fitness

Assistive devices
- Night orthoses to prevent heel cord contractures
- Mobility devices such as manual and/or power wheelchairs, and Hoyer lift for transfers
- Bathroom equipment such as grab bars, elevated toilet seat, tub bench, commode, and shower chair

Surgical
- Posterior spinal stabilization of scoliotic curve greater than 30° if FVC >30% of predicted
- Heel cord release for plantar flexion contractures
- Percutaneous gastrostomy tube (PEG)

Consults
- Cardiology evaluation for cardiomyopathy
- Pulmonology evaluation for restrictive lung disease and nocturnal hypoventilation requiring noninvasive positive pressure ventilation, and/or cough assistance
- Orthopedic evaluation for scoliosis management
- Gastroenterology if PEG placement indicated
- Speech language pathology evaluation

Prognosis
- Chronic progressive disease with shortened life expectancy due to cardiac and respiratory complications

Helpful Hints
- Must offer genetic counseling to daughters of men with BMD as they are obligate carriers, and to mothers and sisters of young men with the disease

Suggested Readings
Birnkrant DJ, Panitch HB, Benditt JO, et al. American college of chest physicians consensus statement on the respiratory and related management of patients with Duchenne muscular dystrophy undergoing anesthesia or sedation. *Chest.* 2007;132(6):1977–1986.

Finsterer J, Stollberger C. Cardiac involvement in Becker muscular dystrophy. *Can J Cardiol.* 2008;24(10):786–792.

Leiden Muscular Dystrophy Pages with reading frame checker at: http://www.dmd.nl/

Muscular Dystrophy: Congenital

Nanette C. Joyce DO

Description

The congenital muscular dystrophies (CMD) are a group of autosomal recessive inherited disorders with clinical heterogeneity. They are characterized by perinatal muscle weakness with hypotonia, joint contractures, and abnormal muscle biopsy.

Etiology/Types

- All have autosomal recessive inheritance patterns; however, reported cases of Ullrich congenital muscular dystrophy with autosomal dominant inheritance from germ line de novo mutations exist
- Multiple classification systems
- The following is based on location of the defective protein and pathogenesis:
  - CMD associated with defects in structural proteins of the basal lamina or extracellular matrix including: merosin deficiency, merosin-positive CMD, and Ullrich disease
  - CMD associated with impaired glycosylation of α-dystroglycan including: Fukuyama CMD, Walker-Warburg syndrome, muscle-eye-brain disease (MEB), CMD 1C, and CMD 1D
  - CMD associated with selenoprotein N1 mutations: Rigid spine syndrome

Epidemiology

- Incidence of all forms: 4 to 6 per 100,000
- Prevalence of all forms: 1 per 125,000
- Affects both sexes equally
- Present at birth or in the first year of life

Pathogenesis

- Merosin deficiency is due to abnormality in the *LAMA2* gene, and comprises 30% to 40% of CMD
- Causative mutation has not been clearly identified in merosin-positive CMD, but considered genetically heterogenous
- Mutations in Ullrich CMD are in the *COL6A1*, *COL6A2*, and *COL6A3* genes. Collagen type VI is markedly reduced in the endomysium and basal lamina
- Alpha-dystroglycan is an integral protein in the dystrophin-glycoprotein complex, which stabilizes the sarcolemmal membrane during contraction/relaxation and if abnormal, leads to increased tears with subsequent necrosis
- Dystroglycan is also expressed in the CNS, retina, and cochlea, playing a role in neuronal migration
- Selenoprotein N1 is found in the endoplasmic reticulum—its function is unknown

Risk Factors

- Familial inheritance
- Spontaneous mutations occur

Clinical Features

- Generalized muscle weakness and hypotonia at birth
- Joint contractures that worsen over time
- Severe hyperlaxity may occur in distal joints
- Eye malformations in MEB, and Walker-Warburg syndrome include: congenital cataracts, fixed pupils, hypoplasia of the optic nerve, and retinal dysplasia
- CNS findings include: hypomyelination, cerebellar hypoplasia, hydrocephalus, flat pons, lissencephaly, and polymicrogyria. Common in subtypes associated with impaired glycosylation of α-dystroglycan
- Possible seizures

Natural History

- Generalized weakness with hypotonia at birth
- Most infants reach independent sitting
- May not stand or ambulate
- Weakness is static or minimally progressive

Diagnosis

Differential diagnosis

- Congenital myotonic dystrophy
- Prader-Willi Syndrome
- Spinal muscular atrophy
- Bethlem myopathy
- Congenital myopathies

History

- Reduced fetal movements may be noted in utero
- Delayed early motor milestones
- May report cognitive developmental delays

Exam

- Varies with CMD
- Diffuse weakness
- Concomitant joint contractures and hyperlaxity
- Ullrich's : enlarged calcanei and keratosis pilaris
- Calf pseudohypertrophy
- Eye abnormalities in Walker-Warburg and MEB
- Cognitive impairments
- Rigid spine

Testing

- Serum creatine kinase; normal to 150 times normal
- Muscle biopsy with immunostaining
- Magnetic resonance imaging of the brain to identify those with normal brain anatomy, malformations, and abnormal neuronal migration, or benign white matter changes
- Electromyography including nerve conduction studies, with normal to mildly abnormal NCS and myopathic MUAPs on needle examination
- Electroencephalography if seizure activity
- DNA testing
- Prenatal testing is available for multiple variants

Pitfalls

- DNA testing for many of the disease subtypes is not commercially available

Red Flags

- May suffer respiratory failure requiring mechanical ventilation

Treatment

Medical

- No definitive treatments available
- Antiseizure medications may be required

Therapeutic exercises

- Range of motion exercises to reduce contractures and improve mobility

Assistive devices

- Orthoses to prevent contractures
- Mobility devices: stroller seating system, manual or power wheelchair, stander, Hoyer lift for transfers
- Bathroom equipment: tub bench, commode, and shower chair

Surgical

- Posterior spinal stabilization for progressive scoliosis
- Contracture releases and corrective foot surgery
- Percutaneous gastrostomy tube (PEG)
- Tracheostomy

Consults

- Cardiology evaluation for cardiomyopathy
- Pulmonology evaluation for respiratory insufficiency and nocturnal hypoventilation requiring noninvasive positive pressure ventilation, mechanical ventilation via tracheotomy, and/or cough assistance
- Orthopedic evaluation for scoliosis management, joint contracture releases, and foot deformities
- Gastroenterology if PEG placement indicated
- Ophthalmology
- Neurology for seizure management
- Speech language pathology

Prognosis

- Morbidity and mortality rates depend on type of CMD; often associated with respiratory insufficiency
- Some children die in infancy while others live into adulthood with little disability

Helpful Hints

- For DNA test availability: http//www.genetests.org

Suggested Reading

Muntoni F, Voit T. 133rd ENMC International workshop on congenital muscular dystrophy (IX international workshop) January 2005, Naarden, the Netherlands. *Neuromuscul Disord.* 2005;15(11):794–801.

Muscular Dystrophy: Congenital Myotonic

Jay J. Han MD ■ Gregory T. Carter MD

Description

Myotonic muscular dystrophy is a hereditary myopathy with additional multisystem effects on the heart, eye, endocrine system, and central nervous system. There are two subtypes of myotonic dystrophy, DM1 and DM2 (dystrophia myotonica type 1 and 2). Severity of the disease can span a continuum from mild to severe. Congenital form of myotonic dystrophy represents the most severe phenotype with hypotonia at birth and respiratory insufficiency. The primary characteristics of myotonic muscular dystrophies include muscle weakness and wasting, myotonia, cataracts, cardiac conduction problems, restrictive lung disease, cognitive impairment, and increased risk for diabetes.

Etiology/Types

- DM1: (autosomal dominant) abnormal expansion of CTG trinucleotide repeats in the DMPK gene on chromosome 19q13.3
- DM2/PROMM (proximal myotonic myopathy): (autosomal dominant) abnormal expansion of CCTG repeats in the ZNF9 gene on chromosome 3q21
- Congenital myotonic dystrophy: most severe DM1

Epidemiology

- DM1 incidence estimated at approximately 1 per 10,000 and accounts for 98% of myotonic dystrophy
- DM1: most common muscular dystrophy in adults
- Congenital myotonic dystrophy: 10% to 15% of DM1

Pathogenesis

- Exact disease mechanism is unclear; toxicity from transcribed CTG or CCTG RNA repeats postulated
- DMPK: loss in protein function thought to result in abnormal calcium homeostasis and altered excitation-contraction coupling; highest amounts in skeletal and heart muscles
- ZNF9: thought to be involved in sterol synthesis
- Abnormal CTG and CCTG repeats in RNA result in abnormal splicing of chloride channel RNA
- DM1: likelihood and severity of disease correlates with increased number of CTG repeats

- DM2: CCTG repeat expansion in intron 1 of ZNF9 gene ranges from 75 to 11,000, average of 5000 repeats

Risk Factors

- Genetic anticipation: expansion of CTG repeats in successive generations with more severe phenotype
- Congenital myotonic dystrophy in about 25% of offspring from mothers with DM1

Clinical Features

- Facial features: frontal balding, ptosis, temporal and masseter wasting; often described as "hatchet" face
- Myotonia: state of delayed relaxation or prolonged contraction of muscle
- DM1: more distal than proximal weakness; finger and wrist flexors, ankle dorsiflexors
- DM2/PROMM (proximal myotonic myopathy): as the name implies more proximal weakness pattern
- Cardiac: about 75% of patients show electrocardiographic (EKG) or echocardiographic abnormalities; prolonged PR interval, abnormal axis, brady or tachyarrhythmias, and cardiomyopathy later in disease course
- Endocrine: increased insulin resistance and likelihood of diabetes, as well as hypogonadism
- Pulmonary: progressive restrictive lung disease, aspiration, and nocturnal hypoventilation
- Cataracts are common with disease progression
- Mental retardation in congenital DM1 (50%–60%)
- Cognitive deficits can be mild to severe
- Smooth muscle and gastrointestinal: constipation and dysphagia
- Neuromuscular scoliosis in congenital DM1

Natural History

- Variability of disease severity within family
- Symptom onset approximately 29 years earlier in child compared with parent
- DM1: early disease involving distal limb weakness and later involving neck, shoulder, and hip girdle muscles as well as the diaphragm

- Causes of death: pneumonia and respiratory insufficiency (>30%); cardiac arrhythmia and sudden death (30%)

Diagnosis

Differential diagnosis
- Limb-girdle muscular dystrophies
- Facioscapulohumeral muscular dystrophy
- Distal myopathies
- Myotonia congenita (Thomsen or Becker disease)
- Paramyotonia congenita
- Congenital myopathies

History
- Family history, grip and percussion myotonia (inability to let go; failure to relax after contracting)
- Tripping over toes and fall history
- Cardiac: palpitations, presyncope and syncope, poor exercise tolerance, and congestive heart failure
- Congenital myotonia: floppy infant

Exam
- DM1: distal > proximal weakness
- DM2: proximal > distal weakness
- Grip myotonia
- Percussion myotonia over thenar muscles
- Cardiac arrhythmias
- Absent or reduced muscle stretch reflexes
- Normal sensation

Testing
- DNA testing for number of CTG or CCTG repeats
- Serum creatine kinase: normal or usually mildly elevated
- Needle electromyography revealing myotonia distal > proximal; found in mother more frequently than baby
- Cataract, diabetes, and testosterone level screen
- Muscle biopsy showing myopathic changes
- Prenatal DNA testing is available

Pitfalls
- Cardiac involvement may be presenting symptoms
- Medications to avoid: statins, amitriptyline, procainamide, digoxin, propranolol, and sedatives
- Caution with surgeries/procedures and anesthetics

Red Flags
- Cardiac conduction problems typically progress and require careful follow up by a cardiologist
- Sudden death can occur

Treatment

Medical
- No specific treatment for progressive weakness
- Limited efficacy of mexilitine and carbamazepine for myotonia symptoms
- Annual EKG; echocardiogram and 24-hour Holter monitoring per cardiology recommendation
- Annual check: diabetes, cataracts, and hypogonadism
- Treatment of diabetes and thyroid dysfunction
- Hormone replacement therapy for low testosterone

Therapeutic exercises
- Stretching and moderate intensity aerobic exercises

Assistive devices
- Ankle foot orthosis for foot drop
- Walking aides such as canes and walkers
- Assistive devices: commodes and tub benches
- Bilevel positive airway pressure or cough assist machines

Surgical
- Pacemaker or automatic internal cardiac defibrillator placement
- Cataract removal
- Ptosis corrective surgery as needed

Consults
- Cardiology
- Ophthalmology
- Pulmonology
- Genetics counseling
- Neurology

Prognosis
- Cardiac and pulmonary involvement is major determinant of prognosis and death
- Normal life expectancy in the absence of significant cardiac or pulmonary involvement
- Rarely individuals require wheelchair for mobility

Helpful Hints
- Hallmarks of disease are myotonia and progressive muscle weakness with typical facial features, cataract, insulin insensitivity, and cardiac involvement

Suggested Reading
Schara U, Schoser BG. Myotonic dystrophies type 1 and 2: a summary on current aspects. *Semin Pediatr Neurol.* 2006;13(2):71–79.

Muscular Dystrophy: Duchenne

Dennis J. Matthews MD

Definition

Duchenne muscular dystrophy (DMD) is a neuromuscular disease (dystrophinopathy) characterized by a progressive loss of strength affecting the muscles of the hips, pelvic area, thighs, and shoulders, with onset in early childhood, 2 to 6 years old.

Etiology

- X-linked recessive. Xp21
- Ninety-six percent with frame shift mutation
- Thirty percent with new mutation
- Ten percent to 20% of new mutations are gonadal mosaic

Epidemiology

- 1:3500 to 1:6000 male births

Pathogenesis

- An absence of dystrophin, a structural protein that bridges the inner surface of the muscle sarcolemma to the protein F-actin
- Other membrane proteins
  - Sarcoglycans: reduced
  - Aquaporin 4: reduced

Risk Factors

- Family history
  - X-linked recessive pattern

Clinical Features

- Generalized weakness and muscle wasting first affecting the muscles of the hips, pelvic area, thighs, and shoulders
- Calves are often enlarged
- Boys begin to show signs of muscle weakness as early as age 3
- The disease gradually weakens the skeletal or voluntary muscles, those in the arms, legs, and trunk

Natural History

- Distribution of weakness is proximal > distal, symmetric, affecting legs and arms, and eventually affecting all voluntary muscles
- There is reduced motor function by 2 to 3 years

- Steady decline in strength after 6 to 11 years
- Obesity is common starting at age 10 years
- Malnutrition with rapid onset near end of life
- Cardiomyopathy is seen with tachycardia: >100 beats per minute; common even <10 years of age
- Dilated cardiomyopathy: May develop after period of hypertrophy; increased frequency with age; symptomatic in 57% by age 18
- Conduction system abnormalities; electrocardiography changes in 60%
- By the early teens or earlier, the boy's heart and respiratory muscles also may be affected
- Survival is rare beyond the early 30s
- Death is most common between 15 and 25 years without respiratory support, usually due to respiratory or cardiac failure
- Life prolonged by 6 to 25 years with respiratory support

Diagnosis

Differential diagnosis
- Muscular dystrophy
- Congenital myopathy

History
- Family history
- Frequent falls
- Difficulty with stairs
- Slower than peers
- Speech delays

Exam
- Gowers sign: using hands to push up on knees to arise
- Toe walking
- Symmetrical leg weakness
- Calf pseudohypertrophy
- Decreased/no reflexes

Testing
- Creatine kinase elevated 5 to 100 times normal
- Genetic: *Xp21* deletion, duplication, small mutation, point mutation
- Muscle biopsy
  - Dystrophin: Absent staining
- Electrodiagnosis: myopathic patterns, nonspecific

- Respiratory care includes routine evaluation of respiratory function: forced vital capacity (FVC), forced expiratory volume in one second, maximal inspiratory pressure, maximum expiratory pressure, peak cough with airway clearance: cough assist, vest
- Polysomnography: hypoventilation with noninvasive ventilation: bilevel positive airway pressure, continuous positive airway pressure, or invasive ventilation

Pitfalls
- Frequently seen by GI for increased liver enzymes (muscle fraction of transaminases)
- Early baseline screening for cardiomyopathy
- Morning headaches, behavior changes, and decreased school performance may indicate hypoventilation

Red Flags
- FVC <1 liter
- Rapid weight loss

Treatment

Medical
- Nutrition: monitor weight and caloric intake
- Corticosteroids: demonstrated to have a beneficial effect on muscle strength and function. Monitor benefits and side effects
- Prednisone 0.75 mg/kg/day and deflazacort 0.9 mg/kg/day
- Osteoporosis is seen; use calcium, vitamin D
- End of life directives

Exercise
- Contractures: Ankles, hips, and knees, so use night splints on ankles, passive stretch, and early ambulation after surgery
- Assistive device: wheelchair, assistive devices for activities of daily living, environmental controls, and ventilation

Surgical
- Scoliosis: surgical instrumentation
- Contracture release

Consults
- Cardiology
- Pulmonary

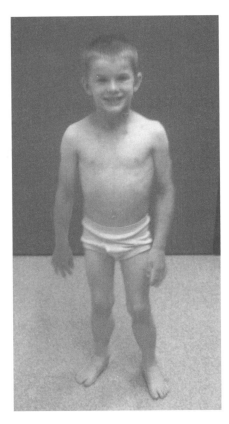

Five-year-old boy with difficulty going up stairs and falling more frequently, enlarged calves, and flexed hips and knees.

- Orthopedic surgery
- Genetics

Prognosis
- Progressive, steady decline in strength: 6 to 11 years
- Death 15 to 25 years of age without respiratory assistance

Helpful Hints
- Family support
- Genetic counseling
- End of life directives

Suggested Readings
Biggar WD. Duchenne muscular dystrophy. *Pediatr Rev.* 2006;27:83–87.

Dubowitz V. *Muscle Disorders in Childhood.* London, England: Saunders; 1995.

Muscular Dystrophy: Emery-Dreifuss

Andrew J. Skalsky BS MD ■ Jay J. Han MD ■ Gregory T. Carter MD

Description

Emery-Dreifuss muscular dystrophy (EDMD) is a hereditary myopathy. The primary characteristics of the disease include contractures of the elbows, posterior neck, and ankles; muscle weakness and wasting; and cardiac disease, including arrhythmias and cardiomyopathy.

Etiology/Types

- EDMD1—X-linked recessive inheritance because of mutation in the emerin gene on chromosome Xq28
- EDMD2—autosomal dominant or recessive inheritance due to mutation in the lamin A/C gene (LMNA) on chromosome 1q21.2
- EDMD3—autosomal dominant inheritance due to mutation in the synaptic nuclear envelope protein 1 gene (SYNE1 or nesprin-1) on chromosome 6q25
- EDMD4—autosomal dominant inheritance due to mutation in the synaptic nuclear envelope protein 2 gene (SYNE2 or nesprin-2) on chromosome 14q23

Epidemiology

- EDMD1 most common
- Prevalence not known but estimated at 1 per 100,000

Pathogenesis

- EDMD1 and EDMD2—disorder of lamin A/C-emerin nuclear protein complex which provides framework for nuclear envelope
- EDMD3 and EDMD4—results in loss of protein that binds lamin A and emerin

Risk Factors

- Familial inheritance
- Spontaneous mutation risk factors are unknown

Clinical Features

- Severe joint contractures, especially elbows, posterior neck (into extension), and ankles
- In EDMD1, contractures often more disabling than weakness
- Symmetrical humero-peroneal distribution of weakness predominately affecting the biceps and triceps as well as the scapular stabilizers with sparing of the deltoids; lower leg muscles affected later in course
- Winged scapulae
- Biceps and triceps wasting
- Cardiac disease including atrial paralysis and dilated cardiomyopathy

Natural History

- Onset neonatal to third decade
- Joint contractures in first two decades of life
- Slowly progressive muscle weakness
- Loss of ambulation by the 4th decade in autosomal dominant variants; however, loss of ambulation rare in X-linked form
- Contractures may limit ambulation, resulting in wheelchair use
- Onset of cardiac symptoms usually after second decade
- Usually require pacemaker by age 30
- Increased risk for sudden cardiac death and cerebral emboli resulting in sudden death

Diagnosis

Differential diagnosis

- Several conditions with muscle weakness and contractures or cardiac disease but none with the triad
- Limb-girdle muscular dystrophies with cardiac involvement
- Myotonic muscular dystrophies (DM1 and DM2)
- Collagen VI related myopathies
- Facioscapulohumeral muscular dystrophy

History

- Toe walking in childhood
- Contractures that are congenital or begin in early childhood
- Cardiac involvement manifesting as palpitations, presyncope and syncope, poor exercise tolerance, and congestive heart failure
- Family history

Exam

- Severe joint contractures, especially elbows into flexion, posterior neck into extension, and ankles

145

- Symmetric elbow flexion and extension weakness with sparing of shoulder abduction
- Winged scapulae
- Biceps and triceps wasting
- Rigid spine
- Cardiac arrhythmias and/or murmurs
- Absent or reduced muscle stretch reflexes
- Normal sensation

Testing
- DNA testing
- Serum creatine kinase can be normal to elevated up to 10 × upper limit of normal, usually mildly elevated
- Needle electromyography revealing myopathic units
- Magnetic resonance imaging of posterior calf shows soleus involvement but gastrocnemius sparing
- Muscle biopsy showing nonspecific dystrophic changes; immunoflurescence and/or western blot of muscle tissue may yield diagnosis
- Immunodetection of *emerin* by immunoflurescence and/or western blot in various tissues in EDMD1
- Immunodetection of *lamin A/C* by immunoflurescence and/or western blot in various tissues in EDMD2

Pitfalls
- Muscle biopsy may be nondiagnostic
- Cardiac involvement may be presenting problem

Red Flags
- Cardiac involvement is invariable
- Sudden death can occur

Treatment

Medical
- Antiarrhythmics
- Afterload reduction agents
- ACE-inhibitors
- Angiotensin II receptor blockers

Therapeutic exercises
- General strengthening and stretching

Assistive devices
- Orthoses to compensate for foot drop
- Walking aides such as canes and walkers
- Wheelchair for longer distance mobility
- Household assistive devices such as commodes and tub benches

Surgical
- Achilles tenotomy
- Pacemaker placement

Consults
- Cardiology
- Occupational and physical therapy
- Neurology

Prognosis
- Cardiac involvement is major determinant of prognosis
- Normal life expectancy in the absence of significant cardiac involvement
- Rarely individuals can no longer ambulate

Helpful Hints
- Hallmarks of disease are triad of joint contractures in early childhood, slowly progressive muscle weakness and wasting, and cardiac involvement

Suggested Readings
Helbling-Leclerc A, Bonne G, Schwartz K. Emery-Dreifuss muscular dystrophy. *Eur J Hum Genet.* 2002;10(3):157–161.
Muchir A, Worman HJ. Emery-Dreifuss muscular dystrophy. *Curr Neurol Neurosci Rep.* 2007;7(1):78–83.

Muscular Dystrophy: Facioscapulohumeral

Andrew J. Skalsky BS MD

Description

Facioscapulohumeral muscular dystrophy (FSHD) is the third most common muscular dystrophy, resulting in the slow progression of weakness, mainly involving the facial and shoulder girdle muscles followed by leg, thigh, and hip girdle weakness.

Etiology/Types

- Autosomal dominant inheritance
- Reduction in D4Z4 repeats on 4q35
- 10% to 30% of cases are new mutations

Epidemiology

- Prevalence: 1 to 5 per 100,000
- Males often more symptomatic than females

Pathogenesis

- Pathophysiology of muscle weakness and wasting remains unknown
- Postulated mechanism is transcriptional misregulation of neighboring genes, especially DUX4
- Size of chromosome 4q35 deletion and earlier onset of symptoms correlate with disease severity

Risk Factors

- Familial inheritance
- Spontaneous mutation risk factors are unknown

Clinical Features

- Facial muscle weakness followed by shoulder girdle muscle weakness
- Marked winging of the scapulae
- Hip girdle, thigh, and lower leg muscle weakness later in disease course
- Often asymmetric
- Forearm muscles relatively spared
- Predominantly asymptomatic high frequency hearing loss, but can require hearing aids
- Mainly asymptomatic retinal telangiectasias, but can be severe, resulting in retinal detachment (Coat's syndrome)
- Bulbar muscles generally spared

Natural History

- Onset can be congenital to late in life
- Slowly progressive muscle weakness
- Often normal life expectancy
- 20% of individuals become dependent on wheelchair

Diagnosis

Differential diagnosis

- Limb-Girdle muscular dystrophies
- Emery-Dreifuss muscular dystrophy
- Acid maltase deficiency (Pompe disease)
- Inclusion body myositis
- Polymyositis
- Becker muscular dystrophy
- Mitochondrial myopathy
- Proximal myotonic myopathy (DM2)

History

- Inability to whistle or drink from a straw
- Sleeping with eyes open which may cause irritation due to dry eyes
- Slowly progressive weakness
- Family history

Exam

- Widened palpebral fissures
- Diminished facial expression
- Inability to purse lips
- Dysarthria
- Winged scapulae
- Increased lumbar lordosis
- Protuberant abdomen
- Wasted upper arms and relatively spared forearms resulting in cartoon character Popeye appearance
- Weak shoulder girdle, leg, thigh, hip girdle, and trunk muscles
- Absent or reduced muscle stretch reflexes
- Normal sensation

Testing

- DNA testing
- Serum creatine kinase can be normal to 5 times upper limit of normal, usually mildly elevated

147

- Needle electromyography revealing myopathic units
- Muscle biopsy with nonspecific dystrophic changes

Pitfalls

- Muscle biopsy may be nondiagnostic and rarely needed

Red Flags

- Screening fluorescein angiography to determine severity of retinal telangiectasias
- Five percent can have cardiac conduction abnormalities

Treatment

Medical

- Oral albuterol has been shown to increase muscle mass but limited effect on muscle strength

Therapeutic exercises

- General stretching and strengthening, avoiding fatigue, which may strengthen strong muscles and delay weakness

Assistive devices

- Orthoses to compensate for foot drop
- Walking aides such as canes and walkers
- Wheelchair for longer distance mobility
- Household assistive devices such as commodes and tub benches

Surgical

- Scapular fixation or scapulothoracic arthrodesis may place upper limb in more functional position and reduce pain

Consults

- Audiology for hearing evaluation
- Ophthalmology for retinal telangiectasia screening
- Cardiology evaluation if cardiac conduction abnormalities present
- Speech language pathology evaluation for dysarthria and dysphagia
- Neurology

Prognosis

- Normal life expectancy in the absence of significant cardiac, respiratory, or bulbar involvement
- Twenty percent of individuals become full-time wheelchair users

Helpful Hints

- Slowly progressive but marked weakness of facial muscles and scapular stabilizers, resulting in winged scapulae, are hallmarks of disease
- Avoid fatigue

Suggested Readings

Fisher J, Upadhyaya M. Molecular genetics of facioscapulohumeral muscular dystrophy (FSHD). *Neuromuscul Disord.* 1997;7(1):55–62.

Tawil R, Van Der Maarel SM. Facioscapulohumeral muscular dystrophy. *Muscle Nerve.* 2006 Jul;34(1):1–15.

Muscular Dystrophy: Limb-Girdle

Nanette C. Joyce DO

Description

The limb-girdle muscular dystrophies (LGMD) are a phenotypically and genotypically heterogenous group of disorders classically characterized by progressive weakness involving proximal shoulder and pelvic girdle muscles while sparing muscles of the face.

Etiology/Types

- Two categories classified by mode of inheritance
  - Autosomal dominant inheritance: LGMD 1
  - Autosomal recessive inheritance: LGMD 2
- Further alphabetical subclassification based on genotype includes LGMD 1A-F and LGMD 2A-N

Epidemiology

- Prevalence: 8 to 70 per million
- Equal occurrence in males and females
- Reported in races and countries throughout the world

Pathogenesis

- Protein defects occur affecting multiple substrates in the normal biologic function of muscle
- Gene defects have been identified that encode proteins associated with the sarcolemma, contractile apparatus, and enzymes involved in muscle function
- Though the primary genetic defect has been identified in many LGMDs, the mechanism leading to dystrophic changes often remains unknown
- Affected proteins include calpain 3, dysferlin, sarcoglycan, telethonin, TRIM32, fukutin-related protein, titin, *O*-mannosyl transferase-1, fukutin, and myotilin

Risk Factors

- Familial inheritance
- Spontaneous mutations have been identified but frequency rates remain unknown

Clinical Features

- Proximal upper and lower limb weakness
- Scapular winging
- Calf hypertrophy or hypotrophy
- Few variants with distal greater than proximal limb weakness. Most common variants presenting with distal weakness; LGMD 2B, LGMD 2G, and LGMD 2J

- Cardiac disease including cardiomyopathy, conduction abnormalities, and arrhythmias
- Rare variants with dysarthria, dysphagia, myoglobinuria, and rippling muscles

Natural History

- Onset from early childhood to late adult life
- Age of onset varies among differing mutations and within families with the same mutation
- Rate of progression of weakness is variable
- Life expectancy is variable, dependent on the extent of respiratory and cardiac involvement, ranging from premature death to normal life span
- May have slowly progressive scoliosis, particularly in LGMD 2

Diagnosis

Differential diagnosis

- Duchenne muscular dystrophy
- Becker muscular dystrophy
- Acid maltase deficiency (Pompe disease)
- Spinal muscular atrophy type III
- Emery-Dreifuss muscular dystrophy
- Proximal myotonic myopathy

History

- Family history
- Toe walking if onset in childhood
- Difficulty climbing stairs and with overhead activities

Exam

- Proximal weakness with muscular atrophy in the shoulder and hip girdle
- Winging scapula
- Joint contractures
- Hypertrophy or hypotrophy of the calf muscles
- Severely increased lumbar lordosis
- Wide-based Trendelenburg gait
- Sensation intact

Testing

- Serum creatine kinase may be normal to 100 times upper limit of normal
- Needle electromyography reveals myopathic units

149

- Magnetic resonance imaging to identify affected muscles
- Muscle biopsy
- DNA testing
- Electrocardiography (EKG) to evaluate for conduction defects
- Echocardiogram

Pitfalls
- Muscle biopsy may be nondiagnostic
- Genetic testing may not identify causative mutation

Red Flags
- Cardiac conduction abnormalities with increased risk for sudden cardiac death
- Early respiratory failure due to diaphragmatic weakness may be presenting symptom
- Potential increased risk and adverse outcome with anesthesia

Treatment

Medical
- Some anecdotal evidence of improvement with corticosteroid treatment, but large therapeutic trials have not been performed
- Small number of patients have shown modest strength improvement with short courses of creatine monohydrate dosed at 5 to 10 g/day
- Angiotensin-converting enzyme inhibitors inhibition and/or β-blocker treatment in patients identified with impaired cardiac function

Therapeutic exercises
- Small trial showed no increase in serum creatine kinase with mild to moderate exercise
- General strengthening and stretching to prevent contractures; avoid fatigue

Assistive devices
- Orthoses to treat heel cord contractures, stabilize shoulder function, and for scoliosis management
- Mobility devices such as walking aids (cane and walkers), scooter, and manual or power wheelchair
- Bathroom equipment such as grab bars, elevated toilet seat, tub bench, commode, and shower chair

Surgical
- Posterior spinal stabilization of scoliotic curves greater than 30°
- Scapular fixation or scapulothoracic arthrodesis may reduce pain and position the upper limb in a more functional position
- Implantation of cardiac defibrillator for patients with conduction abnormalities who are at risk for sudden cardiac death
- Percutaneous gastrostomy tube in those with significant dysphagia resistant to swallowing techniques and dietary changes

Consults
- Cardiology evaluation for cardiomyopathy and cardiac conduction abnormalities
- Pulmonology evaluation for restrictive lung disease and nocturnal hypoventilation requiring noninvasive positive pressure ventilation, and/or cough assistance
- Orthopedic evaluation for scoliosis management
- Gastroenterology, if percutaneous endoscopic gastrostomy placement indicated
- Speech-language pathology evaluation, if symptoms of dysarthria or dysphagia
- Neurology

Prognosis
- Morbidity and mortality vary; however, an early onset often predicts a more rapid course
- Patients may become wheelchair users in their early teens and die from respiratory complications in their late teens
- Patients with slowly progressive LGMD may remain ambulatory throughout a normal life span

Helpful Hints
- Monitor EKG and cardiology status

Suggested Readings
Gulieri M, Straub V, Bushby K, Lochmuller H. Limb-girdle muscular dystrophies. *Curr Opin Neurol.* 2008;21:576–584.
Straub V, Bushby K. Therapeutic possibilities in the autosomal recessive limb-girdle muscular dystrophies. *Neurotherapeutics.* 2008;5(4):619–626.

Myasthenia Gravis

Supreet Deshpande MD

Description

A disorder of the neuromuscular junction (NMJ) with defect in the proteins required for neuromuscular transmission or autoantibodies to the nicotinic acetylcholine receptors at the NMJ. Both lead to abnormal neuromuscular transmission leading to fluctuating muscle weakness and fatigability.

Etiology/Types

- Neonatal myasthenia gravis (NMG) due to transfer of antibodies from mother
- Congenital myasthenic syndromes (CMS), which are inherited disorders
- Acquired myasthenia gravis (MG) is an autoimmune disorder

Epidemiology

- NMG is a transient disorder in 10% to 15% of babies born to mothers with MG
- CMS is rare, prevalence of 1:500,000, with postsynaptic defects making up to 75%
- Acquired MG is more common with incidence of 2:1,000,000 and prevalence of 100/1,000,000. More common in females

Pathogenesis

- CMS—autosomal recessive inheritance with defective or absent presynaptic, synaptic, or postsynaptic proteins required for neuromuscular transmission
- Acquired MG—autoimmune disorder with production of antibodies against nicotinic acetylcholine receptors at the NMJ
- Eighty percent have thymic involvement. In early-onset, generalized disease, thymus is more often hyperplastic and produces acetylcholine receptor antibodies. In late-onset disease, thymomas are more common

Risk Factors

- Maternal myasthenia for NMG
- Parents with MG for CMS
- Other autoimmune conditions and female for acquired MG

Clinical Features

- Weakness that improves with rest
- Ptosis and diplopia
- Dysphagia
- Dysphonia
- Respiratory involvement
- Proximal muscle weakness
- No sensory, bowel, or bladder involvement

Natural History

- NMG—flat facies, dysphagia, respiratory weakness, which may require mechanical ventilation; generally these improve in 2 weeks and 90% fully recover by 2 months
- CMS—variable, may develop scoliosis, dysphagia, and respiratory problems
- GMG—presents with ocular symptoms but progresses to generalized myasthenia gravis (GMG). GMG more severe in first few years

Diagnosis

Differential diagnosis

- Botulism
- Tick paralysis
- Acute inflammatory demyelinating polyradiculoneuropathy.
- Mitochondrial neuromuscular disorders
- Motor neuron diseases involving oropharangeal weakness
- Lambert Eaton syndrome

History

- NMG—history of MG in the mother
- CMS—family history, early onset of symptoms
- Acquired MG onset time variable
- All present with weakness, which improves with rest
- May have diplopia, dysphagia, dysphonia, respiratory difficulties, and trouble with overhead activities and stairs
- In CMG, initial symptoms may be weak cry and suck, and hypotonia

Exam

- Asymmetric weakness of extraoccular muscles, which cannot be attributed to a single cranial nerve

- Ptosis with sustained upward gaze
- Inability to close mouth after sustained downward pressure on jaw
- Difficulty with whistling, blowing
- Inability to push tongue into cheek and/or protrude it
- Dropped head
- Difficulty with bringing arms above head

Testing

Congenital myasthenic syndromes
- Absence of serum acetylcholine receptor antibodies, a prerequisite
- Repetitive stimulation on electrodiagnostic exam varies in the different subtypes
- Muscle biopsy predominance of type 1 fibers and reduced acetylcholine receptors at the NMJ
- Genetic testing can be confirmatory

Acquired MG
- Pharmacologic—Edrophonium/tensilon-immediate improvement in fatigued muscle
- Electrophysiologic—At least 10% decrement with 2 to 3 Hz repetitive nerve stimulation and increased jitter and blocking on single-fiber electromyography
- Immunologic—serum for acetylcholine receptor antibodies
- Miscellaneous—ice pack test (place ice pack over an eyelid with ptosis for 2 minutes; may see improvement since neuromuscular transmission improves at cooler temperatures) and muscle biopsy

Pitfalls

- MG cannot be ruled out just by the absence of ocular symptoms as it can present without ocular symptoms
- Several common medications can cause exacerbation of symptoms. Some of the most common medications are antibiotics—aminoglycoside and macrolides, cardiovascular drugs such as β-blockers, angiotensin-converting enzyme inhibitors, quinidine, lidocaine, and procainamide, central nervous system drugs like phenytoin, antirheumatics-chloroquine, D-penicillamine, and prednisone

Red Flags

- Myasthenic crisis, an exacerbation of myasthenic symptoms that is sufficient to necessitate ventilatory support. It is often accompanied by bulbar involvement. This (due to insufficient medication) must be differentiated from cholinergic crisis (excess medication). Myasthenic crisis is often triggered by fever, infection, and adverse effects to medications or stress

Treatments

Medical
- Acetylcholinesterase inhibitors, works for CMS too
- Immunosuppression
  - Corticosteroids
  - Azathioprine
  - Cyclosporine
  - Cyclophosphamide
- Temporary treatment—used in situations of rapidly progressing weakness/impending bulbar symptoms
  - Plasma exchange
  - Intravenous immune globulin

Exercise
- Not well studied; avoid fatigue
- May benefit from strength training
- Teach energy conserving techniques
- Scheduled rest breaks between activities
- Inspiratory muscle training and breathing retraining found to be beneficial

Surgical
- Thymectomy—accepted treatment but still controversial
- Most beneficial in early onset, seropositive, GMG
- Also indicated in thymomas, even when benign, as may become malignant. In this case, surgery may not alter the course of MG

Consults
- Neurology

Complications
- Cholinergic crisis
- Medication-related side effects

Prognosis
- NMG complete resolution
- In CMG, depends on subtype. Most often symptoms do not progress but improve over time. Exacerbation with intercurrent illness common. Life span not affected

Helpful Hints
- Surveillance for spinal complications in CMS
- Respiratory distress can occur

Suggested Readings
Hantai D, Richard P, Koenig J, Eymard B. Congenital myasthenic syndromes. *Curr Opin Neurol.* 2004;17(5):539–551.
Nicolle MW. Myasthenia gravis. *Neurologist.* 2002;8(1):2–21.

Myelodysplasia/Spina Bifida

Mary McMahon MD

Description

Myelomeningocele (MMC) is a developmental birth defect of the neural tube, resulting in an open spinal cord lesion, most often in the lumbar or sacral spine. This is often called spina bifida.

Types of Neural Tube Defects

- Anencephaly occurs when the cephalic end of the neural tube fails to close, resulting in absence of a large portion of the brain, skull, and scalp
- Spina bifida occulta is a defect of the posterior bony elements of the spine only and is almost always asymptomatic
- Meningocele is protrusion of the meninges through the bony defect, without accompanying nervous tissue
- MMC is a spinal deformity involving the spinal cord, nerve roots, meninges, vertebrae, and skin

Epidemiology

- The incidence of live neural tube defect (NTD) births in the United States has decreased from 2.62 to 1.90 per 10,000, in part due to a mandatory fortification of grains with folate in 1998
- The rates of NTD differ by geographic region and race, with lower rates in the Asian and African American populations
- There is an increased rate of NTDs in subsequent pregnancies after a prior pregnancy with an NTD

Pathogenesis

- MMC is caused by a failure of closure of the embryonic caudal neural tube in the first 4 weeks of gestation
- Most cases of NTD occur sporadically and are felt to have a multifactorial etiology, with a mix of maternal and environmental factors
- Up to 10% of cases will have an associated chromosomal abnormality

Risk Factors

- Maternal folic acid deficiency
- Maternal obesity
- Maternal diabetes
- Maternal hyperthermia
- Maternal medication use (valproic acid, carbamezapine)

Clinical Features

- Hydrocephalus (>90%)
- Arnold Chiari II (AC II) malformation (>90%)
- Variable cognitive deficits with greater difficulty with visual perceptual skills, executive functioning and attention, and a relative strength in verbal skills
- Neurogenic bowel and bladder in approximately 90% to 95%
- Weakness associated with impaired mobility and decreased independence with self-care skills
- Increased risk for a wide variety of musculoskeletal disorders, including scoliosis, hip dislocation, flexion contractures of the hips and knees, foot abnormalities, and rotational deformities
- Variable sensory deficits and increased risk for pressure sores
- Increased incidence of osteoporosis, associated with pathological fractures
- Increased incidence of obesity and short stature
- Variable sexual dysfunction and fertility
- Increased incidence of depression
- High incidence of latex allergy

Natural History

- The majority of pregnancies, with an isolated NTD, will be uneventful with delivery at term
- At least 75% to 85% of children born with MMC can be expected to live into adulthood

Prenatal Diagnosis

- Maternal serum α-fetoprotein
- Prenatal ultrasound
- Amniocentesis can confirm abnormal results on above

History

- Headaches, cognitive changes, nausea, or vomiting
- Pain
- Functional status
- Bowel and bladder function
- Brainstem dysfunction: feeding, swallowing, stridor, aspiration pneumonia, and apnea related to AC II malformation

Exam

- Neurologic exam: fundoscopic exam, cranial nerves, mental status, sensation, strength, tone, and gait
- Musculoskeletal exam: spine, shoulders, hips, knees, and feet
- Skin

Testing

- Urodynamics, serum creatinine, and kidney ultrasound
- Spine films to evaluate scoliosis
- Magnetic resonance imaging of spine to evaluate for brainstem compression (C-spine), syrinx, or tethered cord (entire spine)
- Brain computed tomography to evaluate hydrocephalus
- Neuropsychological testing

Red Flags

- Apnea, stridor, or severe dysphagia may indicate syrinx, tethered cord, AC II manifestation, or shunt malfunction
- Pain
- Headaches or increasing difficulty in school
- Rapidly advancing scoliosis
- Change in strength, tone, or sensation
- Change in bladder function or symptoms

Treatment

Medical

- Anticholinergic medications to increase bladder capacity
- Stool softeners, suppositories, and enemas

Therapy

- Communication, feeding, and cognition
- Fine motor and self-care skills
- Gait training and transfers
- Develop a home program to include stretching, strengthening, and aerobic exercise
- Education on joint protection and proper wheelchair propulsion

Injections

- Rare botulinum toxin for bladder or legs

Surgical

- MMC repair within the first few days
- Approximately 90% will require a shunt for hydrocephalus

- A minority will require an occipitocervical decompression for symptomatic Chiari malformation, a tethered cord release, or shunting of a syrinx
- Spinal fusion for progressive scolioisis
- Appendicovesicostomy or augmentation cystoplasty to facilitate urinary continence
- Appendicostomy or cecostomy for antegrade colonic enema to treat severe constipation

Equipment considerations

- Orthotics: hip-knee-ankle-foot orthoses, reciprocating gait orthoses, knee-ankle-foot orthoses, ankle-foot orthoses, ground reaction ankle-foot orthoses, supramaleolar orthoses, and spinal orthosis
- Twister cables or derotational straps
- Mobility aides: walkers, forearm crutches, and canes
- Standers: static or mobile
- Wheelchairs (manual or power)
- Knee or ankle splints for prolonged stretch
- Bath or commode chairs

Consults

- Neurosurgery
- Orthopedic surgery
- Urology

Complications

- Hydrocephalus and shunt malfunctions
- Syringomyelia or tethered cord
- Bladder infection, renal calculi, and renal dysfunction

Prognosis

- The majority of patients with iliopsoas strength grade ≤ 3 will be nonambulatory
- The majority of patients with iliopsoas and quadriceps strength grade 4 to 5 will be community ambulators

Helpful Hint

- Individuals with MMC are underemployed and are less likely to live independently. Increased independence with mobility and daily activities increases the probability of employment

Suggested Readings

Dicianno BE, Kurowski BG, Yang JMJ, et al. Rehabilitation and medical management of the adult with spina bifida. *Am J Phys Med Rehabil.* 2008;87:1026–1050.

McDonald CM, Jaffe KM, Mosca VS, et al. Ambulatory outcome of children with myelomeningocele: effects of lower-extremity muscle strength. *Dev Med and Child Neuro.* 1991;33:482–490.

Myopathies: Congenital

Maureen R. Nelson MD

Description

These are a heterogeneous group of muscle disorders presenting primarily in early infancy with hypotonia and weakness, with resultant delayed developmental milestones. There is genetic abnormality of muscle development.

Etiology/Types

- Central core (CC)
- Centronuclear (CN)/myotubular
- Nemaline (NR)
- Minicore (multicore) (MM)

Epidemiology

- Incidence is estimated at 6/100,000 live births
- Prevalence estimated at 3.5–5/100,000 pediatric population
- CC is the most common form

Pathogenesis

- Type I fiber predominance
- Type I fiber hypotrophy
- Characteristic structural abnormalities in subtypes:
  - NM: rod-like bodies in longitudinal section of muscle; multiple genetic mutations lead to abnormality of muscle thin filaments
  - CC: areas of reduced oxidative activity; absent mitochondria; mutations of skeletal muscle *RYR1* gene on chromosome 19q13.1
  - CN: large numbers of muscle fibers with centrally located nuclei that show similarities to fetal myotubes
  - MM: atrophic type I fibers predominate, but also type II; multiple foci of myofibrillar degeneration; focal decrease in mitochondria

Risk Factors

- Variable inheritance patterns
- Spontaneous mutation risk factors are unknown

Clinical Features

- Muscle weakness, especially proximally
- Hypotonia and hyporeflexia
- Dysmorphic facies
- High arched palate
- Scoliosis
- Joint contractures
- Central core
  - Musculoskeletal abnormalities, including congenital hip dislocation, foot deformities, and kyphoscoliosis
- Nemaline
  - Diaphragm may be weak
  - Weakness of face, foot dorsiflexors, toe extensors, neck and trunk flexors; limb girdle and distal limb muscles
- Centronuclear
  - Ptosis
  - Bulbar/extraocular movement (EOM) involvement
  - Elongated face
- Minicore/multicore
  - Opthalmoplegia
  - Diaphragm weakness (risk of nocturnal hypoventilation)
  - Spinal rigidity

Natural History

- Variable
- Generally slow progressive or stable
- CN may show severe respiratory difficulty with early death or ventilator dependence

Diagnosis

Differential diagnosis

- Congenital myotonic dystrophy
- Spinal muscular atrophy

History

- Decreased intrauterine movement
- Delayed gross motor development
- Family history

Exam

- Muscle weakness, especially proximal
- Hypotonia
- Contractures
- Normal sensation
- Normal cognition

Testing

- Creatine kinase usually normal
- Electromyography: myopathic with small amplitude, short duration polyphasics
  - Fibrillations in CN (less in NM)
  - Myotonic discharges in CN
- Muscle biopsy confirms
- Magnetic resonance imaging of leg muscle

Pitfalls

- Pulmonary risk in NM

Red flags

- Malignant hyperthermia risk in CC

Treatment

Medical

- Monitor pulmonary function

Exercises

- General strengthening, endurance, and stretching, including aquatic program

Modalities

- Can be used with stretching

Injection

- Possible for contracture treatment

Surgical

- Orthopedic procedures for contractures and scoliosis

Consults

- Orthopedic surgery
- Genetics
- Neurology

Complications of treatment

- Postoperative atrophy if not rapidly mobilized
- Exercise-induced myalgia in CC

Prognosis

- Continued function is expected

Helpful Hints

- Malignant hyperthermia is allelic with CC so high risk with anesthesia

Suggested Readings

D'Amico A. Congential myopathies. *Curr Neurol Neurosci Rep.* 2008;8:73–79.

Fujimura-Kiyono C, Racz GZ, Nishino I. Myotubular/centro-nuclear myopathy and central core disease. *Neurol India.* 2008;56(3):325–332.

Quinlivan RM, Muller CR, Davis M, et al. Central core disease: clinical, pathological, and genetic features. *Arch Dis Child.* 2003;88:1051–1055.

Neurofibromatosis

Scott M. Paul BES MD

Description

Neurofibromatosis (NF) is a common genetic disorder, primarily of the peripheral nervous system, that can cause neurologic and also behavioral, cognitive, cardio-vascular, and musculoskeletal disabilities.

Etiology/Types

- Autosomal dominant
- Because of mutations in the NF1 gene at 17q11.2 resulting in abnormal neurofibromin protein, a presumed negative growth regulator
- The related condition NF II ("central type") is a disorder of neurofibromin 2 protein due to an abnormality at chromosome 22q12.2 and is usually limited to central nervous system neurofibromata, and only rarely, cutaneous lesions

Epidemiology

- Incidence of 1 in 2500 to 3000 persons
- Equally distributed by race, gender, and ethnicity

Pathogenesis

- Abnormalities of cells embryologically derived from the neural crest

Risk Factors

- First-degree relative with NF1
- Fifty percent of cases are due to spontaneous mutations

Clinical Features

- Café au lait spots: six or more is significant
- Skinfold freckling
- Multiple cutaneous nodules (dermal NF)
- Learning disabilities (especially visual perceptual)
- Attention-deficit hyperactivity disorder
- Scoliosis
- Long bone bowing with thicker cortices and medullary narrowing
- Pseudoarthrosis
- Joint contractures
- Leg length discrepancy
- Lisch nodules (iris hamartomata)

- Optic pathway gliomas (can affect vision and/or pituitary function)
- Valvular heart disease
- Arterial stenosis (especially renal artery)
- Aneurysm
- Arteriovenous malformations
- Plexiform neurofibromata (benign but invasive tumors which may stem from multiple cranial and/or spinal nerve roots or their branches)
- Peripheral neuropathy
- Malignant peripheral nerve sheath tumors (MPNST)
- Precocious puberty
- Pheochromocytoma
- Gastroendocrine tumors

Natural History

- Freckling and café au lait spots, plexiform NF, and bony dysplasia usually present early in life
- Other features tend to present later in childhood
- Dermal NF usually begin to emerge in adolescence or early adulthood
- 10% risk of development of MPNST over lifetime

Diagnosis

Differential diagnosis

- Proteus syndrome
- McCune Albright syndrome/polyostotic fibrous dysplasia
- NF II
- Schwannomatosis

History

- Comprehensive developmental/family history
- Comprehensive history of current function
  - Weakness
  - Limitations in range of motion (ROM)
  - Problems with coordination
  - Difficulties with walking
  - Pain and sensation
  - Academic performance
  - Attention and behavior

Exam

- Limitations in ROM related to underlying plexiform NF
- Weakness, often proximal
- Scoliosis
- Leg length discrepancy
- Check heart rate and blood pressure since pheochromocytoma is possible
- National Institutes of Health criteria—two or more of the following:
  - Six or more café au lait spots
  - Axillary or inguinal fold freckling
  - One or more plexiform NF or two or more of any kind of NF
  - Two or more Lisch nodules on slit lamp examination
  - Distinctive-related osseous lesion
  - First-degree relative who meets above criteria

Testing

- Whole body magnetic resonance imaging to screen for plexiform NF
- Scoliosis series x-rays if clinical evidence of curve
- Electrodiagnostic study if clinical signs of neuropathy
- Genetic testing is *not* done routinely
- Asymptomatic NF are *not* routinely biopsied

Pitfalls

- Less than thorough history and examination can miss various manifestations of the disease

Red Flags

- Signs or symptoms of MPNST's
  - Persistent pain, especially disturbing sleep
  - New, unexplained neurologic deficits since can cause severe functional deficits
  - Change in consistency or rapid growth of plexiform NF
- Hypertension (sign of pheochromocytoma or renal artery stenosis)

Treatment

Medical

- Experimental chemotherapies through participation in an approved clinical trial (www.clinicaltrials.gov)
- Symptomatic treatment of neuropathic and/or musculoskeletal pain

Exercise

- Stretching will be more successful before a plexiform NF has grown to the degree that it limits joint ROM
- Targeted strengthening exercises
- Overhead reaching and/or suspension exercises
- Aquatic and land-based aerobic activities

Modalities

- Safety of deep thermal modalities and electrical stimulation has not been established
- Superficial heat and cold can be used

Rehabilitation equipment

- Scoliosis bracing may be effective in patients whose curve is not due to plexiform NF
- Shoe lifts and orthoses
- Gait aids
- Wheelchair seating and mobility

Surgical

- Debulking of plexiform NF
- Spinal fusion for scoliosis
- Orthopedic intervention for pseudarthrosis or severe long bone bowing

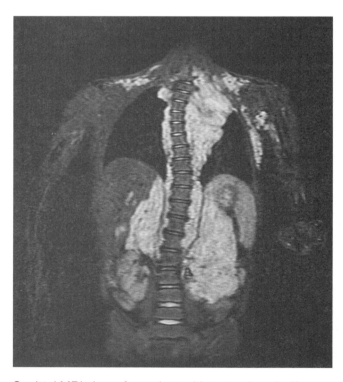

Sagittal MRI view of a patient with extensive plexiform neurofibromata (seen in white) involving bilateral brachial plexi, thoracic, and lumbar roots. Note the associated thoracolumbar scoliosis. Courtesy of Drs. Eva Dombi and Brigitte Widemann, Pediatric Oncology Branch, NCI.

- Vascular intervention for stenosis
- Excision of pheochromocytomata

Consults
- Oncology
- Orthopedic surgery
- Opthalmology
- Audiology
- Dermatology
- Neurology

Complications of treatment
- Dependent on chosen treatment for specific condition

Prognosis
- Highly variable
- Life span, on average, may be shortened by 15 years

Helpful Hints
- More complex cases will benefit from management at a specialty center

Suggested Readings

Ferner RE, Huson SM, Thomas N, et al. Guidelines for the diagnosis and management of individuals with neurofibromatosis 1. *J Med Genet.* 2007;44(2):81-88.

Williams VC, Lucas J, Babcock MA, Gutmann DH, Korf B, Maria BL. Neurofibromatosis type 1 revisited. *Pediatrics.* 2009;123(1):124-133.

Osteogenesis Imperfecta

Melanie Rak MD

Description

Osteogenesis imperfecta (OI) is a heritable disorder of abnormal bone quality or quantity.

Etiology/Types

- Traditionally types I–IV were described, based on an abnormal amount of type I collagen or abnormal structure of type I collagen molecules
- Recently OI types V–VIII were described, which have normal collagen but other genetic mutations and distinct histology
- Numerous genetic mutations can lead to similar phenotypes of OI
- Most are autosomal dominant but some are autosomal recessive; some have unclear inheritance patterns

Epidemiology

- Incidence is approximately 1 in 15,000 to 18,000 births
- Prevalence is approximately 1 in 20,000 population

Pathogenesis

- Abnormal bone predisposes to fractures

Risk Factors

- Familial inheritance
- Spontaneous cases are common; ~35%

Clinical Features

- Fractures, which vary from a few to hundreds
- Sclerae may be normal, blue or gray, or may be colored early and fade to white with time
- Short stature, which tends to be extreme in those with more fractures
- Relative macrocephaly
- Triangular facies
- Hearing loss, conductive from bony abnormalities and/or sensorineural of unknown etiology
- Bony deformities, for example, bowing of long bones
- Scoliosis
- Hypermobility
- Joint malalignment
- Bruising

- Basilar impression, an abnormaility of the occipitovertebral junction, can lead to acute neurologic compromise
- Dentiogenesis imperfecta
- Barrel chest
- Normal intelligence
- Hyperplastic callus (type V)

Natural History

- Hearing loss beginning in the second or third decades in some
- Progressive bony deformities in more severe forms

Diagnosis

Differential diagnosis

- Nonaccidental trauma

History

- Family history of fractures
- Age at first fracture, number of fractures
- Mobility and activities of daily living

Exam

- Height and weight
- Bony angulations
- Strength

Testing

- Skin biopsy for collagen and associated proteins
- Hearing, beginning in childhood and continuing through adulthood
- Intraoperative bone biopsies have been studied, especially when type I collagen is normal. These lead to the description of new types of OI (V–VIII) recently reported

Pitfalls

- Normal collagen does not rule out OI

Red Flags

- Signs of abuse
- Neurologic signs, which can indicate basilar impression
- A fracture may not always be visible on an early radiograph

Treatment

Medical

- Bisphosphonates have been shown to decrease fractures in most studies, though ideal age of treatment onset, dosage, and duration of treatment are being investigated
- Pain management
- Bracing can help with joint alignment and supporting weak muscles
- Immobilization of fractures should use light materials and be as short in duration as possible
- Growth hormone may help with growth and possibly fractures

Exercises

- Careful positioning of infants to encourage active range of motion
- Avoid passive range of motion
- Weightbearing and walking are encouraged
- Aquatic therapy is often helpful and well accepted

Surgical

- Rodding of long bones can decrease fractures but rods can migrate and break
- Scoliosis repair

Consults

- Orthopedic surgery
- Genetics
- Neurosurgery if basilar impression is suspected

Complications of treatment

- Fever and needle phobia with bisphosphonates
- Rodding of long bones can decrease fractures but rods can migrate and break

Prognosis

- Varies by type, from fatal in utero to normal lifespan
- Respiratory infection is a common cause of death
- Adults with OI tend to be well educated and are employed at a much higher rate than the overall rate for people with disabilities

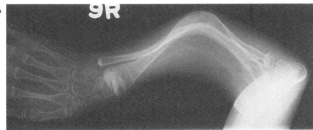
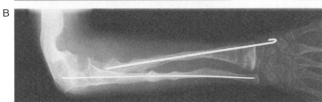
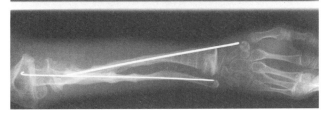

Radiographs showing bowing of radius and ulna before (A) and after (B) fragmentation and rodding surgery.

Helpful Hints

- Physical activity should be encouraged
- The Osteogenesis Imperfecta Foundation has guides for medical management, therapy recommendations, and ratings of risks and benefits for numerous sports and recreational activities

Suggested Readings

Chiasson R, Munns C, Zeitlin L, eds. *Interdisciplinary Treatment Approach for Children with Osteogenesis Imperfecta.* Montreal: Shriners Hospital for Children; 2004.

Cintas HL, Gerber LH, eds. *Children with Osteogenesis Imperfecta: Strategies to enhance performance.* Gaithersburg: Osteogenesis Imperfecta Foundation; 2005.

Wacaster P, ed. *Managing Osteogenesis Imperfecta: A medical manual.* Gaithersburg: Osteogenesis Imperfecta Foundation; 1996.

Osteoid Osteoma

Robert J. Rinaldi MD

Description

Osteoid osteoma (OO) is a benign, solitary tumor of bone characterized by nocturnal pain that is relieved with nonsteroidal anti-inflammatory medications (NSAIDS).

Etiology/Types

- Classification is based on the location of the tumor and includes cortical, cancellous, and subperiosteal types
- The exact etiology and genetic factors, if any, are undefined

Epidemiology

- OO is the third most common benign bone tumor
- Eleven percent of benign bone tumors are OOs; 3% of all bone tumors
- Most commonly seen in the second and third decades of life
- Male to female ratio of 3:1

Pathogenesis

- Tumor nidus surrounded by a thickened, sclerotic cortex
- Nidus consists of osteoid rich tissue, osteoblasts, and fibrovascular stroma
- Surrounding bone sclerosis is variable
- Prostaglandin E2 concentrations are elevated in the nidus
- Nidus osteoblasts demonstrate strong staining for cyclooxygenase-2
- Most commonly located in the diaphyseal or metaphyseal cortices (75%), with more than 50% occurring in the lower extremities

Risk Factors

- None identified

Clinical Features

- Initial presentation of localized bone pain
- Acute or subacute onset
- Pain is worse at night
- Pain can worsen with activity
- Pain dramatically relieved with NSAIDs
- Constitutional symptoms absent

- Spinal tumor sites may show painful scoliosis due to paravertebral muscle spasms
- Intra-articular tumor sites may show pain, decreased range of motion, and joint swelling
- Tumors located near a physis may show limb length discrepancies

Natural History

- No malignant potential
- Little tumor growth
- Frequently self-limited with spontaneous resolution
- May become dormant

Diagnosis

Differential diagnosis

- Osteoblastoma
- Ewing's sarcoma
- Bone or soft tissue trauma
- Osteomyelitis
- Bone metastases
- Bone island
- Growing pains

History

- Acute or subacute onset of focal pain
- Pain worsens at nighttime
- Pain may worsen with activity
- Pain improves dramatically with NSAIDs

Exam

- Focal tenderness
- Structural deformity
- Depending upon the location of the tumor:
  - For spinal column involvement may see paravertebral muscle spasms and scoliosis
  - For intra-articular involvement may see limited range of motion and joint effusion

Testing

- X-rays demonstrate a lucent circular nidus (<1 cm) surrounded by an area of reactive bone with variable sclerotic response
- Computed tomography is useful for definitive diagnosis and accurate tumor/nidus localization

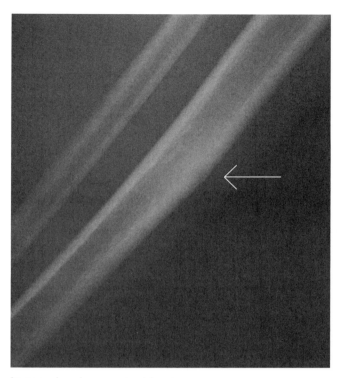

Image showing a osteoid osteoma.

- Technetium bone scanning is most accurate means for tumor localization
- Magnetic resonance imaging is less definitive for diagnosis or localization

Red Flags
- Painful scoliosis
- Decreasing range of motion

Treatment

Medical
- Conservative treatment
- NSAIDs

Exercise
- Range of motion

Surgical
- Nidus removal essential for successful outcome
  - Accurate nidus localization is imperative
- Invasive techniques: En bloc resection, burr-down with nidus curettage
- Noninvasive techniques: percutaneous nidus removal, radiofrequency ablation

Consults
- Orthopedic surgery

Prognosis
- Symptom resolution in 75% to 100% following surgery
- Spontaneous resolution in some conservatively treated cases

Helpful Hints
- Initial conservative management with NSAIDs warranted
- Surgical referral should be made if pain does not resolve or if impairments evolve

Suggested Readings
Lee EH, Shafi M, Hui JHP. Osteoid osteoma: a current review. *Pediatr Orthop.* 2006;25(5):695-700.

Saccomanni B. Osteoid osteoma and osteoblastoma of the spine: a review of the literature. *Curr Rev Musculoskelet Med.* 2009;2:65-67.

Section II: Pediatric Diseases and Complications

Osteoporosis

Susan D. Apkon MD

Description

Children with disabilities are at risk for reduced bone mineral density and subsequent fractures related to minimal trauma. Diagnosis and management of reduced bone mineral density in children with disabilities is a relatively new field with an ever-growing focus on improving the ultimate outcome, which is reduction of the rate of fractures.

Osteoporosis is described as a systemic bone disease characterized by low bone mass and microarchitectural deterioration of bone tissue. Osteoporosis in children with disabilities results in an increase in bone fragility and susceptibility to fractures often related to minimal trauma. The term osteoporosis should not be routinely utilized in children without the presence of a fracture history and low bone mass on dual-energy x-ray absorptiometry (DXA).

Etiology/Types

- Primary osteoporosis: bone loss associated with loss of estrogen (postmenopausal) or aging. This is the most common type of osteoporosis
- Secondary osteoporosis: bone loss associated with other conditions. This occurs in less than 5% of cases but most common in children with disabilities

Epidemiology

- Prevalence of fractures in children with cerebral palsy (CP) reported 5% to 60%
- Prevalence of fractures in boys with Duchenne muscular dystrophy reported as high as 44%
- Prevalence of fractures in children with spina bifida reported 11.5% to 30%

Pathogenesis

- Reduction in bone mass can result from:
  - Failure to produce a skeleton of optimal mass and strength during growth
  - Excessive bone resorption, resulting in decreased bone mass
  - An inadequate formation response to increased resorption during bone remodeling

Risk Factors

- Immobilization or decreased weight bearing
- Neuromuscular conditions including: CP, muscular dystrophy, spinal muscular atrophy, spinal cord injury, and spina bifida
- Medications including corticosteroids and antiepileptics
- Chronic illness including rheumatologic and renal diseases, and cancer
- Poor nutrition

Clinical Features

- Fractures associated with minimal to no trauma
- Fractures more common in lower extremities
- Fractures can be confused with deep vein thromboses (DVT), heterotopic ossification (HO), or infection
- Pain may be present in children with normal sensation
- Pain may not be present in children with spinal cord injuries or spina bifida
- Fractures following casting of an extremity (post-casting phenomenon)

Natural History

- Bone mineral density (BMD) increases as children age, with peak bone mass by third decade.
- BMD accrues at highest rate during puberty
- Children with CP increase BMD/year but have overall decrease compared to able-bodied peers
- BMD decreased in ambulatory boys with Duchenne muscular dystrophy with significant reduction in BMD when child becomes non-ambulatory

Diagnosis

Differential diagnosis

- Primary versus secondary osteoporosis
- Fracture
- Infection
- HO
- DVT

History

- No history of trauma need be obtained or history may be of minimal trauma

- Family history of osteoporosis may suggest primary osteoporosis
- Recent surgery with immobilization or casting
- Medications (antiepileptics, corticosteroids)

Exam
- Pain on palpation over swelling (may not be present in child with spinal cord injury or spina bifida)
- Swelling, erythema, warmth of extremity
- Malalignment of extremity

Testing
- Plain x-ray unable to quantify degree of bone loss
- DXA most common method for evaluation bone density, with a Z-score which is a comparison to sex and aged-matched peers. Z-score must be interpreted with greater clinical picture
- Quantitative computed tomography scan assesses volumetric BMD measurements. Takes into account size of bone
- Laboratory assessment may include serum and urine calcium, phosphorus, parathyroid hormone, and vitamin D metabolites to rule out underlying diseases of bone metabolism

Pitfalls
- DXA is 2-dimensional representation of 3-dimensional bone which may lead to inaccurate determination of BMD in small children
- Inability to assess lumbar spine or proximal femur BMD when orthopedic hardware present
- Size and pubertal status of child impacts DXA results
- The relationship between DXA results and risk of fractures in children with disabilities has not been established

Red Flags
- Recurrent fractures in child with a disability should be further evaluated

Treatment

Medical
- Optimize dietary calcium and vitamin D and consider supplements

- Consider bisphosphonates for recurrent fracture in consultation with bone health specialist

Exercise
- Active weight-bearing exercises as tolerated and able
- Limited benefits of passive standing

Surgical
- Open reduction with internal fixation of long bone when deemed necessary by orthopedic surgery

Consults
- Endocrinology to assess for bone metabolism problems
- Orthopedic surgery when surgical intervention necessary

Complications of treatment
- Bisphosphonates can cause gastrointestinal issues and musculoskeletal pain
- Reports of osteonecrosis of jaw in adults taking bisphosphonates
- Unknown safety and efficacy of bisphosphonate treatment in children with disabilities

Prognosis
- Medications have shown promise in treatment of decreased bone mass in children but further studies are indicated

Helpful Hints
- A comprehensive evaluation with DXA and markers of bone metabolism should be undertaken in children with fractures unrelated to significant trauma

Suggested Readings
Bachrach LK, Ward LM. Clinical review 1: bisphosphonate use in childhood osteoporosis. *J Clin Endocrinol Metab.* 2009;94(2):400-409.

Zacharin M. Current advances in bone health in disabled children. *Curr Opin Pediatr.* 2004;16:545-551.

Pain: Chronic

Joshua Wellington MD MS

Description

Although many children may experience acute pain during their development due to injury, some deal with chronic nonmalignant pain issues that are usually multifactorial and challenging to treat. Psychological components, either underlying or due to the chronic pain, often increase this treatment challenge.

Etiology/Types

- Musculoskeletal
- Neuropathic
- Headache
- Functional (formerly recurrent) abdominal pain

Epidemiology

- Estimated to affect 15% to 20% of children
- Headache 1-year prevalence about 6% in adolescents
- Abdominal pain prevalence about 11% in primary/secondary school age children

Pathogenesis

- Variable depending on type of pain

Risk Factors

- Likely that no risk factors present in most chronic pain
- Prior trauma

Clinical Features

- Musculoskeletal: pain in joint, extremity
- Neuropathic: pain in affected extremity, possible skin/hair changes, possible autonomic signs
- Headache: based on International Headache Society criteria (i.e., migraine, tension-type headache, cluster headache and other autonomic cephalalgias, other primary/secondary headaches)
- Functional abdominal pain: periumbilical pain, autonomic signs may be present

Natural History

- Musculoskeletal: variable
- Neuropathic: associated with peripheral nervous system (PNS)/central nervous system (CNS) injury
- Headache: often begins at school age
- Functional abdominal pain: may be associated with altered bowel habits, nausea/vomiting, and migraine

Diagnosis

Differential diagnosis

- Musculoskeletal: trauma, orthopedic, infection, inflammatory, hematological, metabolic, psychological, cancer, and idiopathic (i.e., growing pains)
- Neuropathic: posttraumatic/surgical peripheral nerve injury, complex regional pain syndrome, metabolic/toxic neuropathies, neurodegenerative disorders, tumor infiltration of PNS/CNS, central pain following CNS injury, mitochondrial disorders, and erythromelalgia
- Headache: migraine, tension-type headache, chronic daily headache, sinusitis, dental (braces), obstructive sleep apnea, increased intracranial pressure, and tumor
- Functional abdominal pain: constipation, gastroesophageal reflux disease, lactose intolerance, *Helicobacter pylori* infection (organic cause found in only ~10%)

History

- Musculoskeletal: aching, dull, throbbing pain in joint, extremity
- Neuropathic: character of pain (i.e., burning, shooting, and electric-like), autonomic changes
- Headache: onset, frequency, duration, and neurological signs/symptoms
- Functional abdominal pain: periumbilical pain at least once per month for 3 consecutive months, accompanied by pain-free periods, severe enough to interfere with normal activities (i.e., school), lasts <1 hour usually and almost never >3 hours, doesn't wake child from sleep

Exam

- A comprehensive and systematic physical examination is critical in evaluating any child with chronic pain

Testing

- Musculoskeletal: x-ray, consider computed tomography or magnetic resonance imaging (MRI)

- Neuropathic: consider electrodiagnosis/ electromyography/nerve conduction studies
- Headache: consider MRI if neurological symptoms
- Functional abdominal pain: complete blood count, erythrocyte sedimentation rate (ESR), urinalysis and culture, and rectal exam with stool guaiac test

Pitfalls
- Ordering unnecessary studies

Red Flags
- Musculoskeletal/neuropathic: progressing pain, loss of function
- Headache: age ≤ 5, morning/nocturnal HA with vomiting, behavioral changes, growth/developmental slowing, rapidly increasing cranial circumference, and persisting or progressing neurological deficits
- Functional abdominal pain: weight loss, dysuria, fevers, anemia, pain awakening child at night, guaiac positive stool, pain far from umbilicus, and elevated ESR

Treatment
Medical
- Nonsteroidal anti-inflammatory drugs; avoid aspirin
- Analgesics
- Adjuvants (antidepressants: tricyclic antidepressants, selective-serotonin reuptake inhibitors; antiepileptics; and topicals)
- Opioids in very select patients; controversial
- 5-HT$_1$ agonists for symptomatic migraine treatment not adequately investigated except sumatriptan, which has promising results
- Prophylactic medication for migraine not shown effective in pediatric clinical trials
- Avoid analgesic overuse (especially those containing caffeine, barbiturates) to prevent refractory headaches

Exercises
- Appropriateness of treatment depends on type/ etiology of pain
- May vary from limited immobilization in certain types of musculoskeletal etiologies to aerobic and strength training for some types of neuropathic pain

Modalities
- Heat
- Ice
- TENS
- Biofeedback
- Relaxation training
- Cutaneous desensitization for neuropathic pain
- Cognitive behavioral therapy
- Acupuncture
- Injections
- Botulinum toxin (for refractory headache), diagnostic nerve blocks, sympathetic plexus blocks

Surgical
- Musculoskeletal etiology with a correctible orthopedic procedure
- Usually not indicated for neuropathic pain, headache, and abdominal pain

Consults
- Neurology
- Orthopedic surgery
- Psychiatry/Psychology

Complications of treatment
- Minimal, if any, as treatments usually conservative
- Impact on family life, school

Prognosis
- Highly variable

Helpful Hints
- A multidisciplinary approach involving physicians, physical/occupation therapists, psychologists, parents, and schools is critical to optimizing the treatment of chronic pain in children so that the highest level of function may be preserved

Suggested Readings
Goodman JE, McGrath PJ. The epidemiology of pain in children and adolescents. *Pain*. 1991;46:247-264.
Schechter NL, Berde CB, Yaster M. *Pain in Infants, Children, and Adolescents*. 2nd ed. Philadelphia, PA: Lippincott Williams & Wilkins; 2003.

Section II: Pediatric Diseases and Complications

Plagiocephaly

Melissa K. Trovoto MD

Description
Plagiocephaly is a term used to describe an abnormal shape of the head resulting from external forces.

Etiology/Types
- Deformational or positional plagiocephaly is an abnormal head shape that is caused by external forces

Prevalence
- Age dependent with peak by 6 months of life

Pathogenesis
- Positional: external forces applied to the infant skull either in utero, at birth, or postnatally

Risk Factors
- Multiple gestation pregnancy
- Assisted delivery
- First-born child
- Male sex
- Prolonged supine positioning
- Infrequent "tummy time"
- Sternocleidomastoid imbalance
- Torticollis
- Slow achievement of motor milestones

Clinical Features
- Positional plagiocephaly may be divided into three subtypes
- One side of the head is misaligned in plagiocephaly. When looking down on the infant's head, it looks as if one side of the head has been pushed forward, often accompanied by malalignment of the ears, forehead, and facial features
- Brachycephaly implies that the back of the head has flattened uniformly. The head takes on a wider and shorter shape and increased head height is common
- Scaphocephaly (dolichocephaly) describes a head with a long, narrow shape and is common in premature babies

Diagnosis

Differential diagnosis
- Craniosynostosis (premature fusion of the sutures)
  - Sagittal synostosis
  - Unilateral coronal synostosis
  - Unilateral lambdoidal synostosis
- Genetic syndromes

History
- Birth history
- Medical history, including family history
- Neck positioning preference for rotation or tilt, especially during sleep
- Time spent with pressure on back of head, including sleep and infant positioners
- Tolerance for "tummy time"
- Time line of asymmetries and pattern of development
- Motor developmental history
- Feeding and sleeping positioning

Exam
- Shape of head, best seen from above
- Malalignment of eyes and ears
- Facial or forehead asymmetry
- Abnormal resting head position
- Impaired active and/or passive neck range of motion

Testing
- Plain x-ray of skull to check for craniosynostosis
- Computed tomography scan of the head with 3D reconstruction if craniosynostosis is suspected, or no improvement is seen with conservative management

Red Flags
- Anterior fontanelle is small or closes earlier than expected
- Associated genetic syndromes
- No improvement seen with growth and conservative management

Treatment

Medical/surgical

- If craniosynostosis is present, neurosurgical evaluation and surgery is indicated to remove the synostosis

Rehabilitative

- Physical or occupational therapy for torticollis or muscle imbalance if present, and to help reinforce repositioning program, provide parent counseling/teaching as infant gains new skills and tolerance for positioning
- Repositioning program
  - Increase amount of supervised "tummy time"
  - Limit use of infant positioners that put pressure on the back of the head such as a bouncy seat or swing
  - Alternate position of head during sleep, feeding, and play
  - Alternate the direction in which infant is placed in the crib/changing table
  - Alternate the arm in which the infant is fed
  - During awake hours minimize the time the infant is on his/her back

Cranial orthosis

- Custom molded cranial shaping helmet, which can be fabricated by an orthotist
- Consider for children with slow improvement, or severe asymmetries, as well as those with associated severe torticollis
- Results are best when prescribed by 9 months of age; however, may be used up to 18 months of age
- Infant wears the orthosis for 23.5 hours per day for average of 3 to 6 months
- Insurance coverage varies

Suggested Readings

Bialocerkowski AE, Vladusic SL, Ng CW. Prevalence, risk factors, and natural history of positional plagiocephaly: a systemic review. *Dev Med Child Neurol.* 2008;50:577-586.

Hutchison BL, Hutchison L, Thompson J, Mitchell ED. Plagiocephaly and brachycephaly in the first two years of life: a prospective cohort study. *Pediatrics.* 2004;114:970-980.

Polio

Michael A. Alexander MD

Description

Poliomyelitis represents the extreme expression of a condition, which in most people presents as an intestinal or pharyngeal infection. In 3%, it presents as a fairly rapid onset of weakness and asymmetric flaccid paralysis associated with pain, with intact sensation.

Etiology/Types

- Enterovirus, an RNA virus, known as a poliovirus (PV)
- There are three of these viruses PV1, PV2, and PV3; the most common is the PV1
- Infection with any one type does not confer immunity to the other two
- Both the Sabin and Salk vaccines contain antigens from all three

Epidemiology

- Seasonal, with a peak in summer and fall
- Incubation is 6 to 20 days (range 3–35 days)
- The mode of transmission is fecal/oral
- It is infectious from 7 to 10 days before onset of symptoms and 7 to 10 days after onset of symptoms
- Endemic in Africa, Afghanistan, and Iraq
- Recently most infections have been from the attenuated live virus in the Sabin vaccine
- Salk vaccine, a dead virus preparation, only used in the United States
- Three percent go on to develop central nervous system symptoms
- Between 1 in 200 and 1 in 1000 develop asymmetric flaccid paralysis

Pathogenesis

- The virus enters the gastrointestinal tract cells and lymphatic cells
- There is a subsequent viremia, which triggers flu-like symptoms
- In a small proportion, it spreads to the neurons with invasion of the virus into the anterior horn cells (AHC)
- The death of the AHC leaves skeletal muscle without the trophic factors that maintain muscle

Risk Factors

- Immune deficiency
- Very young
- Malnutrition
- Tonsillectomy
- Previously injured muscles

Clinical Features

- Asymmetric paralysis of muscles
- Sensitivity to touch
- Muscle pain
- Loss of reflexes
- Constipation
- Difficulty voiding
- Painful muscle spasms
- Bulbar involvement in 2% with weakness
- Headache, neck and back pain, vomiting, extremity pain, fever, lethargy, and irritability

Natural History

- Varies based on whether the AHCs were injured or completely destroyed
- Remaining muscles will hypertrophy and remaining AHC will reinnervate muscles through peripheral sprouting, thus increasing their motor unit territory
- Twenty-five percent to 30% have full functional recovery without atrophy
- Majority show near normal functional recovery with some residual weakness and atrophy
- Eighty percent of those who recover do so in the first 6 months
- Two percent to 5% of children and 15% to 30% of adults with paralysis will die
- Post-polio syndrome: ~40 years after the initial paralysis patients describe loss of strength in muscles they thought were uninvolved, and further loss of strength in muscles that previously had weakness

Diagnosis

Differential diagnosis

- Acute spinal cord malfunction due to hemorrhage, tumor, or myelitis
- Acute motor sensory neuropathies, Guillain Barre

- Botulism
- Rabies
- Tetanus and other encephalopathies

History
- Intestinal or pharyngeal infection followed by weakness

Exam
- Sudden onset of asymmetric flaccid paralysis
- Absent reflexes
- Preservation of sensation
- Post-polio: worsening weakness and atrophy over time

Testing
- The organism can be identified in the stool
- Antibodies in the blood and rarely in the cerebrospinal fluid (CSF)
- CSF: elevated protein and white blood cells
- Electrodiagnosis (EDX) will show a loss of axons and preservation of sensory conductions, with positive waves and fibrillations
- Late EDX findings include large amplitude motor units due to reinnervation

Pitfalls
- The muscles can spasm severely and painfully with dysfunctional positions, producing "contractures" almost over night

Treatment

Medical
- Analgesia is indicated for the muscle pain and headaches
- Close monitoring of pulmonary function and consideration of ventilatory support; often managed with iron lung or other form of negative pressure respiratory support
- In patients with poor control of oral secretions consideration should be given to tracheostomy

Exercises
- Positioning and range of motion
- Frequent mobilization to prevent pressure ulcers, especially on the back of the head in children
- Once the pain phase has resolved, begin active exercises avoiding fatigue
- Bracing for support for walking or sitting
- Occupational therapy for activities of daily living and to provide adaptive devices

Modalities
- Heat modalities, including whirlpool, heated pools, hot packs, and infrared heat lamps

Surgical
- Muscle tendon transfers; anticipate a loss of one muscle strength grade on transfer
- Bony procedures for scoliosis or arthrodesis for joint stabilization

Consults
- Pulmology
- Gastroenterology
- Orthopedic surgery

Complications
- Pneumonia
- Fecal impaction
- Contractures
- Decreased growth of the paralyzed extremities
- Hip dislocation
- Scoliosis

Prognosis
- Bulbar and bulbospinal involvement are associated with highest rate of complications and mortality

Helpful Hints
- Provide electronic control of the environment and consider power mobility early in rehabilitation so that those affected can control their activity

Suggested Readings
Howard RS. Poliomyelitis and the postpolio syndrome. *BMJ*. 2005;330:1314-1318.

Mueller S, Wimmer E, Cello J. Poliovirus and poliomyelitis a tale of guts, brains, and an accidental event. *Virus Res*. 2005;111:175-193.

Section II: Pediatric Diseases and Complications

Prader Willi Syndrome

Maureen R. Nelson MD

Description
Prader Willi syndrome is a multisystem, multigenic disorder characterized by hypotonia, obesity, respiratory difficulties, and intellectual impairments. It is the most common syndromatic cause of obesity.

Etiology/Types
- Multigenic inheritance
- In 75%: a loss of function of paternal gene group on chromosome 15q11.2q13
- In 24%: from abnormal gene expression 15q and from maternal uniparental disomy, which silences paternal alleles
- One percent from imprinting errors

Epidemiology
- Prevalence unknown but thought to be about 1/50,000
- Rare neurogenetic disorder but most common syndromic cause of obesity

Pathogenesis
- Unknown, but a possible hypothalamus connection

Risk Factors
- Familial inheritance

Clinical Features
- Neonatal hypotonia
- Neonatal poor feeding
- Early failure to thrive (FTT)
- Hyperphagia beginning by school age
- Obesity
- Hypogonadism and infertility
- Unusual nasal voice
- Trichotillomania
- Skin picking
- Behavior problems common in teens
- Low IQ

Natural History
- Infantile FTT and poor feeding
- Scoliosis in 30% to 70%; may have kyphosis
- Hyperphagia with obesity as growing
- Oppositional behavior in later childhood onward
- Respiratory risk, including nocturnal hyopoventilation
- Growth hormone insufficiency common
- Low bone mineral density leads to high risk of osteoporosis and fractures
- Twenty-five percent develop diabetes at a mean age of 20 years
- Death frequently from cardiac failure

Diagnosis

Differential diagnosis
- Angelman syndrome
- Fragile X syndrome
- Down syndrome (trisomy 21)
- Familial short stature variants
- Growth hormone deficiency

History
- Neonatal poor feeding and FTT
- Neonatal hypotonia
- Early onset hyperphagia
- Reduced growth velocity
- Learning disabilities
- Deficits in short-term memory and abstract thinking
- Sleep apnea-central and obstructive

Exam
- Obesity
- Short, small hands and feet
- Hypotonia
- Decreased strength and muscle mass
- Hypogonadism
- Thin upper lip and almond-shaped eyes
- Short stature

Testing
- DNA methylation analysis is the only test that can both confirm and reject the diagnosis

Pitfalls
- Behavioral problems can lead to both medical problems due to obesity and to social problems

Red Flags
- Obesity leads to high rate of metabolic syndrome and to cardiac risk

Treatment

Medical
- Growth hormone improves height and body composition but optimal dose and age to treat are still being studied
- Strict nutritional guidelines to minimize obesity are critical
- Medications to promote anorexia have not been found to be effective
- Majority require hormones for puberty
- Behavioral management to minimize behavioral problems

Exercises
- Regular exercise for strength and caloric expenditure

Modalities
- N/A

Injection
- N/A

Surgical
- Rarely for scoliosis, if curve is >70%
- Gastric banding does not show long-term positive effects

- Adenotonsillectomy does not consistently improve sleep apnea

Consults
- Genetics
- Nutrition
- Endocrinology
- Psychiatry/Psychology/Behavioral counselors

Complications of treatment
- Medication side effects, especially steroids

Prognosis
- Can improve muscle mass, decrease obesity, and minimize health risks with careful nutrition and exercise program

Helpful Hints
- Prevention of obesity can limit cardiopulmonary risks in adulthood

Suggested Readings

Brambilla P, Crino A, Bedogni G, et al. Metabolic syndrome in children with Prader-Willi syndrome: the effect of obesity. *Nutr Metab Cardiovasc Dis.* 2010 Jan 18, 2010, Epub.

Goldstone AP, Holland AJ, Hauffa BP, et al. Recommendations for the diagnosis and management of Prader-Willi syndrome. *J Clin Endocrinol Metab.* 2008;93:4183-4197.

Section II: Pediatric Diseases and Complications

Rett Syndrome

Aga Julia Lewelt MD

Description

Rett syndrome is a postnatal progressive neurodevelopmental disorder that manifests in girls during early childhood. It is characterized by normal early development followed by acquired microcephaly, loss of purposeful hand movements and communication skills, social withdrawal, gait apraxia, stereotypic repetitive hand movements, seizures, and intellectual disability.

Etiology/Types

- X-linked disorder with mutation in *MECP2* gene mapped to Xq28
- The more *MECP2* gene mutated X chromosomes are inactivated (Barr bodies) in the girl, the less severely she is affected; since boys have only one X chromosome, all are active and it is fatal
- Atypical/variant

Epidemiology

- Affects one in every 10,000 to 20,000 live female births
- The No. 2 genetic cause of intellectual disability in females

Pathogenesis

- Mutation occurs in the *MECP2* gene that encodes the protein methyl cytosine binding protein 2 so the brain cannot develop normally
- Diffuse cerebral atrophy
- Reduced neuronal size
- Decreased length and complexity of dendritic branching
- Reduced number of Purkinje cells in cerebellum

Risk Factors

- Female sex
- 99.5% cases are sporadic from de novo mutations
- The incidence of familial cases is higher than expected by chance

Clinical Features

- Normocephaly at birth followed by acquired microcephaly with age
- Stereotypic hand movements, such as hand wringing, clapping, and mouthing
- Gait and truncal apraxia
- Seizures
- Dystonia, spasticity, and/or contractures
- Scoliosis
- Growth retardation
- Decreased body fat and muscle mass
- Breathing dysfunction
- Irritability, agitation, and/or anxiety
- Chewing and/or swallowing difficulties
- Hypotrophic small and cold feet or hands
- Peripheral vasomotor disturbances

Natural History

There are four stages of Rett syndrome:

- Stage I—early onset, begins between 6 and 18 months of age
  - May be somewhat vague, infant may begin to show less eye contact and interest in toys; delays in gross motor skills
- Stage II—rapid destructive stage, usually begins between ages 1 and 4 and may last for weeks or months
  - Acquired microcephaly is usually noticed during this stage
  - Purposeful hand use and expressive language skills are lost
  - Characteristic hand movements begin to emerge
  - Breathing irregularities
  - Autistic-like symptoms
  - General irritability
  - Ataxic gait and apraxia
- Stage III—the plateau or pseudo-stationary stage, usually begins between ages 2 and 10 and can last for years
  - Apraxia, motor problems, and seizures
  - Possible improvements in behavior, alertness, attention span, and communication
  - Many girls remain in this stage for most of their lives
- Stage IV—the late motor deterioration stage can last for years or decades
  - Decreased mobility with possible loss of ambulatory function
  - Muscle weakness, rigidity, spasticity, dystonia, and scoliosis

– No decline in cognition, communication, or hand skills
– Repetitive hand movements may decrease, and eye gaze usually improves

Diagnosis

Differential diagnosis
- Autism
- Cerebral palsy
- Angelman syndrome
- Spinocerebellar degeneration

History
- Normocephaly at birth followed by acquired microcephaly with age
- Girls have apparently normal development until 6 to 18 months of age, followed by developmental regression
- Loss of purposeful hand movements between 6 and 30 months, with communication dysfunction and social withdrawal
- Autistic-like behaviors
- Intellectual disabilities and learning difficulties
- Loss of normal sleep patterns
- Loss of social engagement
- Abnormal breathing
- Constipation
- Gastroesophageal reflux disease (GERD)

Exam
- Microcephaly
- Hypotonia
- Scoliosis
- Stereotypic hand movements, such as hand wringing, clapping, and mouthing
- Gait apraxia, toe walking
- Truncal ataxia
- Severely impaired receptive and expressive language

Testing
- Genetic testing for MECP2 mutation on X chromosome

- Neuroimaging shows progressive cortical atrophy and hypoplasia of the corpus callosum

Pitfalls
- Atypical cases can present early in infancy with seizures

Treatment

Medical
- There is no cure
- Symptomatic treatment of spasticity, seizures, constipation, GERD, behaviors, and sleep difficulty
- Regular exam and x-ray for scoliosis
- Supplemental feedings via gastrostomy tube

Modalities
- Weight bearing exercises
- Hydrotherapy, music therapy
- Daily stretching and orthotics

Injection
- Some may benefit from botulinum toxin and phenol

Surgical
- May need for correction of scoliosis
- May need gastrostomy tube

Consults
- Pediatric neurology or developmental pediatrics

Prognosis
- The time course and severity vary
- Typically, it slowly progresses until teenage; then, symptoms may improve
- Most individuals continue to live well into middle age and beyond

Suggested Reading
Ben Zeev GB. Rett syndrome. *Child Adolesc Psychiatr Clin N Am.* 2007;16:723–743.

Websites for Families
http://ghr.nlm.nih.gov/condition=rettsyndrome
http://www.ninds.nih.gov/disorders/rett/detail_rett.htm

Scoliosis: Congenital

Elizabeth Moberg-Wolff MD

Description

Scoliosis is defined as a frontal plane deformity of the spine of >10°, with frequent concurrent rotational deformity in the sagittal or transverse plane. Congenital scoliosis accounts for 20% of all scoliosis. It is diagnosed in infancy, frequently at birth. It differs from infantile scoliosis, neuromuscular scoliosis, and idiopathic scoliosis.

Etiology/Types
- Cervical, thoracic, or lumbar levels
- Kyphoscoliosis

Epidemiology
- Siblings have 5% to 10% risk
- Anomalies of the tracheal, esophageal, gastrointestinal, pulmonary, cardiac, and renal systems commonly coexist

Pathogenesis
- Formation deficit of vertebra (hemi vertebra, wedge vertebrae, and fused vertebra)
- Segmentation deficit of vertebra (fused vertebra and unilateral bar)
- Tethered spinal cord
- Syrinx
- Diastematomyelia
- Lipoma
- Myelomeningocele
- Intraspinal tumor

Risk Factors
- Intraspinal pathology
- Sibling diagnosis
- Klippel-Feil syndrome, congenital synostosis of some or all cervical vertebrae
- VATERL, a syndrome characterized by vertebral, anal, cardiovascular, tracheal, esophageal, renal, and limb bud deformities
- Spinal dysraphism, or incomplete bony development of the spine
- Thoracic insufficiency syndrome

Clinical Features
- Rotational and flexion/extension limitations
- Rib hump seen when looking at the back on forward bending (Adams test)
- Asymmetric pelvis
- Torticollis in infants due to limited neck range of motion
- Leg length discrepancy
- Curves over 100° associated with restrictive lung disease
- Kyphosis most common at the T10–T11 level

Natural History
- Pulmonary insufficiency/restrictive lung disease
- Pain and osteoarthritis
- Fifty percent require surgical intervention

Diagnosis

Differential diagnosis
- Infantile scoliosis (see Scoliosis: Idiopathic chapter)
- Intraspinal pathology (tumor, syrinx, diastematomyelia, tethered cord, etc.)
- Muscle spasm
- Leg length discrepancy

History
- Sibling history
- Usually noticed within first year of life
- Decreased function and mobility
- Pulmonary insufficiency
- Pain—indicative of discitis or tumor
- Webbed neck, skin dimples, café au lait spots indicative of concurrent disorders (Klippel Feil, myelomeningoceole, and neurofibromatosis)

Exam
- Limitations in flexion, extension, or rotation of the spine
- Rib hump on forward bending
- Asymmetric shoulder or hip heights
- Leg length discrepancy
- Pelvic obliquity
- Asymmetric gait

- Lumbosacral spine hairy patch or skin dimple
- Pain

Testing
- Anteroposterior and lateral x-rays with Cobb angle measurement every 3 to 6 months
- Computed tomography scan to evaluate anatomy of curve and of possible nearby organ abnormalities
- Magnetic resonance imaging study to evaluate for intraspinal anomalies if neurologic abnormalities present or preoperatively
- Motor and sensory evoked potentials used to assess cord compression intraoperatively
- Renal ultrasound—10% to 20% have concurrent anomalies

Pitfalls
- Failure to monitor the curve frequently can result in unnoticed significant progression
- Failure to appropriately surgically intervene may result in spinal cord trauma
- Presence of kyphosis increases risk of spinal cord compression

Red Flags
- Quadriplegia
- Pulmonary insufficiency
- Bowel or bladder incontinence
- Sensory changes
- Progressive weakness

Treatment

Medical
- A trial of bracing may be helpful for back pain but for curvature reduction it is typically ineffective

Exercises
- General strengthening and stretching to maintain mobility and developmental progress

Modalities
- Transcutaneous electrical nerve stimulation has not been found to be helpful

Injection
- Botulinum toxin injections to the muscles on the concave side of the curve may temporarily reduce curve measurement

Surgical
- Perioperative nutrition, pain control, and pulmonary toilet essential

- Vertical expandable prosthetic titanium rib implant spans iliac crest to rib and is lengthened every 6 months
- Growth-sparing expandable instrumentation without fusion allows further truncal growth
- Hemi vertebra resection
- In situ fusion
- Hemi fusion on the convex side
- Intraspinal anomaly correction
- Full spine fusion, for whatever levels required, from T1–pelvis
- Cord untethering

Consults
- Neurosurgery or orthopedic-spine surgery
- Genetics

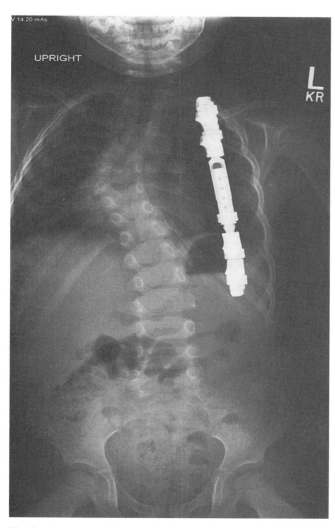

Vertical expandable prosthetic titanium rib implant in a child with congenital scoliosis.

- Cardiology
- Urology

Complications of treatment
- Spinal cord injury
- Persistent pain
- Rib fracture
- Infection
- Pseudoarthrodesis
- Attenuated truncal growth
- Crankshaft deformity occurs when the posterior column of an immature back is fused but the anterior spine continues to grow at both ends of the fusion

Prognosis
- Continued function is possible if assessed early, followed closely, and in most cases, surgically treated

Helpful Hints
- Infantile scoliosis also occurs in young children but is not associated with underlying pathology, and resolves spontaneously in 90% of cases

Suggested Readings

Arlet V, Odent T, Aebi M. Congenital scoliosis. *Eu Spine J.* 2003;12:456–463.

Hedequist DJ. Surgical treatment of congenital scoliosis. *Orthop Clin North Am.* 2007;38:497–509.

Scoliosis: Idiopathic

Elizabeth Moberg-Wolff MD

Description

Scoliosis is defined as a frontal plane deformity of the spine of >10°, with frequent concurrent rotational deformity in the sagittal or transverse plane. Scoliosis is the most common pediatric spine deformity, and idiopathic scoliosis accounts for 80% of cases.

Etiology/Types

- Infantile—<3 years
- Juvenile—age 3 to 10 years
- Adolescent—>age 10, most common

Epidemiology

- Present in 2% to 3% of all children
- Boys and girls equally affected
- Concurrence among twins >50%
- Positive family history 30%
- Juvenile form—up to 20% have associated intraspinal abnormalities
- Adolescent form —25/1000 teens
- School screening of adolescents is controversial and mandated by <50% of states
- Curve progression depends on age of onset, curve size, skeletal maturity, and gender

Pathogenesis

- Multifactorial etiology with familial patterns
- Growth hormone, melatonin production, connective tissues structure, osteopenia, and environmental interactions postulated

Risk Factors

- Infantile scoliosis: European males, with plagiocephaly, hip dysplasia, and torticollis
- Juvenile: genetic predisposition
- Adolescent: genetic predisposition
- Increased curve progression associated with immature Tanner pubertal staging, low Risser classification (0–5) (measure of calcification of the pelvis, indicating the amount of growth remaining), large curve magnitude, and female gender
- Thoracic curves over 50° tend to continue to progress even after growth is complete

Clinical Features

- Torticollis and hip dysplasia in infants
- Rib hump seen when looking at the back on forward bending (Adams test)
- Asymmetric pelvis
- Leg length discrepancy
- Left thoracic curves predominate in infantile scoliosis
- Right thoracic curve predominant in adolescents
- Double curves may be present
- Juvenile—asymptomatic hydromyelia is common
- Progression often related to growth spurts
- Rotational and flexion/extension limitations

Natural History

- Infantile: 90% of cases resolve spontaneously
- Juvenile: 70% require treatment, of which 50% is typically surgical
- Adolescent: 10% require surgical intervention

Diagnosis

Differential diagnosis

- Intraspinal pathology (tumor, syrinx, diastematomyelia, tethered cord, etc.)
- Muscle spasm
- Leg length discrepancy
- Herniated disc
- Hemiplegia
- Myelomeningoceole
- Vertebral anomaly

History

- Positive family history
- Infantile: truncal asymmetry noticed within first year of life
- Decreased function and mobility
- Muscle spasm or pain rare

Exam

- Adam's test: Rib hump seen when child bends forward reaching both hands toward the feet
- Leg length discrepancy
- Pelvic obliquity
- Asymmetric shoulder or hip heights
- Asymmetric gait
- Limitations in flexion, extension, or rotation of the spine
- Lumbo-sacral spine hairy patch or skin dimple possible when underlying pathology present
- No point tenderness unless underlying pathology

179

Testing

- Anteroposterior, lateral and forward bending x-rays with Cobb angle measurement every 3 to 12 months
- Risser classification, an estimation of skeletal maturity defined by the amount of calcification present in the iliac apophysial radiograph
- Tanner staging by pubertal development
- Computed tomography scan to evaluate anatomy of curve if significant rotation or kyphosis present
- Magnetic resonance imaging study to evaluate for intraspinal anomalies if neurologic abnormalities present or if curve 20° in juvenile onset
- Motor evoked potentials and somatosensory evoked potentials are used to assess cord compression intraoperatively

Pitfalls

- Failure to correct large leg length discrepancy may result in secondary pain
- Failure to monitor curves frequently can result in significant progression, limiting treatment options
- Failure to surgically intervene when necessary may result in spinal cord trauma
- Presence of kyphosis increases risk of spinal cord compression and requires monitoring

Red Flags

- Back pain
- Pulmonary insufficiency
- Progressive weakness, sensory change, or bowel and bladder incontinence

Treatment

Medical

- Observation of curves <25° until after skeletal maturity
- Thoracolumbosacral orthosis bracing for curves <40° with apex at T7 may be attempted, 16 to 24 hour daily wear until growth complete, but questionable effectiveness
- Infantile: bracing can interfere with development and is avoided unless the curve is >25° and the child is >1 year of age
- Juvenile: aggressive curve progression is typical. Bracing may potentially prolong period before surgical intervention is required. Utilized in 50% of patients
- Adolescence: bracing results are equivocal

Exercises

- General strengthening and stretching to maintain flexibility may be beneficial in preventing curve progression

Modalities

- Transcutaneous electrical nerve stimulation has not been found to be clinically helpful

Surgical

- Perioperative nutrition, pain control, and psychological support essential
- Size, location, and skeletal maturity impact surgical decisions
- Posterior spine fusion for thoracic curves <50°
- Anterior spine fusion for thoracolumbar or lumbar curves often utilized
- Anterior-posterior fusions utilized for large or rigid curves
- Lumbar lordosis preserved whenever possible
- Growth-sparing instrumentation without fusion done commonly in juveniles

Consults

- Neurosurgery or orthopedic-spine surgery

Complications of treatment

- Spinal cord injury
- Persistent pain
- Infection
- Attenuated truncal growth
- Rib fracture
- Crankshaft deformity occurs when the posterior column of an immature back is fused but the anterior spine continues to grow at both ends of the fusion

Prognosis

- Progression after growth is complete is uncommon unless curve is >50°
- Large untreated curves may cause pain, cosmetic deformity, and pulmonary problems when aging

Helpful Hints

- Reassurance, support and inclusion of the adolescent is an essential part of effective management
- Kyphosis may be associated with scoliosis and complicates bracing and surgical intervention
- Pain is not typical in scoliosis and may indicate a neoplasm, herniated disc, or infection
- A left thoracic curve in a teenage male is unusual and should trigger an investigation of secondary cause

Suggested Readings

Murphy K. Scoliosis: current management and trends. *Phys Med Rehabil.* 2000;14:207–219. Review.
Peele MW, Luhmann SJ. Management of adolescent idiopathic scoliosis. *Neurosurg Clin N Am.* 2007;18:575–583.

Scoliosis: Neuromuscular

Elizabeth Moberg-Wolff MD

Description

Scoliosis is defined as a frontal plane deformity of the spine of >10°, with frequent concurrent rotational deformity in the sagittal or transverse plane. Neuromuscular scoliosis accounts for 20% of all scoliosis and is commonly seen in children with cerebral palsy, neuromuscular disease, spinal cord injury, and genetic syndromes.

Etiology/Types

- Long, sweeping C-shaped thoracolumbar curves involving the pelvis are common
- Double curves

Epidemiology

- Onset is younger than idiopathic scoliosis, less responsive to orthotic management, and more likely to require surgical intervention
- Up to 90% of children with neuromuscular disease affected (dystrophies, upper motor neuron disorders, myopathies, and mitochondrial disorders)
- Up to 70% of children with cerebral palsy and significant motor impairment
- Up to 60% of children with Friedrich's ataxia
- Up to 86% of children with familial dysautonomia
- Up to 100% of children with spinal cord injury occurring prior to skeletal maturity
- Up to 90% of children with L1 or higher myelomeningocoele
- Boys and girls equally affected

Pathogenesis

- Multifactorial due to interactions of the following:
  - Weak truncal musculature
  - Coronal and sagittal malalignment
  - Sensory feedback impairments
  - Asymmetric paraplegia
  - Congenital and intraspinal anomalies

Risk Factors

- Onset or injury at young age
- Prolonged nonambulatory status
- Weak truncal musculature
- Rib cage deformities
- Spasticity and hypotonia

Clinical Features

- Pelvic obliquity resulting in poor positioning
- Rib hump noted on forward bending with both hands reaching for the feet, called the Adams test
- Left-sided curves predominate
- Leg length discrepancy
- Hyperlordosis
- Rotational and flexion/extension limitations
- Progression exacerbated during growth spurts

Natural History

- Curves >50° often continue to progress at 1.5° per year after skeletal maturity
- Curves are largely unresponsive to bracing
- Poor sitting tolerance, pulmonary compromise, cardiac compromise, skin breakdown, pain, and progressive neurologic deterioration may accompany large untreated curves
- Decline in forced vital capacity is predictive of progression in Duchenne muscular dystrophy (DMD)

Diagnosis

Differential diagnosis

- Intraspinal pathology (tumor, syrinx, diastematomyelia, tethered cord, etc.)
- Muscle spasticity
- Leg length discrepancy
- Herniated disc
- Hemiplegia
- Vertebral anomaly
- Congenital scoliosis

History

- Presence of spinal injury, cerebral palsy, neuromuscular disease (Marfan's syndrome, Freidrich's ataxia, and muscular dystrophy), achondroplasia, spinal muscular atrophy, etc.
- Decreased function and mobility
- Pulmonary function decrease
- Muscle spasm or pain
- Poor sitting balance or sitting tolerance
- Insensate skin may be part of primary disorder
- Contractures of the hip or knee

Exam

- Observe sitting, standing, and walking if possible
- Rib hump on forward bending
- Leg length discrepancy
- Pelvic obliquity—note if hip dysplasia present
- Asymmetric shoulder or hip heights
- Asymmetric gait
- Hyperlordosis
- Limitations in flexion, extension, or rotation of the spine
- Lumbosacral spine hairy patch or skin dimple possible when underlying pathology present
- No point tenderness unless underlying pathology

Testing

- Anteroposterior and lateral x-rays with Cobb angle measurement every 3 to 12 months
- Pulmonary function tests in muscular dystrophies
- Electrocardiography and echocardiogram for dystrophy patients
- Computed tomography scan to evaluate anatomy of curve if significant rotation or kyphosis present
- Magnetic resonance imaging study to evaluate for intraspinal anomalies if neurologic abnormalities present
- Risser classification, an estimation of skeletal maturity defined by the amount of calcification present in the iliac apophysial radiograph
- Tanner staging by pubertal development
- Motor evoked potentials and somatosensory evoked potentials used to assess cord compression intraoperatively

Pitfalls

- Improperly fitting thoracolumbosacral orthoses (TLSOs) can compromise feeding, gastrointestinal (GI), and pulmonary status
- Failure to monitor curves frequently can result in significant progression, limiting treatment options
- Failure to surgically intervene may result in spinal cord trauma
- Presence of kyphosis increases risk of spinal cord compression and needs monitoring

Red Flags

- Back pain
- Pulmonary compromise
- Progressive weakness, sensory change, or bowel and bladder incontinence

Treatment

Medical

- Steroid treatment in DMD slows the progression of scoliosis and prolongs ambulatory status
- Observation of curves <25° until after skeletal maturity
- TLSO bracing for ambulatory patients with short curves <40° may delay surgery until further growth achieved—requires 16 to 24 hour daily wear
- Bracing ineffective in preventing progression in muscular dystrophy

Exercises

- General strengthening and stretching to maintain flexibility may be beneficial in maintaining health

Modalities

- Transcutaneous electrical nerve stimulation has not been found to be clinically helpful

Injection

- Botulinum toxin injections into the muscles on the concave side of the curve may temporarily reduce curve measurement

Surgical

- Perioperative nutrition, pain control, skin protection, GI motility, and pulmonary toilet essential
- Size, location, and skeletal maturity impact surgical decisions
- Posterior spine fusion for thoracic curves <50°
- Anterior spine fusion for DMD thoracolumbar curves increases morbidity
- Anterior-posterior fusions utilized for large or rigid curves
- Lumbar lordosis preserved whenever possible
- Growth-sparing instrumentation without fusion done commonly

Consults

- Neurosurgery or orthopedic-spine surgery
- Pulmonology
- Nutrition and gastroenterology

Complications of treatment

- Loss in function due to reduced spinal flexibility, lumbar lordosis, and lateral sway
- Increased energy consumption during gait
- Spinal cord injury
- Pain
- Infection
- Pseudoarthrodesis

- Attenuated truncal growth
- Pulmonary compromise if preoperative forced vital capacity less than 30%
- Crankshaft deformity occurs when the posterior column of an immature back is fused but the anterior spine continues to grow at both ends of the fusion

Prognosis

- Large untreated curves may cause discomfort, cosmetic deformity, and pulmonary problems with aging

Helpful Hints

- Kyphosis complicates bracing and surgical intervention.
- TLSO bracing may be beneficial for truncal positioning, even if ineffective in delaying the progression of a curve

Suggested Readings

Berven S, Bradfrod D. Neuromuscular scoliosis: causes of deformity and principle for evaluation and management. *Semi Neurol.* 2002;22:167–178.

Murphy N, Firth S, Jorgensen T, Young P. Spinal surgery in children with idiopathic and neuromuscular scoliosis. What's the difference? *J Pediatr Orthop.* 2006;23:211–220.

Seizures

Pamela E. Wilson MD

Description

Seizure

Sudden, transient disturbance of brain function manifested by changes in sensory, motor, psychic, or autonomic function. Symptoms are based on the area of the brain involved.

Epilepsy

Repeat seizure activity without an acute cause.

Status epilepticus

Ongoing seizure activity or repeat seizures without regaining consciousness for 30 minutes or longer.

Etiology/Types

- Symptomatic—identifiable cause (vascular, traumatic, tumors, infectious)
- Cryptogenic—undetermined etiology, congenital CNS abnormalities
- Idiopathic—genetic
    Based on the International League Against Epilepsy classification
- Partial—originate in a small area of cortex, usually causing focal symptoms
- Generalized—both hemispheres are involved and is always associated with a loss of consciousness (LOC)
- Unclassifiable

Epidemiology

- Developed countries—2%
- Bimodal distribution (first few years and then in the elderly)
- Posttraumatic seizures: all types of traumatic brain injury (TBI) 2% to 2.5%

Pathogenesis

- Varies between traumatic and nontraumatic etiology, as well as focal and generalized
- Abnormal intermittent but sustained discharge of groups of neurons in focal seizure
- Abnormal generalized discharge of entire cortex simultaneously in generalized seizure

Risk Factors

- Structural abnormalities, infections, family history, trauma, and cerebral palsy
- Immunizations are unlikely to cause seizures except for febrile type

Clinical Features

Partial

- Simple—no LOC and generally short duration; can have sensory, motor, autonomic, or psychic symptoms
- Complex—classically has an aura, associated with an impaired level of consciousness and automatisms
- May progress to generalized

Generalized

- Tonic/clonic (grand mal)—usually has an associated aura, LOC, tonic/clonic movement patterns, and a postictal phase
- Tonic—presents as tonic muscle contraction
- Clonic—jerking motion is noted and can by asymmetric
- Atonic—drop attacks, usually characterized by a loss of muscle tone, impaired consciousness but lasting only a few seconds, and head may drop forward
- Absence or petite mal—classic absence is characterized by a sudden lack of awareness and lack of motor activity, although tone is preserved, they seem to just "space out," while atypical tend to be longer in duration with incomplete LOC
- Myoclonic—a brief sudden contraction of muscle or group of muscles

Natural History

- Single seizure has a 50% chance of recurrence with no treatment indicated
- Antiepileptic drugs (AEDs) are continued until person is seizure free for 1 to 2 years
- Seizure prophylaxis is recommended for children at high risk for seizures for 1 week after TBI
- Seizure prophylaxis does not prevent development of late seizures after a TBI

Diagnosis

Differential diagnosis
- Neurologic: migraines, transient ischemic attack, transient global amnesia, breath holding, benign paroxysmal vertigo, and tics
- Cardiac: syncope, vasovagal episode, and cardiac arrhythmias
- Pseudoseizures/conversion disorders, sleep disorders, narcolepsy, and parasomnias

History
- Description of the seizure
- Family history

Exam
- Neurologic exam
- Head circumference in baby/toddler

Testing
- Electroencephalography (EEG): sleep-deprived may be requested to increase risk of seizure activity; transition to/from sleep and sleep may activate an EEG change, as may photic stimulation with flashing strobe lights, or hyperventilation
- Metabolic lab: glucose, calcium, magnesium, electrolytes, blood urea nitrogen/creatinine, thyroid-stimulating hormone, toxicology screen to look for treatable cause
- Lumbar puncture if infection suspected
- Imaging: magnetic resonance imaging first choice

Treatment

Medical
- Adrenocorticotropic hormone is given for infantile spasms
- AED:
  - Carbamezepine—10 to 30 mg/kg/day up to 1000 to 2000 mg/day
  - Felbamate—45 to 60 mg/kg/day up to 2400 to 3600 mg/day
  - Gabapentin—30 to 100 mg/kg/day
  - Lamotrigine—1 to 15 mg/kg/day up 300 to 500 mg/day
  - Levetiracetam—40 to 100 mg/kg/day, up to 1200 to 2400 mg/day
  - Phenobarbitol—2 to 6 mg/kg/day, up to 60 to 120 mg/day
  - Phenytoin—4 to 8 mg/kg/day, up to 200 to 600 mg/day
  - Topirimate—5 to 25 mg/kg/day, up to 100 to 400 mg/day
  - Valproic Acid—20 to 60 mg/kg/day, adult level 750 to 1500 mg/day
  - Zonisamide—4 to 10 mg/kg/day, up to 200 to 600 mg/day

Exercises
- Protective helmet when up
- No drastic changes in activity levels

Modalities
- Ketogenic diet is sometimes tried—high in fats and low in protein and carbohydrates; initially may see hypoglycemia and acidosis

Injection
- N/A

Surgical
- Vagal nerve stimulator—is an implantable device which attaches to the left vagus nerve with a goal to prevent or interrupt a seizure
- Neurosurgery—used for medically intractable seizures or seizures resistant to medication, and requires identification of epileptiform focus

Consults
- Neurology/neurosurgery

Complications of treatment
- Gingival hyperplasia from prolonged use of some AEDs

Helpful Hints
- Driving—usually permitted if no seizures within 1 year and under the care of a physician
- Sports—swimming with a buddy, no height (climbing or parachuting) or scuba activities

Suggested Readings

Nabbout R, Dulac O. Epileptic syndrome in infancy and childhood. *Curr Opin Neurol.*2008;21:161-166.

Tuxhorn I, Kotagal P. Classification. *Semin Neuro.* 2008;28:277-288.

Section II: Pediatric Diseases and Complications

Sensory Integration Deficits

Rajashree Srinivasan MD

Description

Sensory integration (SI) is the organization of sensation for use. The information obtained from the surroundings and the physical conditions of our body is streamlined by the brain. It has been described as the most important type of sensory processing.

Sensory integration disorders (SIDs) are described as the result of poor integration of sensation by the brain. Hence, the disorders are thought to be due to the brain not being able to put information together. This is not recognized as a diagnosis in *Diagnostic and Statistical Manual of Mental Disorders, 4th ed., Text Revision* or *The International Statistical Classification of Diseases and Related Health Problems, 10th Revision*, but is commonly reported.

Etiology/Types

Described as three types of SIDs:
- Type I—Sensory modulation disorder: over or under responding to sensory stimuli. Child may have fearful or anxious behaviors, negative or stubborn behaviors, self-absorbed behaviors or constantly seeking attention
- Type II—Sensory-based motor disorder: disorganized motor output due to incorrect processing of sensory information
- Type III—Sensory discrimination disorder: sensory discrimination or postural challenges seen. Dyspraxia, inattentiveness, disorganization, or poor school performance are seen
- These children reportedly usually have average or above average intelligence
- Multifactorial
- Genetic
- Environmental

Epidemiology

- It has been theorized that 5% to 10% of children have some type of problem with SI
- Boys more than girls

Pathogenesis

- Unknown
- Difficult as there is no way to measure the disorder in the brain at present

- Theoretically, children classically obtain sensory stimulation from regular play and do not need therapy. However, in a child with sensory integrative dysfunction, the neurologic problem prevents the processing of sensations of play, precluding the development of adaptive responses that organize the brain
- The different senses involved in SI are the auditory system, vestibular system, proprioceptive, tactile, and visual input
- These senses help to develop the ability to concentrate, organize, and can contribute to the capacity for abstract thought and reasoning, self-confidence, self-control, and self-esteem

Clinical Features

- Often hyperactive
- Disturbed by excess sensory input—sound, sight, or touch
- Difficulty being touched
- Inconsolable

Natural History

- Variable

Diagnosis

Differential diagnosis

- Behavioral disorders
- Autism
- Cerebral palsy
- Fetal alcohol syndrome
- Fragile X syndrome
- Brain injury

History

- Some infants have delayed motor milestones
- Later they may have trouble learning to tie shoe laces, riding a bicycle without training wheels, and so on
- Awkward running, clumsiness, frequent falls, or stumbling
- Delay in language development; problems with listening may be seen
- Difficulty coloring between lines or cutting with scissors may be seen

- Some children may get anxious and angry when touched
- Problems may be more apparent when entering school
- The stress of following two step commands, in addition to dealing with learning new information, can make school problematic

Exam
- Intolerance to touch and sound
- Clumsy, poor balance
- Lack of variety in play

Testing
- Sensory profile evaluation by certified therapists (auditory, visual, and touch)

Pitfalls
- Lack of uniformly accepted specific criteria

Red Flags
- N/A

Treatment

Medical

SI therapy
- Therapy aims to provide and control sensory input from vestibular system, muscles, joints, and skin in a way to attempt to guide the child to form the adaptive responses needed to integrate the responses
- SI therapy is a specialty of occupational therapy, which emphasizes human behavior from a neurologic viewpoint
- SI therapy focus is on integrating function, including activities like finger painting and play-doh activities

Modalities
- To provide sensory input

Injection
- N/A

Surgery
- N/A

Consultations
- Developmental pediatrics
- Neurology

Complications
- N/A

Suggested Readings

Ayres AJ. *Sensory Integration and the Child: 25th Anniversary Edition.* Los Angeles, CA: Western psychological Services; 2005.

Greenspan S. The development of the ego: biological and environmental specificity in the psychopathological developmental process and the selection and construction of ego defenses. *J Am Psychoanal Assoc.* 1989;37:605–638.

Section II: Pediatric Diseases and Complications

Sialorrhea

Elizabeth Moberg-Wolff MD

Description
Sialorrhea, ptyalism, or drooling is the unintentional loss of saliva from the mouth. This affects up to 40% of children with neurologic impairment.

Etiology/Types
- Drooling may occur anteriorly or posteriorly in the mouth; the latter is more likely to cause aspiration by going down the throat
- Poor oral motor control (impaired swallow, poor lip closure) is typically the cause in neurologic disorders such as cerebral palsy, rather than excessive salivation
- Medications, disease, or poisons may cause excessive production of saliva

Epidemiology
- Normal until age 4
- Wide variation in severity

Pathogenesis
- Muscarinic receptors in the sublingual, submaxillary glands, and parotid glands are controlled by the cholinergic system
- Parotid glands produce the majority of saliva and react mainly when stimulated
- Submandibular and sublingual glands produce 70% of unstimulated salivation
- Saliva is vital to assisting with swallowing, remineralizing tooth enamel, buffering cariogenic acids, removing food residue, and inhibiting bacterial growth

Risk Factors
- Neurologic disease
- Dysphagia
- Poor head and trunk positioning
- Medication use

Clinical Features
- Wet chin
- Rash on chin
- Tongue thrusting
- Poor lip closure
- Choking
- Poor head control

Natural History
- Normal while teething, up to 4 years
- Wide variability in severity

Diagnosis

Differential diagnosis
- Teething
- Epiglotittis
- Medication side effect or overdose (L-dopa pilocarpine, etc.)
- Poisoning (insecticides, arsenic, mercury, etc.)
- Parotiditis/mumps
- Macroglossia
- Sialadenitis (salivary gland infection)
- Worsening neurologic disease
- Rabies
- Glandular tumor

History
- Increasing symptoms with oral motor stimulation
- Increasing symptoms with focused activities
- Recent dental problems

Exam
- Excessive pooling of saliva in the anterior mouth
- Poor lip closure
- Tongue thrusting
- Chin redness or rash

Testing
- Drooling Scale—Five-point scale of severity, and four-point scale of frequency of drooling
- Swallow study
- pH study for gastroesophageal reflux
- Radionucleotide salivagram study
- Milk scan—drink milk with dye and evaluate for aspiration

Pitfalls
- Missed tumor
- Overtreatment can cause dental decay and dysphagia

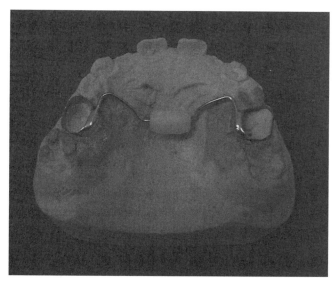

Dental "bead" retainer aids lip closure and tongue movement to direct saliva toward the pharynx.

Red Flags

- Facial rash
- Asymmetric gland swelling: infection/tumor
- Social stigmatization
- Worsening neurologic dysfunction

Treatment

Medical

- Anticholinergic medications such as scopalamine (patch, gel, and pills), glycopyrrolate (liquid, pill), and trihexylphenidyl (liquid, pill) may be effective. Their ease and frequency of use must be correlated with the severity and frequency of sialorrhea
- Antireflux medications (proton pump inhibitors, H_2 antagonists) may reduce saliva production by reducing stimulus in some patients

Exercises

- Oral motor strengthening
- Head and trunk positioning

Modalities

- Dental "bead" retainer—aids lip closure and tongue movement to direct saliva toward the pharynx; only useful in those that tolerate oral hygiene (see figure)
- Biofeedback

Injection

- Botulinum toxin injections into glands with ultrasound guidance may reduce production for several months

Surgical

- Ductal ligation
- Ductal rerouting
- Gland excision
- Salivary denervation (transtympanic neurectomy)

Consults

- ENT
- Neurology
- Dental

Complications of treatment

- Dysphagia from excessive dryness
- Dental decay
- Infection
- Sialocele
- Facial nerve paralysis

Prognosis

- Highly variable

Helpful Hints

- Dental bead retainer and botulinum toxin injections provide treatment options

Suggested Readings

Blasco PA, Allaire JH. Drooling in the developmentally disabled: management practices and recommendations. Consortium on Drooling. *Dev Med Child Neurol.* 1992;34:849-862.

Erasmus CE, VanHulst K, Rotteveel LJ, Jongerius PH, VanDenHoogenFJ, Roeleveld N, et al. Drooling in cerebral palsy: hypersalivation or dysfunctional oral motor control? *Dev Med Child Neurol.* 2009;51(6):454–459.

Section II: Pediatric Diseases and Complications

Sickle Cell Disease

Maurice Sholas MD PhD

Description

Sickle cell disease is an inherited hemoglobinopathy that distorts red blood cells and inhibits its ability to carry oxygen. It shortens the red cell life span and leads to vascular occlusion. There is a chronic hemolytic anemia and intermittent vaso-occlusive pain crises.

Etiology

- The etiology of the disease is a mutation in the hemoglobin B gene, a substitution of valine for glutamine that causes production of hemoglobin S. The error makes the hemoglobin change shape under situations of low oxygen tension. This conformational change makes the red blood cell less compliant and not able to flow through small blood vessels
- Two sickle genes are required for sickle disease
- Autosomal recessive transmission pattern

Epidemiology

- Sickle cell anemia (SCA) is the most common heritable blood disorder in the United States
- Incidence is 1 in 500 blacks in America
- Incidence is 1 in 1000 to 1400 Hispanics
- Eight percent of black American population has at least one sickle gene (carrier status)

Pathogenesis

- There is a substitution of valine for glutamate which makes hemoglobin less soluble when oxygen tension is low or when there is increased acidity, thus the hemoglobin crystallizes
- Dehydration, increased acidity, and low oxygen levels lead to this phenomenon on a large scale
- Red blood cells with crystallized hemoglobin do not deform normally to allow flow through small capillaries
- Red blood cells with sickle hemoglobin carry less oxygen
- The decreased oxygen-carrying capacity combined with the obstructed blood flow leads to infarcts
- The location of the infarcts determines the symptoms

Risk Factors

- Genetic inheritance
- Black, Mediterranean, or Hispanic origin

Clinical Features

- Fatigue and anemia
- Pain crises
- Dactylitis and arthritis
- Bacterial infections
- Failure to thrive
- Growth retardation

Natural History

- Initial symptoms do not present until older than 5 months of age as there is presence of protective fetal hemoglobin in the postnatal period
- Does not resolve with time
- There are varying severities of expression of the disease process due to various genetic modulators
- The pain crises recur and require hydration and aggressive narcotics for pain control
- Over time, these patients become asplenic (from trapping misshapen blood cells in the spleen, causing anemia and swelling, and eventual autoinfarction of the spleen) and susceptible to bacterial infection, particularly encapsulated ones
- Those with the worst prognosis have strokes
- Twenty-five percent of those with SCA will have a stroke

Diagnosis

Differential diagnosis

- Iron deficiency anemia
- Thalassemia
- Aplastic anemia
- Leukemia
- Nutritional deficits

History

- Fatigue
- Failure to thrive
- Recurrent pain episodes
- Recurrent infections
- Swelling/inflammation of hands and/or feet
- Priapism
- Recurrent pneumonia
- Familial risk factors

Exam
- Small frame or small for age
- Absent spleen
- Liver enlargement
- Scleral icterus
- Heart murmurs
- Leg ulcers
- Retinal hemorrhage
- Pain with weight bearing to large joints or decreased range of motion

Testing
- Hemoglobin electrophoresis is the gold standard
- Low oxygen prep blood smear
- X-rays to look for signs of joint arthritis, aseptic necrosis, or bone infarcts
- Brain magnetic resonance imaging for evidence of old infarcts

Pitfalls
- Undertreating pain crisis
- Overexertion-induced crises

Red Flags
- Recurrent infection
- Pathological fracture
- Chest crisis—new infiltrate on chest x-ray and fever, cough, sputum production, dyspnea, or hypoxia; acute chest syndrome is the leading cause of death
- Recurrent cerebrovascular accidents
- Failure to thrive

Treatment

Medical
- Hydroxyurea
- Pneumococcal vaccine
- Analgesics
- Exchange transfusions
- Bone marrow transplant

Exercises
- Avoid high dynamic activities
- Avoid exercise to the point of exhaustion
- Maintain hydration status in warm environment/exercise

Modalities
- Moist heat
- Ice

Surgical
- Surgical stabilization of unstable fractures
- Joint replacement

Consults
- Hematology/oncology
- Pain service
- Genetics

Complications
- Progressive pain and dysfunction
- Cerebral infarcts
- Joint inflammation and pain
- Osteomyelitis
- Osteopenia
- Bone infarcts with pathological fractures
- Hepatomegaly and jaundice
- Pneumonia
- Extremity ulcers
- Priapism
- Retinal hemorrhage and detachment
- Blindness

Prognosis
- With optimal management life span is into the fourth decade
- Bacterial infection is most common cause of death
- Progressive tissue and organ damage
- Recurrent pain crises negatively impacting quality of life

Helpful Hints
- Pain control and monitoring for sequelae of bone or joint destruction is most often overlooked
- Heterozygous sickle cell carriers are thought to have selective advantage against malaria

Suggested Reading
Bunn HF. Pathogenesis and treatment of sickle cell disease. *N Engl J Med.* 1997;337:762–769.

Sleep Apnea: Central

Anne May MD ■ Mark Splaingard MD

Description

Sleep apnea is the cessation of airflow during sleep for 20 seconds or two respiratory cycles, associated with a drop in oxygen saturation ≥4% from baseline, electrocortical arousal, or awakening. Sleep apnea may be divided into two broad categories based on specific characteristics: obstructive sleep apnea and central sleep apnea.

Etiology

- Central sleep apnea is due to inappropriate nervous system signaling or ineffective feedback due to cardiopulmonary disease (i.e., congestive heart failure [CHF])

Pathogenesis

- Hyperventilation
  - Obstruction or hypoxia stimulates increased respiratory rate (hyperventilation), causing decreased pCO_2, with cessation of respiratory drive and resultant central apnea
  - Central apnea persists until pCO_2 rises above "set point" when ventilation resumes
- Hypoventilation
  - Reduced drive to breathe causes either central apnea or increased pCO_2
  - pCO_2 "set point" is altered with metabolic compensation
  - At onset of sleep, the wake control of breathing is lost, and central apnea becomes more frequent
- Causes include
  - Sedatives, narcotics, antiepileptics
  - Medullary/pontine/massive cortical injury
  - Arnold Chiari malformation

Risk Factors

- Brain injury or tumor
- Stroke

Epidemiology

- Occurs in 80% of preterm infants at 30 weeks' gestational age
- Disappears in most infants by 46 weeks' gestational age
- Common in brain injury, Chiari malformations, and heart failure

Clinical Features

- Pauses in breathing without respiratory effort, cyanosis, and gasping
- Morning headaches
- Seizures

Natural History

- Depends on successful treatment of underlying etiology

Diagnosis

Differential diagnosis

- Seizure activity, congenital central hypoventilation syndrome
- Cheyne-Stokes respiration
  - Crescendo/decrescendo respiratory pattern seen in patients with CHF and neurologic disease

History

- Cyanotic episodes
- Daytime sleepiness or agitation
- Snorting may be heard with arousal and resumption of breathing
- Morning headaches
- ALTE (acute life-threatening event)

Exam

- Abnormal neurologic examination, cerebral palsy, and myelomeningocele

Testing (polysomnography)

- Absent or reduced airflow without evidence of thoracoabdominal movement for 10 seconds with oxygen desaturation (or 15–20 seconds without desaturation)

Red Flags

- Morning headaches
- Daytime sleepiness
- Seizures
- Cyanosis
- ALTE

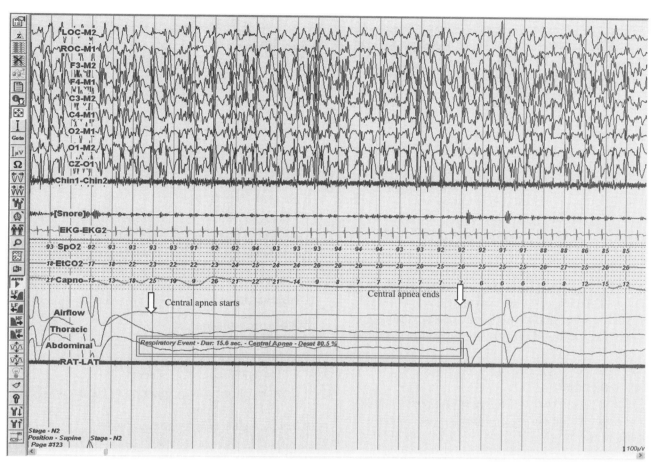

Eleven-year-old with CP, abnormal generalized spike wake activity and central apneas (30-second tracing).

Treatment
- Varies with etiology
- Respiratory stimulants
  - Caffeine in preterm infants, theophylline
- Bilevel positive airway pressure with back up rate
- Tracheostomy with positive pressure ventilation and rate during sleep

Consults
- Pulmonology

Complications
- Seizures

Prognosis
- Symptoms resolve and long-term complications avoided with adequate treatment of underlying disease
- Monitoring for compliance is needed

Helpful Hints
- Compliance with continuous positive airway pressure (CPAP)/bilevel positive airway pressure (BiPAP) can be improved with appropriate delivery; multiple methods available to maximize comfort
- CPAP/BiPAP via tracheostomy should not be standard, since these devices are not FDA approved in pediatrics. Home mechanical ventilators preferred

Suggested Readings
Fauroux B. What's new in paediatric sleep? *Paediatr Resp Rev.* 2007;8:85-89.

Robet D, Argaud L. Non-invasive positive ventilation in the treatment of sleep-related breathing disorders. *Sleep Med.* 2007;8:441-452.

Section II: Pediatric Diseases and Complications

Sleep Apnea: Obstructive

Mark Splaingard MD ■ Anne May MD

Description

Sleep apnea is the cessation of airflow during sleep for 20 seconds or two respiratory cycles, associated with drop in oxygen saturation ≥4%, electrocortical arousal, or awakening. Sleep apnea may be divided into two broad categories based on specific characteristics: obstructive sleep apnea (OSA) and central sleep apnea.

Etiology

- In OSA, decrease in muscular tone and/or airway diameter leads to obstruction of airway, resulting in decreased airflow despite respiratory efforts during sleep

Pathogenesis

- Onset of sleep leads to decreased pharyngeal muscle tone, worsening during random eye movement (dream) sleep
- Decreased pharyngeal musculature tone causes airway narrowing
- Partially narrowed airways due to enlarged tonsils, adenoids, tongue, or small jaw are more easily obstructed.
- Obstruction leads to frequent O_2 desaturations, which resolve with arousals (partial awakenings from sleep) that causes sleep fragmentation
- Sleep fragmentation may cause cognitive, behavioral, and mood problems

Epidemiology

- Ten percent of 5-year-olds snore, with 2% to 3% having OSA

Risk Factors

- Obesity
- Neurologic or craniofacial abnormalities with narrow airway
- Family history

Clinical Features

- Daytime hyperactivity, irritability, or less frequently, sleepiness
- Nocturnal restlessness or awakening

- Gasping, snoring (usually inspiratory), cessation of breathing, sweating during sleep, or unusual sleeping posture (neck extended or head down)

Natural History

- Mild OSA may worsen with normal adenotonsillar growth between ages 2 and 6 years
- Untreated OSA can lead to pulmonary hypertension, cor pulmonale, systemic hypertension, and death

Diagnosis

Differential diagnosis

- Fixed airway obstruction (subglottic stenosis, vocal cord paralysis, and subglottic hemangioma). Noise will be while awake or asleep
- Primary snoring (snoring without OSA), which is typically inspiratory
- Tracheomalacia/laryngomalacia
  - Tracheomalacia is usually an expiratory noise; laryngomalaica is typically inspiratory
  - Noise generally increases with effort or stress, and often varies with position

History

- Daytime sleepiness or hyperactivity
- Nocturnal enuresis, especially new onset
- Snoring/gasping during sleep
- Morning headaches

Exam

- Enlarged tonsils/adenoids, nasal polyps
- Obesity
- Craniofacial anomalies, micrognathia

Testing (Polysomnography)

- Apnea/hypopnea index (AHI) >1.5 (more than 1.5 events/hour) in children; (AHI) >5 in adults
- Absent or reduced airflow accompanied by evidence of thoracoabdominal movement

Red Flags

- Morning headaches
- Markedly increased daytime sleepiness
- Cyanosis
- Acute life-threatening event

Treatment

- Adenotonsillectomy
- Continuous positive airway pressure (CPAP) or bilevel positive airway pressure (BiPAP)
- Tracheostomy is generally curative, unless lower airway pathology; ventilation is not routinely needed with tracheostomy

Prognosis

- Seventy percent of children with OSA improve/resolve after adenotonsillectomy
  - Decreased cure rate in children with obesity, craniofacial abnormalities, and neurologic disorders such as cerebral palsy.
- Symptoms resolve and long-term complications are avoided with adequate treatment

- Monitoring for compliance is needed—CPAP compliance may be only 40%

Helpful Hints

- Compliance with CPAP/BiPAP can be improved with appropriate delivery; multiple methods are available to maximize comfort
- CPAP/BiPAP via tracheostomy should not be standard, since these devices are not FDA approved in pediatrics; home ventilators should be preferred

Suggested Readings

Dayyat E, Kheirandish-Gozal L, Gozal D. Childhood obstructive sleep apnea: one or two distinct disease entities? *Sleep Med Clin.* 2007;2(3):433–444.

Robet D, Argaud L. Non-invasive positive ventilation in the treatment of sleep-related breathing disorders. *Sleep Medicine.* 2007;8:441–452.

Section II: Pediatric Diseases and Complications

Small Stature/Achondroplasia

Andre N. Panagos MD

Description
Achondroplasia is the most common form of dwarfism, resulting in a characteristically large head with frontal bossing and a long narrow trunk with short limbs.

Etiology/Types
- Autosomal dominant inheritance
- Fibroblast growth factor receptor 3 gene (FGFR3) point mutation causes 95% of cases
- Eighty percent of cases are new mutations

Epidemiology
- Achondroplasia is the most common form of dwarfism
- Occurs in 1 in 10,000 to 30,000 live births
- Affects 250,000 individuals worldwide

Pathogenesis
- Decreased endochondral bone growth

Risk Factors
- Familial inheritance
- Spontaneous mutation risk factors are unknown

Clinical Features
- Large head with frontal bossing
- Hypoplastic midface
- Long narrow trunk with short limbs
- Joint hyperextensibility affecting the hands and knees
- Restricted elbow rotation and extension
- Thoracolumbar gibbus may develop by 4 months of age leading to a fixed kyphoscoliosis
- Exaggerated lumbar lordosis
- Infants may develop respiratory distress due to cervical medullary compression
- Motor development may be delayed due to narrowing of the foramen magnum
- Tibial bowing affects 42% of the population
- Neurogenic claudication and spinal stenosis are common in older children and adults

Natural History
- Cervical and lumbar spinal stenosis with aging
- Increasing back pain due to spinal stenosis, exaggerated lumbar lordosis, and spondylosis
- Ten percent of affected individuals have neurogenic claudication by 10 years of age
- Eighty percent of affected individuals have neurogenic claudication by 60 years of age

Diagnosis

Differential diagnosis
- Hypochondroplasia
- Severe achondroplasia with developmental delay and acanthosis nigricans
- Thanatophoric dysplasia type I and II
- Other causes of short stature include familial short stature, genetic disorders (Turner syndrome), chronic disease, malnutrition, endocrine disorders (growth hormone [GH] deficiency), and constitutional delay

History
- Increasing neck or low back pain
- Increased weakness
- Decreased function and mobility
- Assessing birth length, weight, and fronto-occipital circumference
- Final height and weight of parents and siblings

Exam
- Short stature
- Large head with frontal bossing
- Hypoplastic midface
- Long narrow trunk with short limbs
- Lower motor neuron or upper motor neuron findings
- Fixed kyphoscoliosis or exaggerated lumbar lordosis

Testing
- Serum levels of insulin-like growth factor (IGF-1) and IGF-binding protein-3
- Serum levels of GH
- DNA testing
- X-rays demonstrate normal height and width of vertebral bodies with short, thickened pedicles throughout the spine
- X-rays to assess growth plates
- Narrowed central spinal canal
- Exaggerated lumbar lordosis

- Computed tomography is used to assess for medullary compression due to craniocervical stenosis
- Somatosensory-evoked potentials may be used to assess cervical cord compression
- Electrodiagnostic studies to assess radicular symptoms

Pitfalls

- Repetitive nerve compression injuries may result in irreversible muscle atrophy and loss of mobility

Red Flags

- Tetraplegia
- Cauda equina syndrome

Treatment

Medical

- Nonsteroidal anti-inflammatory drugs
- A trial of bracing may be helpful for back pain and curvature reduction
- Recombinant human GH; used to stimulate growth, if deficient GH levels
- Recombinant IGF-1; used to stimulate growth, if normal stimulated GH levels

Exercises

- General strengthening and stretching

Modalities

- Heat, cold, ultrasound, and transcutaneous electrical nerve stimulation have been used for symptomatic relief of pain and muscle spasms.

Injection

- Trigger point injections for symptoms of myofascial pain
- Epidural steroid injection for radicular symptoms

Surgical

- Five percent to 10% of patients have cervical medullary decompression surgery as early as infancy
- Extensive decompressive laminectomy may need to be performed, which may involve the entire spine
- Reoperation may be required within 8 years

Consults

- Physical medicine and rehabilitation
- Neurosurgery or orthopedic spine surgery
- Neurology
- Pediatric endocrinologist
- Psychologist to focus on peer acceptance and eating disorders

Complications of treatment

- Syringomyelia
- Tetraplegia
- Persistent and severe sciatica
- Cauda equina syndrome
- Delayed diagnosis of occult chronic disease

Prognosis

- Continued function is possible if assessed early and surgically treated

Helpful Hints

- Repetitive nerve compression injuries may result in irreversible muscle atrophy and loss of mobility so early treatment is important

Suggested Readings

Boguszewski CL, Carlsson B, Carlsson LM. Mechanisms of growth failure in non-growth-hormone deficient children of short stature. *Horm Res.* 1997;48:19-22.

Horton WA, Hall JG, Hecht JT. Achondroplasia. *Lancet.* 2007;370:162-172.

Lee MM. Clinical practice. Idiopathic short stature. *N Engl J Med.* 2006;354:2576-2582.

Section II: Pediatric Diseases and Complications

Spasticity

Judith L. Gooch MD

Description

Hypertonia: abnormally increased resistance to externally imposed movement about a joint. It may be caused by spasticity, dystonia, rigidity, or a combination of factors. In spasticity or spastic hypertonia, resistance to externally imposed movement increases with increasing speed of stretch and varies with the direction of stretch.

Etiology

- Upper motor neuron disorder
- Spasticity can result from injury along the pathway connecting the primary motor and premotor cortex to the spinal circuitry
- Patients with stroke, cerebral palsy, traumatic brain injury, and spinal cord injury typically develop spasticity

Epidemiology

- Related to the epidemiology of the underlying neurological conditions

Pathogenesis

- Pathophysiology incompletely understood
- Mechanisms may vary with location of injury
- Main hypotheses include: increased stretch induced stimulation of muscle spindles in less extensible muscles, increased excitability of alpha motor neurons, and increased excitability of spinal interneuronal pathways

Risk Factors

- Injury to the pyramidal motor system leading to the upper motor syndrome

Clinical Features

- Hypertonia which increases with speed of stretch and varies with the direction of joint movement
- Resistance to stretch rises rapidly above a threshold speed or joint angle
- Varies with state of alertness, position, emotional state, and activity level
- Typically affects flexor, adductor, and internal rotator muscles more than antagonists
- Children with extrapyramidal injury often manifest with dystonia and/or athetosis; dystonia may show

hypertonicity exacerbated by voluntary movements, independent of posture and speed
- Children with cerebral palsy often have both spasticity and dystonia
- Contractures

Natural History

- Often evident by 1 year of age, but may be present earlier in children with severe neurologic impairment
- Effects of spasticity often worsen as a child grows, with prolonged muscle contraction leading to contractures and joint deformities

Diagnosis

Differential diagnosis

- Contracture
- Hypertonia due to dystonia or rigidity

History

- Limb tightness
- Decreased function, pain, and difficulty with activities of daily living (ADLs)

Exam

- Hypertonia
- Spastic catch: a sudden resistance to rapid passive stretching
- Affects flexor, adductor, and internal rotator muscles most

Testing

- Clinical exam: palpation of the muscle at rest, measure resistance to movement at different speeds and positions
- Ashworth scale (see Ratings Scales chapter)
- Tardieu scale compares occurrence of a catch at low and high speeds (see Ratings Scales chapter)
- Assess functional abilities to determine whether spasticity has a beneficial or detrimental effect on function

Pitfalls

- May be a useful adaptive response to weakness by increasing muscle activation for facilitating transfers and standing

■ Differentiating from contracture and other types of hypertonia

Red Flags

■ Eliminating spasticity that is beneficial to function

Treatment

Medical

■ Baclofen, benzodiazepines, tizanidine, dantrolene sodium, and gabapentin

Exercises

■ Stretching
■ Strengthening
■ Functional training

Modalities

■ Splints/orthotic devices
■ Serial casting
■ Electrical stimulation

Injections

■ Botulinum toxin
■ Phenol
■ Alcohol

Surgical

■ Intrathecal baclofen pump implantation

■ Selective dorsal rhizotomy
■ Orthopedic intervention

Consults

■ Neurology
■ Neurosurgery
■ Orthopedic surgery

Complications

■ Deformity
■ Pain
■ Difficulties with ADLs
■ Functional limitations

Prognosis

■ Variable, depends upon underlying condition

Helpful Hints

■ Manage early to minimize complications

Suggested Readings

Albright AL. Neurosurgical treatment of spasticity and other pediatric movement disorders. *J Child Neurol.* 2003;18 (suppl 1):S67–S78.

Sanger TD, Delgado MR, Gaebler-Spira D, Hallett M, Mink JW; Task Force on Childhood Motor Disorders. Classification and definition of disorders causing hypertonia in childhood. *Pediatrics.* 2003;111(1):e89–e97.

Spinal Cord Injury: Paraplegia

Ellen S. Kaitz MD ■ Carl D. Gelfius MD

Description
Paralysis of both lower limbs due to an injury or abnormality of the thoracic, lumbar, or sacral spinal cord.

Etiology/Types
- Traumatic: including motor vehicle accident (MVA), falls, sports, and violence
- From hyperflexion injury, compressive injury, expansile lesion, traction/stretch injury, shear injury with/without distraction, burst injury, Chance fracture, and other spinal fracture
- Nontraumatic: including congenital, inflammatory, neoplastic, infectious, vascular, toxic, and radiation
- Spinal cord injury (SCI) without radiographic abnormality (SCIWORA)

Epidemiology
- Pediatric SCIs comprise ~5% of all reported SCIs up to age 15 years, then ~15% for those 16 to 20 years, for an incidence of nearly 500 and 1800 yearly, respectively, for these two groups (in United States)
- Thoracic, lumbar, and sacral SCI account for 20% to 40% of pediatric SCI
- Traumatic pediatric SCI at all levels most commonly results from MVAs, falls, firearm injury/gunshot wounds, and sport-related injury

Pathogenesis
- SCI below the cervical level
- Inflammatory injury
- Infection

Risk Factors
- Male gender (variably reported, up to 2:1 M:F with difference starting in toddlers and greatest in adolescents)
- Age 9 years and older

Clinical Features
- Impaired or absent sensation
- Impaired or absent motor control
- Impaired sitting balance with upper thoracic injury
- Impaired respiratory status with thoracic injury
- Impaired or absent bladder/bowel continence
- Initial areflexia of the lower limbs often followed by hyperreflexia/clonus
- Spasticity of the lower limbs
- SCI level and grade categorized using the American Spinal Injury Association (ASIA) Impairment Scale (see Ratings Scales chapter)
- Abnormal thermoregulation and risk of autonomic dysreflexia for those with high thoracic level injury

Natural History
- Initial spinal shock with loss of reflexes below the level of injury; reflexes return within weeks to months
- Initial ileus and low rectal tone during acute injury phase progress to delayed bowel emptying and rectal tone
- Expected bladder capacity: age in years +2 equals ounces (×30 equals cc)
- Parents initiate bowel/bladder management by age 3
- Patients can begin self-cath and bowel program at developmental age 5 years
- More rostral injuries in skeletally immature individuals can result in scoliosis (up to 98%)
- Restrictive lung disease may result from scoliosis and increase risk for pneumonia
- Hip dislocations may result when injury occurs before 10 years of age (up to 93%)
- Life expectancy for pediatric paraplegic patients is greater than that for pediatric tetraplegic patients; however, adult-onset paraplegic patients have a greater life expectance than pediatric-onset paraplegic patients
- Risk of heterotopic ossification (HO)
- Risk of pressure ulcers
- Risk of frequent urinary tract infections, renal disease, and spasticity
- Risk of late deterioration due to syrinx

Diagnosis

Differential diagnosis
- Transverse myelitis
- Acute inflammatory demyelinating polyneuropathy
- Toxic myelopathy
- Conversion disorder
- Syphilis

History
- Trauma, infection, tumor, as relevant
- Lower limb weakness/paralysis
- Inability to stand/walk, with frequent falls
- Numbness/tingling, and absent sensation
- Constipation
- Urinary retention
- Bowel/bladder incontinence
- Trauma
- Back pain
- Abnormal thermoregulation (in those with injuries above T7)

Exam
- Poor trunk control in many
- Lower limb weakness/paralysis
- Impaired or absent light touch and pin prick sensation of the torso and/or lower limbs
- Lower motor neuron or upper motor neuron findings of the lower limbs
- Absent rectal sensation
- Absent voluntary anal contraction
- ASIA evaluation (see Ratings Scales chapter)

Testing
- X-rays, computed tomography, and/or magnetic resonance imaging
- Renal ultrasound to assess protection of kidneys with neurogenic bladder
- Urodynamic studies to assess optimal care of neurogenic bladder

Pitfalls
- Missing treatable etiology
- Missing hidden concomitant injuries
- Missing HO

Red Flags
- Rostral progression and/or progressive decrease in sensation/strength: risk of syrinx
- Autonomic dysreflexia risk (in those with injuries above T7)

- Hyperphagia, irritability, nausea, vomiting, may indicate hypercalcemia

Treatment

Medical

Early
- Thoracolumbosacral orthosis with or without surgery for 8 to 12 weeks posttrauma
- Evaluation for concomitant traumatic brain injury
- Deep venous thrombosis prophylaxis in pubertal patients
- Monitoring for immobilization hypercalcemia and hypercalciuria
- Incentive spirometry/cough assist

Long term
- Establishment of bladder program
- Establishment of bowel program
- Skin monitoring and pressure relief program
- Spasticity management
- Analgesia
- Monitoring for scoliosis

Exercises
- Comprehensive inpatient rehabilitation
- Strengthening and stretching exercises
- Energy conservation techniques
- Adaptive techniques and equipment use
- Balance, transfers, and mobility
- Wheelchair use and safety

Modalities
- Heat
- Cold
- Electrical nerve stimulation
- Orthoses

Injection
- Trigger point injections
- Epidural steroid injections for radicular pain

Surgical
- Anterior, posterior, or combined anterior-posterior fusion
- Mitrofanoff procedure (see Bladder chapter)
- Bladder augmentation (see Bladder chapter)
- Antegrade continence enema procedure (see Bowel chapter)

Consults

- Neurosurgery or orthopedic spine surgery
- Urology
- Rehabilitation psychology

Complications

- Syringomyelia
- Chronic neuropathic pain
- Upper limb overuse syndromes, including shoulders, elbows, and wrists
- Dermal pressure ulcer

Prognosis

- Good potential for independence/modified-independence with self-care, bowel/bladder management, transfers, and mobility

- Become a community ambulatory if L3 or lower injury and preserved lower limb range of motion

Helpful Hints

- Early education on ergonomics and appropriate modifications may minimize or delay future repetitive motion injuries in the arms

Suggested Readings

Cirak B, Ziegfeld S, Knight VM. Spinal injuries in children. *J Pediatr Surg.* 2004;34(4):607–612.

Vogel LC, Mendoza MM, Schottler JC, et al. Ambulation in children and youth with spinal cord injuries. *J Spinal Cord Med.* 2007;30(1):S158–S164.

Spinal Cord Injury: Tetraplegia

Maria R. Reyes MD ■ Teresa L. Massagli MD

Description

Paralysis of both lower limbs due to an injury or abnormality of the cervical spinal cord. Cervical injury occurs in 30% to 55% of children and adolescents with spinal cord injury (SCI).

Etiology/Types

- Traumatic: motor vehicle, pedestrian, sports, and acts of violence (including nonaccidental trauma)
- Nontraumatic: infection, tumor, juvenile rheumatoid arthritis (JRA), skeletal dysplasias, and transverse myelitis
- Neonatal: torsion or traction

Epidemiology

- Traumatic: male:female ratio similar up to age 3; after age 3, males exceed females
- Neonatal: 1 per 60,000 births
- Children younger than 15 years account for ~5% or 500 of new traumatic SCIs annually, and those from 16 to 20 years are about 15% or 1800 of those injured in the United States

Pathogenesis

- Immature spine (until 8 to 10 years for upper cervical spine; 14 years for lower cervical spine): elastic spinal ligaments, incomplete ossification of vertebrae, relative large head, high fulcrum of flexion extension (C2–C3), and shallow facet orientation
- Insult to cervical spinal cord

Risk Factors

- Improper use of seat belts, car seats, or booster seats
- Down syndrome: atlantoaxial instability
- JRA: synovitis, especially C1–2
- Achondroplasia: narrow foramen magnum

Clinical Features

- 0 to 8 years: 30% of SCI results in tetraplegia; higher incidence C1–C3; 1/3 incomplete
- 9 to 15 years: 53% tetraplegia; more likely C4–C6; 48% incomplete
- Impaired or absent sensation and motor control
- Impaired respiratory status
- Impaired bowel/bladder control
- Impaired autonomic function
- Impaired balance, trunk control, ± head control

Natural History

- Initial spinal shock with loss of reflexes below the level of injury; reflexes return within weeks to months
- Most patients with complete tetraplegia below C4 gain one motor level of function during the first year
- Initial ileus and low rectal tone during acute injury phase progress to delayed bowel emptying and rectal tone
- All levels of tetraplegia at risk for restrictive lung disease, atelectasis, and weak cough
- Intrinsic minus hand can prevent tenodesis grasp
- Scoliosis likely if SCI prior to puberty
- Menarche similar to uninjured population; may have amenorrhea up to 6 months after injury
- Expected bladder capacity: age in years +2 equals ounces (×30 equals cc)
- Initially bladder detrusor is flaccid, then progresses to reflex contractions and detrusor sphincter dyssynergia
- Parents initiate bowel/bladder management by age 3
- Patients can begin self-catheterization and bowel program at developmental age 5 if they can reach perineum
- Transfers: <4 years old dependent; 5 to 7 years old can learn sliding board
- Power mobility: as young as 18 to 24 months, depending on cognition and supervision
- Children <8 years old (and some older children) with injuries at C7 to T1 may not have enough strength to use manual wheelchair in the community

Diagnosis

Differential diagnosis

- Transverse myelitis
- Acute disseminated encephalomyelitis
- Conversion disorder

History

- Mechanism of injury
- Associated traumatic brain injury

- Complete review of systems: especially pain, respiratory, cardiovascular, gastrointestinal, genitourinary, skin

Exam
- The American Spinal Injury Association exam for motor and sensory level, completeness of injury (see Ratings Scales chapter)
- Skin
- Range of motion
- Spasticity assessment
- Chest auscultation
- Abdominal palpation

Testing
- Plain radiographs, computed tomography, magnetic resonance imaging (MRI)
- Spinal cord injury without radiographic abnormality (SCIWORA) in 60% age 0 to 10 years and 20% age 11 to 15 years; usually confirmed with MRI: anterior or posterior longitudinal ligament disruption, disk abnormality, cord injury, and endplate fractures

Pitfalls
- Young children (preschool age) may not be able to report dysreflexia symptoms
- Immobilization hypercalcemia may have insidious onset

Red Flags
- Ascending loss of sensory or motor function: syrinx
- Malaise: hypercalcemia, urinary tract infection (UTI), obstipation, and depression
- Facial sweating: autonomic dysreflexia, syrinx, and hyperthermia
- Urinary incontinence: UTI, detrusor hyperreflexia
- Lower extremity swelling: deep vein thrombosis, heterotopic ossification (HO), fracture, soft tissue hematoma

Treatment

Medical
- Halo orthosis, ± neurosurgery
- Pneumococcal and influenza vaccinations
- Autonomic dysreflexia protocol
- Thromboembolism prophylaxis
- Spasticity medications and stretching
- Hypercalcemia: normal saline, pamidronate, etidronate, and calcitonin

- Orthostatic hypotension: hydration, compression stockings, abdominal binder, and α-adrenergic medications
- Thermoregulation via environment and clothing

Exercises
- Glossopharyngeal breathing (if >7 to 8 years old)
- Incentive spirometry
- Strengthening of innervated muscles
- Range of motion exercises

Modalities
- Phrenic nerve pacing in C1–C3 injuries if intact lower motor neuron
- Spinal orthoses may be used to prevent progression of scoliosis exceeding 20° to 40°
- Hand splints; ankle-foot orthoses to maintain range of motion

Surgical
- Initial spine stabilization
- Spinal fusion for scoliosis
- Bladder augmentation if low capacity
- Continent urinary diversion to allow self-catheterization by those with some hand function
- Antegrade continence enema for bowel program, to enhance independence in patients who cannot do rectal digital stimulation or place suppository
- Upper extremity tendon transfers to facilitate function such as writing

Consults
- Neurosurgery or orthopedic spine surgery
- Urology

Complications
- Scoliosis; may further impair pulmonary function
- Venous thromboembolism
- Immobilization hypercalcemia: males > females
- Osteoporosis; fractures
- HO: incidence lower in children (3%) than adults (10%–20%)
- Hip dislocation
- Neurogenic bladder and bowel
- Pressure ulcers
- Spasticity
- Syrinx
- Chronic musculoskeletal problems

Prognosis

- Life expectancy is less than that for those injured at age < 16 years, possibly due to greater length of exposure to complications
- No data available to compare recovery of function in those younger than 21 years versus adults with tetraplegia

Helpful Hints

- Reassess expected level of function at each visit and as child matures update treatment plan to facilitate independence in activities of daily living and mobility

Suggested Readings

Betz RR, Mulcahey MJ, eds. *The Child with a Spinal Cord Injury.* Rosemont, IL: American Academy of Orthopedic Surgeons; 1996.

Consortium for Spinal Cord Medicine. Clinical Practice Guidelines and Consumer Guides for SCI. Available at http://www.pva.org/site/PageServer

Spinal Muscular Atrophy

Nanette C. Joyce DO

Description

Spinal muscular atrophies (SMAs) are a group of neurodegenerative disorders characterized by progressive symmetric weakness and atrophy due to the loss of anterior horn cells of the spinal cord and motor cranial nerve nuclei V, VII, IX, X, XI, and XII.

Etiology/Types

- SMA is inherited as an autosomal recessive disorder linked to abnormalities on chromosome 5q
- Classification is based on age of onset/disease severity
- SMA I (acute infantile, Werdnig-Hoffman)
- SMA II (chronic infantile, intermediate)
- SMA III (chronic juvenile, Kugelberg-Welander)
- SMA IV (adult onset)

Epidemiology

- Incidence: approximately 1 per 10,000 live births
- Carrier frequency: 1 in 40 to 60 people
- Equal occurrence in males and females
- Reported in races and countries throughout the world

Pathogenesis

- Genetic abnormality located on the long arm of chromosome 5, identified as the SMN (survival motor neuron) gene
- Two genes identified: SMN 1 considered disease causing and SMN 2 disease modifying
- SMN 1 typically encodes full-length protein, however, in SMA exons 7 and 8 are commonly deleted producing a truncated protein
- SMN 2 occasionally encodes full-length protein
- An inverse relationship exists between SMN 2 copy number and disease severity: zero copies induce embryonic lethality; five copies of the SMN 2 gene may result in a normal phenotype
- Approximately 95% of patients have homozygous deletions of exons 7 and 8

Risk Factors

- Familial inheritance
- Spontaneous, de novo, mutations occur in approximately 2% of patients

Clinical Features

- Floppy infant
- Progressive, proximal greater than distal, upper and lower limb weakness
- Evidence of degeneration of anterior horn cells of the spinal cord and motor cranial nerves
- Abnormal motor milestones

Natural History and Prognosis

- SMA I: Onset is birth to 6 months; never sits independently; death usually prior to 2 years, but later in some cases, especially with technology
- SMA II: Onset is 6 to 18 months; will sit but never walk; death most common in the 20s to 30s
- SMA III: Onset older than 18 months; walks independently; may have normal life span
- SMA IV: Onset usually in mid-30s; slowly progressive weakness, transitioning to wheelchair dependence over 20 years; normal life expectancy

Diagnosis

Differential diagnosis

- Central nervous system abnormalities
- Congenital muscular dystrophy
- Infantile acid maltase disease
- Limb girdle muscular dystrophy
- Congenital myasthenia gravis
- Congenital myopathy
- Amyotrophic lateral sclerosis

History

- Hypotonia
- Impaired motor development
- Loss of gained motor skills

Exam

- Mild facial weakness with sparing of extraocular muscles
- Tongue fasciculations and/or poor suck
- Frog-leg positioning with abdominal breathing
- Scoliosis more common in SMA II than III
- Joint contractures
- Wide-based Trendelenburg gait if ambulatory
- Sensation intact

- Fine tremor in the hands
- Decreased muscle tone and bulk with proximal greater than distal atrophy
- Reduced or absent reflexes
- Normal to above normal intelligence

Testing
- Serum creatine kinase: normal to two times normal
- Electrodiagnostic testing reveals spontaneous potentials; fasciculations in SMA II and III; and large amplitude, long duration, polyphasic motor unit action potentials
- Muscle biopsy: grouped atrophy of type I and II fibers with rare angulated large type I fibers
- DNA testing: targeted mutation analysis of SMN 1 for identifying deletions of exons 7 and 8. Sequence analysis to identify intragenic mutations. SMN 2 duplication analysis to quantify gene copies

Pitfalls
- Missed diagnosis of treatable similar disease

Red Flags
- Severe metabolic acidosis may occur during intercurrent illness or fasting. Typically resolves with IV fluids over 2 to 4 days

Treatment

Medical
- No disease-modifying medications available
- Drug trials ongoing to identify treatment to increase transcription of the full-length protein product from the SMN 2 gene

Therapeutic exercises
- Insufficient evidence
- Focus has been on range of motion and contracture prevention

Assistive devices
- Orthoses to address contractures and scoliosis management, though does not halt progression of spinal curvature it helps balance and sitting comfort

- Mobility devices such as power wheelchair, scooter, manual wheelchairs, and Hoyer lift for transfers
- Bathroom safety equipment such as grab bars, infant positioning devices, elevated toilet seat, tub bench, commode, shower chair, etc.
- Respiratory devices such as bilevel positive airway pressure, cough assist, and intrapulmonary percussive ventilator

Surgical
- Posterior spinal stabilization if scoliosis is greater than 50° and forced vital capacity greater than or equal to 40% predicted. Delay until spine is mature to avoid crankshaft deformity, with change above and below surgical site with growth
- Percutaneous gastrostomy tube
- Tracheotomy, if desired, in the setting of severe restrictive lung disease with failure of noninvasive ventilation. Discuss with family in advance of need

Consults
- Pulmonology evaluation for restrictive lung disease and nocturnal hypoventilation requiring noninvasive positive pressure ventialtion, tracheotomy, and cough assistance
- Orthopedic evaluation for scoliosis management
- Gastroenterology if PEG placement indicated
- Speech language pathology evaluation if symptoms of dysarthria or dysphagia
- High-risk obstetrics with pregnancy in SMA II/III
- Genetics

Helpful Hints
- Offer genetic counseling to parents of children with SMA

Suggested Readings
Bosboom WM, Vrancken AF, van den Berg LH, et al. Drug treatment for spinal muscular atrophy type II and III. *Cochrane Database Syst Rev.* 2009;21:CD006282.

Schroth MK. Special considerations in the respiratory management of spinal muscular atrophy. *Pediatrics.* 2009;123:S245–249.

Prior TW. Spinal muscular atrophy diagnostics. *J Child Neurol.* 2007;22:952–956.

Section II: Pediatric Diseases and Complications

Stroke

Edward A. Hurvitz MD

Description

Damage to the brain and subsequent impairment of function due to loss of blood flow (ischemia) or bleeding (hemorrhage). The focus here is on stroke past the neonatal period.

Etiology/Types

- Ischemic
- Congenital heart disease (and associated surgery)
- Sickle cell anemia and other blood dyscrasias
- Thrombophilia (factor V Leiden syndrome, protein C and S deficiency—all lead to hypercoaguability and thrombosis)
- Arteriopathy
  - Congenital malformation
  - Moyamoya syndrome—A congenital constriction of cerebral arteries, especially the internal carotid artery, with collateral circulation that appears like a "puff of smoke (moyamoya in Japanese) in arteriography
- Rheumatologic (e.g., vasculitis, Takayasu's arterities—with arterial inflammation and constriction)
- Infections (meningitis, varicella—lead to arterial inflammation and constriction)
- Metabolic syndromes such as mitochondrial myopathy, encephalopathy, lactic acidosis and stroke (MELAS), and homocystinuria
- Hemorrhagic
- Ruptured aneurysm
- Leukemia

Epidemiology

- Hemorrhagic stroke occurs in 1.4 per 100,000 children
- Ischemic stroke occurs in 0.6 to 7.9 per 100,000 children
- Middle cerebral artery distribution: arm more involved than leg
- Anterior cerebral artery: leg more involved
- More common in males 3:2

Pathogenesis

- Ischemic: due to pump failure (congenital heart disease) or loss of flow (embolism, arterial dissection)
- Emboli from thrombophilia or from poor cardiac flow
- Inflammation and infection (e.g., in moyamoya, meningitis)
- Both pregnancy and oral contraceptives can create a hypercoagulable state

Risk Factors

- Congenital heart disease is involved in 25% to 33% of ischemic strokes
- Sickle cell anemia
- Metabolic syndrome not identified as a risk for pediatric stroke

Clinical Features

- Hemiparesis
- Spastic tone
- Cognitive impairment
- Aphasia
- Visual field loss
- Swallowing problems

Natural History

- Residual deficit is common, especially in ischemic stroke. Outcome in hemorrhagic stroke is often better
- Recurrent strokes have poorer outcomes (e.g., MELAS syndrome, moyamoya)

Diagnosis

Differential diagnosis

- Seizure with post-ictal state
- Brain tumor
- Acute demyelinating encephalitis
- Brain trauma
- Migraine with post headache weakness

History

- New onset of seizure with weakness
- Sudden onset of weakness, visual change, dysphagia, or other neurologic signs
- Headache can be severe and unrelenting
- Recent infections such as varicella
- Use of oral contraceptives, anabolic steroids, or other drugs

Exam

- Hemiparesis
- Cranial nerve deficits—facial weakness, dysphagia
- Aphasia (expressive or receptive) or dysphasia
- Cognitive changes

- Neglect, especially with right hemispheric stroke (left hemiparesis)
- Visual field loss

Testing
- MRI of brain to help with diagnosis, localize lesion, identify need for treatment
- MRA (MR angiography) and CTA first line of vascular imaging. If small vessel disease or moyamoya noted, may need classic angiography
- Moyamoya syndrome shows classic "puff of smoke" appearance on angiography
- Lab evaluation includes blood count, metabolic panel, coagulation studies, studies for specific risk factors, studies for inflammation (ESR, CRP), urine metabolic screen
- Pregnancy test in female teenagers

Pitfalls
- Despite extensive testing, many ischemic strokes undiagnosed

Red Flags
- Changing neurologic picture suggesting repeat stroke
- Cardiac instability associated with the stroke
- Fever suggesting meningitis or other infectious problem

Treatment

Medical
- Recombinant tissue plasminogen activator—less common for children
- Antithrombophilic agents—aspirin
- Anticoagulation for cardiac embolism
- Antispasticity medications such as baclofen, dantrolene, zanaflex
- Medications for attention and concentration
- Seizure medications

Exercises
- Comprehensive inpatient rehabilitation
- Constraint induced therapy or bilateral training therapy for upper extremity function
- Range of motion
- Strengthening
- Gait training
- Developmental stimulation
- Speech and language therapy for communication and cognition
- Swallowing therapy

Modalities
- Ankle-foot orthosis and wrist-hand orthosis

Injection
- Botulinum toxin or phenol to reduce spasticity

Surgical
- Neurosurgery for some hemorrhagic strokes with increased intracranial pressure
- Neurosurgical and vascular intervention for arteriopathies, including moyamoya syndrome
- Intrathecal baclofen pump in those with severe tone

Consults
- Neurology
- Neurosurgery
- Vascular surgery
- Ophthalmalogy
- Neuropsychology
- Hematology or cardiology

Complications
- Aspiration in those with dysphagia
- Recurrent stroke in some ischemic etiologies

Prognosis
- Hemiparesis recovers proximally to distally. Hand and foot/ankle function often have poor recovery, and orthotics are frequently required
- Cognitive and language deficits may remain after motor recovery
- ADL function may be more impaired in children who have stroke at a young age, before they initially learn the skill
- In a long-term follow-up study, all children finished high school, and many went to college. About 60% older than age 16 were employed but only a few were financially independent

Helpful Hints
- Parents are often told that their children's brains are "plastic" and they will recover. They must understand the high risk of residual functional loss
- Early intervention and intensive therapy techniques should be considered

Suggested Readings

Bernard TJ, Goldenberg NA. Pediatric arterial ischemic stroke. *Pediatric Clin N Am.* 2008;55:323-338.

Hurvitz E, Warschausky S, Berg M, Tsai S. Long-term functional outcome of pediatric stroke survivors. *Topics Stroke Rehab.* 2004;11:1151-1159.

Kim CT, Han J, Kim H. Pediatric stroke recovery: a descriptive analysis. *Arch Phys Med Rehab.* 2009;90:657-662.

Section II: Pediatric Diseases and Complications

Torticollis

Joyce Oleszek MD

Description

Torticollis is a neck deformity with shortening of the sternocleidomastoid (SCM) muscle resulting in limited neck rotation and lateral flexion. This results in a head tilt to the affected side and rotation to the contralateral side.

Etiology/Types

Etiology is unknown but several theories have been proposed:

- Intrauterine malposition or crowding, including breech deliveries, twin births, and caesarian section
- Complicated deliveries, including use of forceps or vacuum
- Birth trauma theory, with SCM muscle torn at birth with formation of a hematoma and subsequent development of fibrous mass
- Ischemic hypothesis, with venous occlusion causing ischemic changes in the SCM resulting in a compartment-type syndrome
- Plagiocephaly resulting from in utero or intrapartum cranial molding or postnatally resulting from lack of varied supine positioning; can be perpetuated in the supine position since gravity will force the head to turn to the side of the flattened occiput. Associated torticollis can then result from this persistent unidirectional positioning. Either of these can cause the other one

Epidemiology

- Prevalence 0.3% to 20%
- Male to female predominance of 3:2
- No statistically significant difference in side involved
- Associated plagiocephaly in up to 90%
- Plagiocephaly and acquired torticollis have increased since the American Academy of Pediatrics (AAP) recommended in 1992 that infants be placed supine to sleep

Pathogenenesis

- Unilateral fibrous contracture of the SCM; SCM mass may be present
- Myoblasts in various stages of differentiation and degeneration are found in the interstitium of the mass

- Passive stretching of the SCM provides an adaptable stimulation and favors the normal myogenesis of the mass
- SCM mass resolves in weeks to months

Risk Factors

- Breech delivery
- Caesarean section delivery
- Twin A
- Complicated deliveries
- Birth trauma

Clinical Features

- Head tilted to side of shortened SCM and rotated to contralateral side
- Tight SCM
- SCM mass may be present
- Decreased active rotation to affected side
- Head righting decreased on contralateral side
- Positional plagiocephaly
- Hypertropia on contralateral side suspicious for superior oblique palsy
- The reported concurrence with hip dysplasia varies between 2% and 20%

Natural History

- Most resolve with physical therapy and caregiver education on a home program

Diagnosis

Differential diagnosis

- Superior oblique palsy of the contralateral eye
- Central nervous system tumor
- Vertebral anomaly
- Transient inflammatory illness
- Retropharyngeal abscesses and pyogenic cervical spondylitis
- Sandifer's syndrome—association of gastroesophageal reflux and torticollis

History

- Birth history
- Sleeping and feeding positions

- Use of positioning devices (such as bouncy seats, infant carriers, floor entertainers)
- Amount of supervised prone time
- Abnormal eye movements
- Developmental concerns

Examination
- Head tilted and rotated to opposite side with decreased active rotation to affected side
- Decreased head righting to opposite side
- Possible SCM mass
- Positional plagiocephaly
- Evaluate for hip click or asymmetry
- Evaluate for neurologic abnormality

Testing
- Cervical spine x-ray to rule out a vertebral anomaly
- Pelvic x-ray to rule out hip dysplasia
- Hip ultrasound if hip dysplasia suspected in a child less than 4 months

Pitfalls
- Need to rule out nonmuscular causes such as ocular, vertebral, and neurologic

Red Flags
- Dysconjugate gaze, as diplopia may cause this neck positioning
- Acute onset or intermittent torticollis associated with neurologic symptoms may indicate syrinx
- Vertebral anomalies on x-ray as congenital anomalies may be present

Treatment

Exercises
- Home program of stretching the affected neck muscles and strengthening the contralateral side
- Education of caregivers to use daily routines of carrying, positioning, feeding, and play to accomplish the desired postures
- Turning the head of the infant to the nonfavored side while sleeping supine

- Prone play, for skull non-weightbearing allowing more options of neck mobility
- A tubular orthosis for torticollis (TOT collar) is occasionally prescribed

Injection
- Botulinum toxin type-A injections to the affected SCM and/or upper trapezius muscle

Surgical
- SCM release in refractory cases

Consults
- Rarely, ophthalmology, neurosurgery, or plastic surgery

Complications
- Intermittent head tilt—often occurs when the child is fatigued or ill
- Persistent craniofacial asymmetry—can persist despite early and successful treatment of the head tilt
- Scoliosis—often seen in more severe or inadequately treated cases

Prognosis
- Most resolve with a stretching program
- Younger age at diagnosis and less severe rotation or lateral flexion deformities positively influence outcome and treatment duration
- Even if a child requires surgery, studies show a good outcome long term

Helpful Hints
- Caregiver education is the key to treatment as well as prevention

Suggested Readings
Cheng JC, Wong MW, Tang SP, et al. Clinical determinants of the outcome of manual stretching in the treatment of congenital muscular torticollis in infants. A prospective study of eight hundred and twenty-one cases. *J Bone Joint Surg: Am.* 2001;83-A(5):679-687.

Oleszek JL, Chang N, Apkon SD, Wilson PE. Botulinum toxin type A in the treatment of children with congenital muscular torticollis. *Am J Phys Med Rehabil* 2005;84(10):813-816.

Toxic Ingestion

Susan Quigley MD

Description
Toxic ingestion of poisonous substances affects children in primarily two age peaks, related to their developmental level. Children younger than 5 years are often exploring their world and encounter poisons inadvertently, whereas adolescents may encounter poisons more purposefully.

Etiology/Types

Nonpharmaceutical
- Cosmetics/personal care products
- Cleaning products
- Plants, including mushroom, and tobacco
- Insecticides, pesticides, and rodenticides

Pharmaceutical
- Analgesics
- Cough and cold preparations
- Topical agents
- Vitamins
- Antimicrobials

Epidemiology
- Poisoning involves 2 million children younger than 5 years of age each year
- Third most common injury treated in emergency departments for all children younger than 16 years
- More children younger than 4 years die from poisonings than from unintentional firearm injuries in the home
- Approximately 4 million people in the United States are poisoned each year and 60% of those are children younger than 6 years

Pathogenesis
- Varies depending on poisoning agent

Risk Factors
- Developmental level: infant and toddlers in oral phase
- Poorly marked containers of dangerous chemicals
- Changes in routine or environment: moving day
- Medications not stored safely enough: childproof caps may not be sufficient
- Adolescent issues: poor coping strategies and increased stressors

Clinical Features
- Aspirin poisoning: tinnitus, vomiting, prolonged bleeding time, hepatotoxicity, inhibits Krebs cycle, tachypnea, tachycardia, and fever, breath odor: wintergreen
- Acetaminophen poisoning: insidious hepatotoxicity, nausea/vomiting, pallor, and diaphoresis, antidote: N-acetylcysteine (NAC, mucomyst)
- Iron poisoning: colicky abdominal pain, vomiting and diarrhea, gastric scarring and stricture, and shock, antidote: deferoxamine
- Tricyclic antidepressant poisoning: seizures, electrocardiography abnormalities-QRS prolongation, and dysrhythmias, antidote: bicarbonate
- Lead poisoning: pica, abdominal discomfort, lethargy, anemia, basophilic stippling of red blood cells, and neurologic deficits/encephalopathy, antidote: EDTA, DMSA, BAL
- Hydrocarbon poisoning/kerosene: aspiration pneumonia, central nervous system (CNS) depression, and acute respiratory distress syndrome

Breath odors from toxic ingestion

Odor	Substance
Wintergreen	aspirin
Bitter almond	cyanide
Fruity	ethanol, or acetone, or chloroform, or isopropyl alcohol
Peanuts	rat poison
Garlic	arsenic, organophosphates, thallium
Fishy	zinc or aluminum phosphide
Mothballs	camphor

Diagnosis

Differential diagnosis
- Trauma
- CNS pathology
- Infectious etiology
- Diabetes

History
- Suspected time of ingestion
- Possible ingestion agent
- Quantity of agent consumed

Exam
Pupillary findings
- Miosis (pinpoint) narcotics, organophosphates, phenylclidine, clonidine, phenothiazines, barbiturates, and ethanol
- Mydriasis (dilated) anticholinergics, atropine, antihistamines, cyclic antidepressants, and sympathomimetics (amphetamines, caffeine, cocaine, LSD, and nicotine)
- Nystagmus barbiturates, ketamine, phencyclidine, and phenytoin

Testing
- X-rays for radio-opaque ingestion agents
- Toxicology screen urine and blood
- Quantitative levels of specific agents: lead, ethanol, and salicylate level (1st level 4 h after ingestion is ideal)

Pitfalls
- Waiting for salicylate levels to come back before initiating NAC treatment if ingestion time is unclear

Red Flags
- CNS depression or respiratory depression

Treatment

Medical
- Emesis/cathartics
  - Syrup of ipecac-out of favor
- Gastric lavage
- Whole bowel irrigation
- Activated charcoal
- Specific antidotes or binding agents
- Chelation therapy

- Dialysis
- Antidotes:

Ingestion/Exposure	Antidote
Acetaminophen	N-acetylcysteine
Anticholinergics	Physostigmine
Benzodiazepines	Flumazenil
Beta blockers	Glucagon
Calcium channel blockers	Calcium, Glucagon
Cyanide	Amyl nitrite
Digoxin	Digibind
Ethylene Glycol	Ethanol, fomepizole, dialysis
Iron	Deferoxamine
Isoniazid	Pyridoxine
Jimson weed	Physostigmine
Lead	EDAT,DMSA,BAL
Methanol	Ethanol
Mercury	Dimercaprol, DMSA
Methemoglobinemic agents	Methylene blue
Opiates	Narcan(naloxone), nalmefene
Organophosphates	Atropine, pralidoxime
Phenothiazines(dystonic reaction)	Diphenhydramine
Tricyclics	Bicarbonate
Warfarin (rat poison)	Vitamin K

Exercise
- Strength and endurance training for deconditioning that can develop during prolonged hospitalization

Modalities
- Aquatic and land based therapy
- Electrical stimulation
- Range of motion

Injection
- N/A

Surgical
If patient is incapacitated
- Gtube/jtube
- Trach
- Central line access

Consults
- Neurology
- Pharmacology
- Nephrology
- ENT
- GI
- Psychiatry
- Surgery

Complications of Treatment
Aspiration pneumonia
- Due to emetics, nausea/vomiting from poison agent, and inhalation of activated charcoal or petroleum products

Fluid overload
- Due to alkalinization or acidification of urine

Acute dystonic reaction
- Due to an antiemetic drug, metoclopramide, or antidopaminergic agent like neuroleptics (treat with benadryl or cogentin)

Prognosis
- May be favorable if intervention is begun early enough and poisoning agent and quantity are known

- Caustic agents can cause esophogeal erosion and stricture with poorer outcomes
- Salicylate poisonings can result in irreparable hepatotoxicity

Helpful Hints
Protect the airway
Ipecac induced vomiting is contraindicated with:
- CNS depression
- Caustic ingestion
- Hydrocarbon/petroleum distillate ingestion
- Potential nervous system depressant ingestion
- Convulsions
- Time elapsed since ingestion >1 hour

Suggested Readings
Emergency medicine. In: Polin RA, Ditmar MF, eds. *Pediatric Secrets.* 3rd ed. Philadelphia: Hanley & Belfus; 2001:150–164.

Hyams JS, Treem WR. Gastrointestinal diseases. In: Dworkin PH, ed. *Pediatrics.* 3rd ed. Williams & Wilkins; 1996:49–57.

Toxic Neuropathies

Gadi Revivo DO

Description

Medications, industrial and environmental agents, and heavy metals can cause acquired peripheral neuropathies. These agents can affect motor, sensory, and autonomic nerves, creating typical patterns of involvement.

Etiology/Types

- Chemotherapeutic agents
- Antiretroviral medication
- Organophosphates
- Heavy metals

Epidemiology

- Account for a small percentage of acquired neuropathies
- Prevalence of lead poisoning highest among urban, low-income children less than 6 years old living in housing built before the 1970s when lead was removed from paint and gasoline
- Since the 1970s decreasing toxicity in the United States but an estimated 310,000 children are currently at risk for elevated lead level exposure
- Children are at higher risk due to incomplete blood-brain barrier giving easier access to the CNS, as well as behavior such as crawling and playing on the floor, which gives more paint chip exposure than to those who are older

Pathogenesis

- Blood-nerve barrier protecting peripheral nerves is less protective than the blood-brain barrier
- Chemotherapeutic agents may impair axonal transport (cisplatin), cause axonal degeneration (vincristine), or inhibit microtubule function (etoposide)
- Nucleoside analogs (stavudine, zalcitabine) inhibit the enzyme DNA polymerase gamma
- Certain organophosphates inhibit an enzyme called neuropathy target esterase, responsible for a delayed polyneuropathy
- Children retain absorbed lead at a rate about 30 times that of adults, and may develop acute encephalopathy, hearing loss, and developmental delay, particularly in language skills
- Unknown mechanism to explain lead neuropathy
- Possible result of abnormal porphyrin metabolism (motor neuropathy type)

Risk Factors

- Decreased drug metabolism, impaired renal or hepatic clearance may exacerbate toxicity
- Pre-existing inherited neuropathies (e.g., Charcot-Marie-Tooth)
- Sickle cell anemia
- Low CD4 count (<100 cells/mm3); these are a subset of T cells that activate other white blood cells for an immune response

Clinical Features

- Commonly bilateral, symmetric distal involvement of axons (affecting the longer sensory fibers) resulting in numbness, dysesthesias, and areflexia
- Pain, paresthesias, areflexia, and autonomic features (hypotension, constipation) common with vincristine
- Dorsal root ganglion affected with cisplatin and etoposide use resulting in proprioceptive loss and motor ataxia
- Painful distal burning, numbness, and areflexia with nucleoside analogs (sensory axonal loss)
- Organophosphate-induced delayed polyneuropathy is a distal sensorimotor peripheral neuropathy that develops weeks after exposure
- Sensorimotor neuropathy with prolonged lead exposure in children produces motor weakness affecting the legs (foot drop) and distal sensory loss

Natural History

- Onset usually within weeks of exposure (medication) or insidious (environmental exposure)
- Severity of neuropathy is often dose and duration dependent (e.g., chemotherapeutics)
- Sensory changes occur prior to weakness
- Neurocognitive decline more common than neuropathy in children with toxic lead levels

Diagnosis

Differential diagnosis

- Acute inflammatory demyelinating polyradiculoneuropathy

- AIDS-related sensory axonal neuropathy
- Paraneoplastic autonomic neuropathy
- Neuromuscular junction disorders (e.g., myasthenia gravis, Lambert-Eaton myasthenic syndrome)
- Diabetic neuropathy

History
- Progressive distal weakness
- Progressive sensory loss
- Loss of balance and motor control
- Abdominal pain, headache, joint tenderness (lead poisoning)

Exam
- Distal sensory loss (light touch, vibration, pinprick, temperature)
- Absent ankle reflexes
- Motor ataxia
- Lead lines at the gum line are rare, seen only with severe and prolonged lead toxicity

Testing
- Blood lead level
- Peripheral blood smear: basophilic stippling (lead toxicity)
- Abdominal X-rays demonstrate flecks of lead
- Low serum cholinesterase (organophosphate toxicity)

Electrodiagnosis/EMG/NCS
- Vincristine: Reduced sensory nerve action potentials (SNAP), compound muscle action potentials (CMAP) amplitudes, and reduced motor unit action potentials (MUAP) recruitment
- Cisplatin: Reduced SNAP amplitude; motor nerve conduction and EMG normal
- Nucleosides: Reduced SNAP amplitude; normal motor nerve conduction velocities; fibrillation potentials and positive sharp waves on EMG
- Lead: Mild sensory and motor slowing; increased MUAP amplitude, duration, and phases

Red Flags
- Screen for hereditary sensory motor neuropathies prior to chemotherapy treatment

Treatment

Medical
- Dose reduction or withdrawal of medication may improve symptoms
- Remove contact with offending environmental, industrial agent
- Antidepressants (tricyclic, SSRIs, SNRIs), anticonvulsants, or topicals (lidoderm, capsaicin) for pain management
- Chelation therapy with pencillamine or EDTA for lead toxicity, which works by binding heavy metals

Exercises
- Physical therapy for strengthening and balance

Modalities
- Orthoses for foot drop
- Adaptive equipment for safe ambulation, bathing
- Heat
- Cold soaks
- Dietary supplementation with alpha lipoic acid, evening primrose, and vitamin E

Consults
- Environmental medicine
- Neurology

Complications
- Coasting (or worsening of) symptoms weeks after agent is removed before recovery begins

Prognosis
- Dependent on dose and time of exposure

Helpful Hints
- A thorough history with early identification and removal of the causative medication or agent may limit the neuropathy, allowing for greater recovery

Suggested Readings
Dumitru D, Amato AA, Zwarts M. *Electrodiagnostic Medicine.* Philadelphia: Hanley & Belfus; 2002.
Pratt RW, Weimer LH. Medication and toxin-induced peripheral neuropathy. *Seminars Neurol.* 2005;25(2):204-216.

Transverse Myelitis

Frank S. Pidcock MD

Description

Transverse myelitis (TM) is typically a monofocal monophasic inflammatory disorder of the spinal cord.

Etiology/Types

- Idiopathic
  - 10% to 45% of cases
- Disease associated
  - Connective tissue disorders
  - Sarcoidosis, Behcet's disease, Sjogren's syndrome, systemic lupus erythematosis
  - Central nervous system infection
  - Lyme disease, HIV, mycoplasma, herpes virus, leukemia/lymphoma virus-1, syphilis
- Recurrent
  - 10% to 25% of cases
  - Multiple sclerosis eventually diagnosed in 6% to 43% of multiphasic cases

Epidemiology

- 1400 new cases diagnosed in the United States per year
- 20% to 30% occur under the age of 18 years
- Affects all ages from infancy through adolescence with bimodal peaks
  - 0 to 3 years
  - 10 to 18 years

Pathogenesis

- Inflammatory attack on the spinal cord
  - Perivascular infiltration by lymphocytes and monocytes
- Demyelination and atrophy may both occur
  - Postinfectious process hypothesized
  - Shared immunologic recognition sites between microbes and spinal cord by molecular mimicry
  - Lymphocyte activation by microbial super antigen

Clinical Features

- Acute or subacute onset of neurologic dysfunction related to the spinal cord
  - Motor—rapidly progressive paraparesis that may involve arms as well as legs
  - Sensation—distinct level of sensory loss usually in mid thoracic area for adults but may be cervical, especially in children
- Pain—burning/tingling, numbness, or both
- Autonomic—urinary urgency, bowel or bladder incontinence, inability to void, constipation, sexual dysfunction

Natural History

- Initial phase—from onset to maximum deficit
  - 2 to 5 days (range 1–14)
- Plateau phase—time spent with the maximum deficit
  - 6 days (range 1–26)
- Recovery phase—from onset of motor recovery to ultimate neurologic level of function may occur over months to years

Diagnosis

Differential diagnosis

- Noninflammatory myelopathies
- Radiation-induced myelopathy
- Ischemic vascular myelopathy
- Compressive myelopathies
- Neoplasms, hematomas, other masses
- Trauma
- Acute inflammatory demyelinating polyradiculopathy
- Multiple sclerosis
- Neuromyelitis optica

History

- Preceding febrile illness within 3 weeks of onset—47% of children
- Antecedent trauma at an average of 8 days before onset—13% of children
- Relationship of preceding immunization to TM is unclear

Exam

- Back, trunk, or limb pain
- Weakness or paralysis of legs (and arms in some cases)
- Anesthesia corresponding to a spinal cord level
- Loss of sphincter control

Testing
- **First priority**—determine etiology
  - Rule out compressive spinal cord lesion
  - Gadolinium-enhanced **spine** magnetic resonance imaging (MRI)
  - Assess for spinal cord inflammation
  - Lumbar puncture—cerebrospinal fluid (CSF) analysis for white blood cells
  - Gadolinium-enhanced spine MRI
  - Determine whether infectious cause exists
  - CSF and serum assays for infectious agents
- **Second priority**—define extent of demyelination
  - Gadolinium-enhanced **brain** MRI
  - Visual-evoked potential

Treatment

Medical
- Intravenous high-dose steroids for 5 days then taper
- Plasma exchange if no improvement after 5 to 7 days of intravenous steroids for moderate to severe TM (unable to walk, impaired autonomic functions, sensory loss in legs)
- Immunomodulatory treatments such as intravenous cyclophosamide may be considered for aggressive or nonresponsive TM with progression despite intravenous steroid therapy

Rehabilitative
- Spasticity management
  - General strengthening and stretching
  - Appropriate orthoses and wearing schedule
  - Antispasticity drugs—oral, injections, pumps
- Bowel incontinence
  - High-fiber diet and adequate fluids
  - Medications that regulate bowel emptying
  - Regular bowel movement regimen
- Bladder dysfunction
  - Urodynamic evaluation
  - Intermittent catheterization as needed
  - Medications that treat problems of storage or emptying
  - Prompt treatment of urinary tract infections
- Pain
  - Range of motion exercises
  - Analgesic medications
- Early focus on community reentry including communication with the school system to insure appropriate educational accommodations

Consults
- Urology
- Neurology

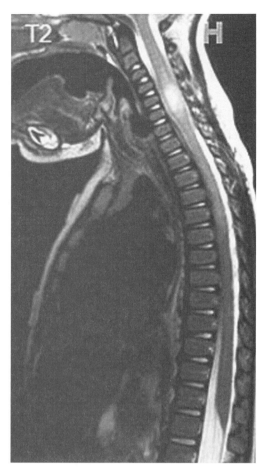

Sagittal T2-weighted MRI image showing hyperintense lesion in the affected cervical spinal cord at arrow. Courtesy of Thierry Huisman, MD.

- Family or individual counseling

Prognosis
- Most patients experience some spontaneous recovery within 6 months with additional improvement up to 2 years
- Moderate to severe impairment may persist
- Ambulation: approximately 44%
- Bladder dysfunction: approximately 40%
- Approximately 1 out of 3 patients have little or no neurologic sequleae
- Age at onset under 3 years is associated with a worse outcome

Suggested Readings
Krishnan C, Kaplin A, Pardo C, Kerr D, Keswani, S. Demyelinating disorders: update on transverse myelitis. *Curr Neurol Neurosci Reports.* 2006;6:236–243.

Pidcock FS, Krishnan C, Crawford TO, Salorio CF, Trovato M, Kerr DA. Acute transverse myelitis in childhood. *Neurology.* 2007;68:1474–1480.

Traumatic Brain Injury: Anoxic

Thomas E. McNalley MD ■ Teresa L. Massagli MD

Description

Anoxic brain injury/Hypoxic ischemic encephalopathy occurs as a result of interrupted blood flow or oxygen supply to the brain. This chapter excludes birth trauma.

Etiology/Types

- Near-drowning
- Cardiopulmonary arrest
- Suffocation/choking
- Inhalation injury/carbon monoxide poisoning
- Asthma
- High altitude
- Drug overdose
- Electrical shock
- Septic shock
- Status epilepticus

Epidemiology

- Rate of near drownings: 5 per 100,000, ages 0–19 years
- Higher rates in ages 1 to 4 years (14 per 100,000) and under 1 year (10 per 100,000)
- Nonfatal suffocation rate 22 per 100,000; but in children under 1 year, 150 per 100,000

Pathogenesis

- Interruption of either oxygen or blood supply to the brain, resulting in hypoxia or ischemia. Neuronal ATP depleted within 3 to 5 minutes of anoxia
- Areas of greatest susceptibility: vascular end zones ("watershed" infarctions) and areas with highest metabolism, including hippocampus, cerebellum (Purkinje cells), insular cortex, and basal ganglia.
- Hypothermia may be protective in a near-drowning experience

Risk Factors

- Nonfenced pools
- Congenital cardiac disease
- Boating/water sports, combined with alcohol use
- Higher risk for blacks, younger children, males (near drowning)

Clinical Features

- Optic and cerebral atrophy
- Seizure
- Altered level of consciousness
- Cognitive dysfunction, dementia, attention deficits
- Aphasia
- Ataxia
- Spastic tetraplegia
- Extrapyramidal syndromes
- Cortical visual impairment

Diagnosis

Differential diagnosis

- Nonaccidental causes: suicide attempt, child abuse

History

- Type of anoxia (near-drowning, cardiopulmonary arrest)
- Duration of anoxia
- Type and length of resuscitation
- Body temperature
- Glasgow Coma Scale at presentation
- Duration of time to following commands
- Seizure before or after event
- Associated trauma
- Drug or alcohol ingestion

Exam

- Brainstem function: corneal, pupillary, doll's eye, and gag reflexes
- Level of alertness
- Latent or absent response to verbal or tactile stimuli
- Aphasia
- Posturing
- Choreoathetoid movement
- Dystonia
- Visual impairment
- Spasticity and increased tone
- Weakness

Testing

- Carboxyhemoglobin
- Arterial blood gas (ABG) pH
- Blood glucose
- Cardiac and liver enzymes
- Coagulation studies
- Renal function studies
- Drug/toxicology screen
- Chest radiograph

- Cervical spine and extremity imaging if trauma
- Brain magnetic resonance imaging (MRI)
- Somatosensory evoked potentials (SEPs)
- Electroencepholography

Red Flags
- Look for signs of spinal cord injury if diving injury (spinal shock, paralysis, and priapism)
- Secondary causes, including neglect and abuse, should be ruled out

Treatment

Medical
- Resuscitation and respiratory support
- Survey for other injuries
- Control hyperglycemia
- Induce hypothermia; avoid hyperthermia
- Protect range of motion (ROM)
- Mobilize early
- Anticonvulsants if history of seizure

Exercises
- General stretching and strengthening
- Balance and gait training

Injections
- Botulinum toxin for spasticity
- Intrathecal baclofen for severe spasticity

Consultations
- Neurosurgery if associated blunt head trauma or spine trauma
- Cardiology for dysrhythmia
- Neurology for prognosis and seizure management
- Physical, occupational, and speech/language therapy
- Psychology for neuropsychological evaluation and behavior management

Complications
- Cerebral edema
- Acute respiratory distress syndrome
- Autonomic instability (storming)

- Myocardial dysfunction
- Multiorgan system failure
- Aspiration
- Dysphagia
- Weakness and reduced mobility
- Cognitive impairment
- Impaired ROM/contracture
- Persistent vegetative state/minimally conscious state
- Heterotopic ossification

Prognosis
- Data are better at indicating mortality and severe disability than good recovery
- Findings associated with poor outcome includes the following:
  - Ongoing cardiopulmonary resuscitation (CPR) on arrival to emergency department (ED)
  - Absent brainstem reflexes at 24 hours
  - Anoxia >25 minutes
  - Water temperature >10°C
  - Initial GCS <4; GCS <5 at 24 hours
  - ABG pH < 7.1
  - Blood glucose >250 mg/dL
  - Coma persisting >24 hours
  - Absent N20 waves on SEPs
  - Diffusion restriction in basal ganglia and cortex on MRI
- No single test conclusive; tests and exams most predictive when performed >24 hours after event
- Findings associated with better outcome
  - Anoxia <10 minutes
  - Pulse present on arrival to ED
  - Spontaneous ventilation immediately after CPR

Suggested Readings
Abend NS, Licht DJ. Predicting outcome in children with hypoxic ischemic encephalopathy. *Pediatr Crit Care Med.* 2008;9:32–39.

Ibsen L, Koch T. Submersion and asphyxial injury. *Crit Care Med.* 2002;30:S402–S408.

Traumatic Brain Injury: Encephalopathic

Stacy J. Suskauer MD ■ Joshua Benjamin Ewen MD

Description

Inflammatory (infectious, parainfectious, paraneoplastic, or primary inflammatory) diseases of the brain manifest by neurologic dysfunction

Etiology/Types

- Infectious: enteroviruses (>80% of cases), arboviruses, herpesviruses
- Parainfectious: acute demyelinating encephalomyelitis (ADEM)

Epidemiology

- Estimated incidence of viral encephalitis in the United States is 3.5 to 7.4 cases per 100,000 persons per year, with most cases occurring in children and young adults
- Enteroviral infection is spread from person to person; cases tend to occur in the summer and fall
- Arboviruses are often zoonotically spread
- Incidence of ADEM: 0.4/100,000 children/year

Pathogenesis

- Neurologic damage results from hematogenous or neurologic spread of viral agent to the brain followed by direct invasion and destruction of neural tissue by the virus or due to host reaction to viral antigens
- Cross-reactivity of viral antigens with normal tissue is proposed in ADEM

Risk Factors

- Geographic and animal exposures
- Viral exposure
- Recent infection or vaccination (ADEM)

Clinical Features

- Mild febrile illness to severe brain injury and death
- Gastrointestinal (GI) symptoms from GI involvement or increased intracranial pressure (ICP)
- Upper respiratory symptoms
- Headache
- Irritability, lethargy, and/or mental status changes
- Seizures
- Weakness/flaccid paralysis; spasticity or movement disorders later in course
- Sensory impairments
- Neuropathy (e.g., with West Nile virus), myelopathy

Natural History

- Sensorineural hearing loss may occur
- Prognosis varies based on viral etiology of infection
- Herpes encephalitis: without treatment, death occurs in 70% of cases
- ADEM: typically uniphasic course with good likelihood of recovery, but variants can be lethal
- Patients later diagnosed with multiple sclerosis may be thought to have ADEM at first presentation

Diagnosis

Differential diagnosis

- Bacterial meningitis
- Collagen vascular disorders
- Toxic/metabolic encephalopathies
- Focal neurological disorders (e.g., tumor, stroke, and abscess)
- Multiple sclerosis or other demyelinating disease

History

- Nonspecific febrile viral prodrome
- Progressive central nervous system symptoms

Exam

- Fever
- Rash (enteroviruses)
- Focal neurologic findings
- Flaccid paralysis
- Alteration in consciousness

Testing

- Cerebrospinal fluid (CSF)—pleocytosis. Polymerase chain reaction may isolate viral agent. In ADEM, CSF is often nonspecifically abnormal
- Magnetic resonance imaging of brain—T2/FLAIR hyperintensities; in herpes, bilateral hippocampal T2 hyperintensities
- Blood—elevated inflammatory markers
- Urine and nasal aspirates—for virus identification
- Brain tissue—may reveal etiology
- Electroencephalography (EEG)—diffuse, high-voltage delta slowing in viral encephalitis. Periodic lateralized epileptiform discharges in herpes encephalitis

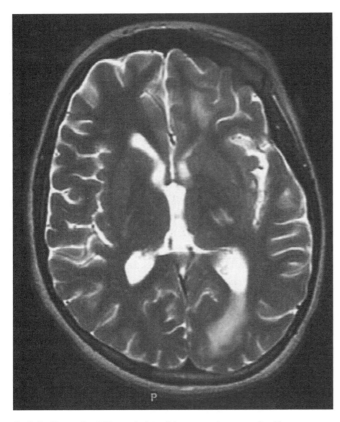

Axial slice of a T2-weighted image demonstrating multiple areas of abnormal hyperintensity in an 11-year-old boy with ADEM.

- ADEM—may have high-voltage slowing or normal EEG

Pitfalls
- Optic neuritis may indicate non-ADEM demyelinating disease

Red Flags
- An apparent second episode of ADEM should prompt consideration of alternative diagnoses (e.g., multiple sclerosis or neurodegenerative disease)

Treatment

Medical
- Supportive care: management of ICP and seizures
- Herpes encephalitis: Acyclovir
- ADEM: High-dose steroids, intravenous immune globulin, plasmapheresis
- Tone/movement disorder management
- Medication for attention/behavioral impairments

Exercises
- Stretching/positioning to maintain range of motion
- Intensive physical, occupational, and/or speech therapy for acquired deficits

Modalities
- As indicated for motor or sensory deficits

Injection
- Botulinum toxin or phenol, if needed to manage tone

Surgical
- Brain biopsy may be required for diagnosis

Consults
- Neurology
- Neurosurgery (ICP management or biopsy)
- Infectious disease/immunology
- Nutrition
- Audiology
- Neuropsychology
- Education
- Behavioral management

Complications
- Hearing loss
- Epilepsy
- Spasticity or movement disorders
- Cognitive impairments
- Behavioral disorders

Prognosis
- Prognosis varies by etiology, ranging from severe chronic impairment to significant recovery
- Rate of functional recovery is variable but typically slower than that observed in traumatic brain injury and stroke
- Neuropsychologic deficits frequently persist

Helpful Hints
- Acyclovir and antibacterial antibiotics should be initiated empirically
- LP should be held until cleared by CT from the risk of supratentorial herniation

Suggested Readings
Silvia MT, Licht DJ. Pediatric central nervous system infections and inflammatory white matter disease. *Pediatr Clin North Am.* 2005;52:1107–1126.

Starza-Smith A, Talbot E, Grant C. Encephalitis in children: a clinical neuropsychology perspective. *Neuropsychol Rehabil.* 2007; 17:506–527.

Traumatic Brain Injury: Inflicted (Shaken Baby Syndrome, Nonaccidental Trauma)

Linda J. Michaud MD

Description

Inflicted traumatic brain injury (iTBI) in children is,

- Definite—when physical examination and radiographic evidence is distinct, consistent, and convincing (with or without consistent history)
- Probable—when combined evidence from physical and radiographic examinations and history is preponderant and noninflicted injury is unlikely to explain the constellation of findings
- Questionable—when some evidence from the physical and radiographic examinations and history suggest inflicted injury, but information about etiology is incomplete
- It is commonly called shaken baby syndrome or nonaccidental trauma.

Etiology/Types

- Shaking
- Shaking-impact
- Battered child with iTBI
- Penetrating injuries including gunshot wounds are beyond the scope of this chapter

Epidemiology

- Incidence of about 17 per 100,000 in children <2 years of age; highest occurrence in first year of life
- Males more affected

Pathogenesis

- Angular deceleration leading to subdural hematomas—shaking, inflicted impact
- Cerebral swelling—may have loss of gray-white matter differentiation
- Contact injuries—scalp hematomas, skull fractures, brain contusions
- Upper cervical or cervicomedullary injury—mechanism not completely understood

Risk Factors

- Male
- Prematurity
- Young mothers
- Multiple births
- Weak association with child physical disability

Clinical Features

- Retinal hemorrhages
- Marks or bruises in unusual locations
- Irritability
- Altered mental status
- Apnea/respiratory compromise
- Seizures
- Poor feeding
- Lethargy
- Skull or other fractures
- Other bodily trauma

Natural History

- Recovery is variable, but outcomes are generally worse in infants after iTBI in comparison to unintentional TBI
- Neurobehavioral deficits may not be appreciated for years, until higher level functions mediated by area(s) of injured brain mature

Diagnosis

Differential diagnosis

- Birth and other nonintentional trauma
- Congenital malformations
- Genetic conditions
- Metabolic conditions
- Hematologic disorders
- Infectious diseases
- Toxins
- Complications of surgical interventions
- Vasculitides
- Oncologic conditions
- Nutritional deficiencies

History

- Report of events leading to evaluation
- If fall reported, fall height details
- Details about timeline of symptoms
- Birth, past medical and trauma history
- Family history, especially of bleeding disorders

- Social history—identify caregivers and their relationship with the child
- Signs/symptoms as above per clinical features

Exam

Entire body, especially,
- Neurologic
- Head, including ophthalmologic
- Skin
- Abdomen
- Bones

Testing

- Brain computed tomography (CT)/MRI
- Skeletal survey to evaluate for fractures; follow-up radiography of suspicious lesions and age of fractures

Pitfalls

- Perpetrators often do not provide accurate history
- CT may not detect early cerebral edema, skull fractures, and shear injury

Red Flags

- Absent, inconsistent, or evolving history
- Developmentally or mechanistically implausible history
- Delay in seeking care

Treatment

Surgery

- Neurosurgery if needed for subdural hematoma evacuation or intracranial pressure monitoring

Consults

- Neurosurgery if concern for need for surgical intervention
- Interdisciplinary child abuse team

Complications

- Hydrocephalus
- Poor brain growth—microcephaly

- Epilepsy
- Motor impairment—quadriplegia, hemiplegia
- Visual impairment
- Hearing impairment
- Feeding problems
- Cognitive deficits
- Behavior problems
- Unstable social environment

Prognosis

- Variable in survivors, ranging from absence of functional deficits to severe physical and/or cognitive impairments; mortality 11% to 33%
- About 2/3 with subdural hematomas have neurologic deficits.

Helpful Hints

- Prevention programs that teach parents and caregivers coping skills, including a focus on the stresses of infant crying
- Parenting and caregiver support—advocacy/home visiting programs
- Programs focused on prevention of subsequent injury to children who have been abused
- Early identification of mental health, family violence, and substance abuse issues
- Perpetrators are most commonly male (2.2:1); first father, then mother's boyfriend, then female babysitter, then mother, in that order
- Further efforts needed to identify effective prevention strategies targeting others beyond mother and father

Suggested Readings

Chiesa A, Duhaime AC. Abusive head trauma. *Pediatr Clin North Am.* 2009;56:317–331.

Reece RM, Nicholson CE, eds. *Inflicted Childhood Neurotrauma.* Elk Grove Village, IL: American Academy of Pediatrics, 2003.

Traumatic Brain Injury: Mild

Linda J. Michaud MD ■ Brad G. Kurowski MD MS

Description

Concussion or mild traumatic brain injury (mTBI), as defined by the American Academy of Neurology is a "trauma-induced alteration in mental status that may or may not involve a loss of consciousness (LOC)." Glasgow Coma Scale score ≥13 without neuroimaging abnormalities defines mTBI.

Etiology/Types

- Falls (most common)
- Motor vehicle accident
- Sports related injuries
- Bicycle related head injury
- Assaults

Epidemiology

- Overall, 100,000 to 200,000 pediatric head injuries per year with a rate of 193 to 367 per 100,000 mTBI
- Males more affected than females (2–4 males:1 female)
- 80% of pediatric TBIs are mild
- mTBI (all ages) ~ 500/100,000 population
- mTBI in children younger than 5 years old ~ 1115/100,000 population
- Peak incidence in early childhood (ages 0–4) and mid to late adolescence (ages 15–19)

Pathogenesis

- Impact, rotational, acceleration, or deceleration forces produce strain and distortion in brain tissue, axons, cerebral vasculature, or other neural elements
- Primary injury refers to injury imparted due to direct forces (e.g., diffuse axonal injury, contusions, epidural hematomas, subdural hematomas, etc.)
- Secondary injury refers to the subsequent pathophysiologic response to the TBI

Risk Factors

- Male
- Not using protective equipment (e.g., no helmet)
- History of previous head injury

Clinical Features

- Headache and dizziness (most common), brief (<30 minutes) LOC, amnesia, confusion, disorientation, slurred speech, incoordination, emotional lability, irritability, memory deficits, nausea, balance deficits, feel like in a "fog", feeling slowed down, blurred vision

Natural History

- Recovery is variable, but most will fully recover over weeks to months. A small subset may have persistent symptoms

Diagnosis

Differential diagnosis

- Intracranial injury/pathology
- Seizures
- Intoxication
- Migraines or other headache disorder
- Cervical spine/whiplash injury

History

- History of head trauma
- Altered mental status with or without LOC
- Signs/symptoms as above per clinical features

Exam

- Confusion
- Amnesia for event
- Memory deficits
- Nonfocal neurologic exam

Testing

- Brain imaging normal
- X-rays of cervical spine to evaluate for fractures
- Head CT/MRI to evaluate for intracranial pathology/injury
- Utility of more advanced imaging modalities (fMRI, MRS, DTI, DWI, PET, and MEG) is being evaluated
- Neuropsychological screening
- Standard and computerized testing are used

Pitfalls

- Denial of symptoms by the individual
- Young children are at higher risk for complications
- Normal exam does not totally exclude the possibility of intracranial pathology/injury
- No consensus on indications for imaging

Red Flags

- Focal neurologic deficits
- Mental status deterioration
- Seizures
- Significant vomiting
- Dramatic worsening of headache
- Skull fracture or scalp hematoma
- History of high velocity trauma
- Age less than 12 months
- Prolonged LOC

Treatment

Medical

- Symptomatic

Exercises

- Rest followed by graded return to school and other activities

Surgical

- Neurosurgery if concerned about more severe injury

Consults

- Neurosurgery if concerned about more severe injury

Complications

- Postconcussion syndrome
  - Persistent symptoms: headache, lightheadedness, memory problems, poor concentration, easy fatigability, irritability, visual disturbances, difficulty concentrating, poor school performance, behavior changes, or sensitivity to light/noise
  - Can persist for 3 months and longer post injury
  - May be associated with impaired cognitive function and social disability
  - Related to the interaction of biological effects of injury and psychological and psychosocial factors
- Second impact syndrome
  - Second head trauma while still symptomatic
  - Disruption of the brain's blood supply autoregulation causing vascular engorgement, diffuse cerebral swelling, increased intracranial pressure, and brain herniation, leading to coma and death
- Increased risk of developing hyperactivity, inattention, conduct-disordered behavior in early adolescence if injured before age 5

Prognosis

- Good, most make full recovery—small subset do not

Helpful Hints

- Best treatment is prevention (e.g., helmet)
- Individualize care—involve the individual, family, and school in management and recovery
- Currently, no consensus on concussion grading schemes and return to play guidelines
- Do not return to activity unless asymptomatic physically, cognitively, and behaviorally

Suggested Readings

Kirkwood MW, Yeates KO, Wilson PE. Pediatric sport-related concussion: a review of the clinical management of an oft-neglected population. *Pediatrics.* 2006;117(4):1359–1371.

Meehand WP, Bachur RG. Sport-related concussion. *Pediatrics.* 2009;123:114–123.

Thiessen ML, Woolridge DP. Pediatric minor closed head injury. *Pediatr Clin North Am.* 2006;53(1):1–26.

www.cdc.gov/ncipc/factsheets/tbi.htm

Yeates KO, Taylor HG, Rusin J, et al. Longitudinal trajectories of postconcussive symptoms in children with mild traumatic brain injuries and their relationship to acute clinical status. *Pediatrics.* 2009;123(3):735–743.

Traumatic Brain Injury: Moderate–Severe

Linda E. Krach MD

Description

Traumatic brain injury (TBI) is the major cause of death and disability in children greater than 1 year of age. Moderate to severe TBI is defined by Glasgow Coma Score (≤ 8 = severe injury, 9–11 = moderate) and duration of unconsciousness (>24 hours = severe, 1–23 hours = moderate).

Etiology

- Cause of injury varies with age
- Motor vehicle related: 66% in adolescents, 20% in young children
- Falls most common cause of injury under age 4, 39% of cases under age 14
- Nonaccidental trauma responsible for majority of severe TBI under age 4
- Sport: more frequently associated with mild injury

Epidemiology

- Males more likely to sustain injury than females, 1.5:1
- In 2004, a report stated that in,
  - Ages 0 to 4: TBI resulted in 216,000 emergency department visits, 18,000 hospitalizations, and 1035 deaths
  - Ages 5 to 14:188,000 emergency department visits, 24,000 hospitalizations, and 1250 deaths
  - Ages 15 to 17: the incidence of hospitalization for TBI has been reported to be 125 per 100,000 children per year
- Commonly associated with other injuries

Pathophysiology

- Primary injury due to impact, rotational, and deceleration forces influenced in children by the following factors:
  - Relatively large head and small, weak neck
  - Incomplete myelinization
  - High brain water content
  - Children less likely than adults to have extra axial hematomas
  - Diffuse axonal injury
- Secondary injury can be caused by hypotension, hypoxia, vasospasm, infarction, prolonged seizure activity, and diffuse edema resulting in increased intracranial pressure and a decrease in cerebral perfusion pressure
- Cascades of biochemical events initiated by cellular power failure, acidosis, overstimulation of excitatory neurotransmitter receptors, lipid membrane peroxidation, increase in intracellular calcium, and cellular damage by free radicals contribute to both primary and secondary injury
- Children more likely than adults to develop diffuse edema
- Second impact syndrome
  - Severe brain swelling after potentially mild brain injury while individual still symptomatic (perhaps subclinically) from prior concussion
- Penetrating injury usually results in focal, not diffuse injury

Risk Factors

- Attention deficit hyperactivity disorder
- Minority status
- Male

Clinical Features

- At least transient alteration in level of consciousness
- Impaired cognition, memory, and executive functioning
- Impaired motor skills, including balance, coordination, and response speed
- Specifics depend on location of focal injury and/or diffuse injury

Natural History

- Acute moderate to severe TBI requires neurosurgical and pediatric intensivist management
- Frequent assessment necessary to monitor status and determine readiness for rehabilitation intervention
- Plasticity may contribute to poorer prognosis of very young children if it results in the younger brain being more likely to increase apoptosis (programmed cell death), because this is a normal part of brain development, normally providing an advantage during the life cycle
- TBI during childhood interrupts normal development and full consequences might not be apparent until years later

Diagnosis

Differential diagnosis

- Typically evident from history of trauma and acute presentation
- Consider possibility of concomitant hypoxic injury

History

- History of trauma and acute presentation
- Decreased function and mobility
- At least transient alteration of consciousness
- Impaired cognition and/or motor function

Exam

- Variable, depending on the severity of injury, from mild impairment of cognition to unconsciousness. Typical areas of dysfunction include the following:
  - Cognitive: Attention, memory, problem solving, orientation, thought organization, executive function, and communication impairment
  - Motor: Balance, coordination, response speed, and motor tone abnormality
  - Behavior: Impulsivity and emotional lability
- Evaluate for concomitant spinal cord or other injury

Testing

- Neuroimaging
  - Acutely-computed tomography to evaluate for potential neurosurgical need, MRI more sensitive to parenchymal damage and to facilitate long-term prognostication
- Electroencephalogram if clinically indicated
- Consider assessment for associated conditions
  - Neuroendocrine malfunction
  - Hearing or visual impairment
  - Oral motor dysfunction
  - Heterotopic ossification
  - Spasticity
- Multidisciplinary team evaluation
  - Specifics of testing depend upon child's age/developmental status
  - Assess severity of injury—Glasgow Coma Score, Duration of posttraumatic amnesia, Children's Orientation and Amnesia Test
  - Behavior Rating Inventory of Executive Function (BRIEF)

Pitfalls

- Continued use of prophylactic anticonvulsants can cloud cognitive function. Early seizures are not predictive of late seizures in children. Anticonvulsant prophylaxis has not been shown to be helpful in the prevention of epilepsy

- TBI in very young children interrupts their development and can have greater consequences than similar injury in older children

Red Flags

- Deterioration in function after condition stabilized or improvement noted
- Central autonomic dysfunction associated with poor prognosis

Treatment

Medical

- Comprehensive multidisciplinary inpatient rehabilitation
- Monitor nutritional status and supplement as necessary
- Monitor/treat sleep disorders as necessary
- Seizure prophylaxis not recommended
  - Posttraumatic epilepsy defined as two or more seizures post TBI
  - When treatment of seizures needed, use medications with least potential cognitive side effects
- Heterotopic ossification
  - More common in older children
    ○ Signs and symptoms
    ○ Decreased range of motion, pain, warmth, swelling
    ○ Treatment—NSAID, range of motion, no surgical intervention until bone matures

Exercises

- Customized for the child's individual presentation and needs

Modalities

- May use electrical stimulation to assist with strengthening focal weakness

Injection

- Injection of botulinum toxin and/or phenol may be helpful in the management of focal hypertonicity

Surgical

- Numerous neurosurgical procedures may be indicated, including intracranial pressure monitor, craniotomy, evacuation of bleed, and shunt
- Postpone surgical intervention for eye muscle imbalance until at least 1 year post injury
- Postpone orthopaedic intervention for fixed contractures until other interventions are exhausted
- May need gastrostomy tube placement for nutritional support

Consults

- Neurosurgery

Potential complications

- Early intervention to prevent complications of immobility
- Heterotopic ossification
- Contracture and ischemic ulcer

Prognosis

- Depends upon the severity of initial injury
- Relates to Glasgow Coma Scale, duration of unconsciousness, and duration of posttraumatic amnesia
- Improvement can continue for months after injury

Helpful Hints

- Differentiate between loss of brain volume due to scarring and hydrocephalus, which is typically accompanied by clinical deterioration and requires neurosurgical intervention

Suggested Readings

Krach LE, Gormley ME, Ward M. Traumatic brain injury. In: Alexander MA, Matthews D, eds. *Pediatric Rehabilitation: Principles and Practice.* 4th ed. New York, NY: Demos Medical Publishing; 2010. 231–260.

MacGregor DL, Kulkarni AV, Dirks PB, Rumney P, eds. *Head Injury in Children and Adolescents. 2007 International Review of Child Neurology Series.* London, UK: MacKeith Press.

Visual Deficits

Michelle A. Miller MD

Description
Visual impairments are deficits in visual acuity, visual-motor skills, visual fields, visual-perceptual skills, or central processing of visual information.

Etiology/Types
- May result from central or peripheral nerve injury or disease
- May result from direct trauma to the eye

Epidemiology
- Worldwide, with incidence and prevalence related to the underlying trauma or disease process
- Amblyopia, the functional reduction of visual acuity from disuse during visual development, affects 1.6% to 3.6% of both boys and girls

Pathogenesis
- Trauma may result in direct injury to the globe, optic nerve, cranial nerves (III, IV, VI, VII), optic chiasm, tracts, radiations, or cortex
- Cranial nerve injuries result in oculomotor deficits or deficits in control of the eyelid and tearing
- Injuries along the chiasm, tracts or radiations result in visual field cuts
- Visual impairments in cerebral palsy may be due to retinopathy of prematurity, hypoxia with resultant cortical blindness, or tract/radiation injury associated with hemiparesis and a resultant homonymous hemianopsia
- Increased intracranial pressure in a number of disease processes may lead to vision loss
- Direct infection of the eye with cytomegalovirus retinitis

Natural History
- Most cranial nerve injuries as a result of trauma resolve within 6 months. The reminder will likely need surgical intervention for improved function
- Without treatment, hydrocephalus, normal pressure hydrocephalus, and infection can lead to permanent blindness

Diagnosis

Differential diagnosis
- TBI
- Brain tumor

History
- History of prematurity, maternal infection with TORCH (toxoplasmosis, rubella, cytomegalovirus, herpes simplex virus, and others), direct trauma to the eye, face, or head
- Declines in spelling, reading, and reading comprehension
- Bumping into objects or difficulty localizing objects
- Complaints of double and/or skewed vision

Exam
- Strabismus
- Visual acuity and assessment of color discrimination (may be impaired)
- Extra ocular movements are restricted or facial weakness noted
- Inability to open eyelid
- Drawing a picture using only a part of the paper or only partially copying a picture presented to them

Testing
- Ophthalmologic exam
- Visual evoked responses
- Head CT

Pitfalls
- Patient cooperation makes testing difficult

Red Flags
- Rapid deterioration or change in vision

Treatment
Medical
- Treat the underlying cause if possible
- Start anticoagulation therapy if appropriate
- Lubrication for eye if appropriate

Exercises
- Exercise extra ocular muscles, "pencil pushups" for visual-motor deficits

Surgery

- Tarsorrhaphy for incomplete closure of eyelid to prevent ulcerations
- Corrective surgery to balance eye musculature
- Ventriculoperitoneal shunt to manage hydrocephalus

Adaptive equipment

- Corrective lenses for acuity and/or astigmatism
- Magnifying glasses
- Prism glasses for field cuts, including Fresnel lenses
- Occlusive dressing (patch)
- Cane or laser cane for navigating environment
- Assistance dog or other animal

Consults

- Ophthalmology/neurophthalmology
- Optometry
- School vision specialist
- Orientation and mobility instructor
- Occupational therapist/rehabilitation teacher
- Communication/computer specialist for Braille

Complications of treatment

- Prism lenses may cause headaches and some children are unable to adjust to them
- Patching without alternation may lead to amblyopia
- Patching results in monocular vision

Prognosis

- Highly variable, depending on cause
- Early treatment for visual-motor deficits has a good prognosis for recovery

Helpful Hints

- Watch functional behavior such as walking, reading, and drawing/writing to help determine a field cut
- Treat astigmatism/amblyopia early and aggressively

Suggested Readings

Guzzetta A, Mercurio E, Cioni G. Visual disorders in children with brain lesions: visual impairment associated with cerebral palsy. *Eur J Paed Neurol.* 2001;5:115-119.

Khetpal V, Donahue S. Cortical visual impairment: etiology, associated findings and prognosis in a tertiary care setting. *J AAPOS.* 2007;11:235-239.

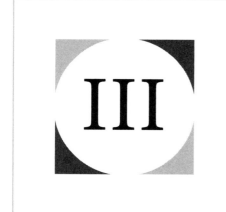

Special Issues

Aging with an Early-Onset Disability

Margaret Turk MD

Description

Typical aging, the last component of the developmental process, involves a natural physiologic decline. Aging with an early-onset disability includes not only typical aging but possibly an accelerated decrease in motor performance and pathologic aging. Some conditions and disabilities have possible later onset medical and health conditions that are disability specific and require vigilance. Secondary health conditions may be seen across disabilities (e.g., pain, fatigue, depression) and require recognition and management. There are also typical health conditions that are commonly seen in an aging population (e.g., hypertension, diabetes), and monitoring and prevention should ensue.

Etiology/Types

- Health concerns and interventions: age-related changes are affected by:
  - Age of onset of disability in relation to developmental maturity (congenital onset vs. adolescent onset)
  - Number of years spent with a disability (hemiparesis noted at birth vs. onset age 17 years)
  - Cumulative effects of medications or treatments (long-term steroid use in Duchenne muscular dystrophy)
  - Era of disability onset (cerebral palsy onset in 1950s vs. 1990s, including different treatments, opportunities, and attitudes)
- Pathologic aging may include seemingly accelerated loss of motor performance
- Pain is a common health condition, no matter what the underlying condition is; common etiologies may be musculoskeletal or neurologic and require evaluation
- There are disability condition-specific health issues that must be monitored

Epidemiology

- Less than 10% of adults with disabilities report onset before the age of 20 years
- About 500,000 children and youth with special health care needs turn 18 years annually

- There are no national surveillance programs that monitor the trajectory of aging with a disability by specific disability condition, by severity, or by age of onset

Health system

- In general, increasing health problems with aging and mortality is related to severity of disability and increased number of existing health impairments
- Health promotion and prevention activities often are not offered to people with disabilities; in particular sexual counseling and medical care are ignored

Pathogenesis

- Fatigue is a common complaint of people with disabilities—the underlying pathology is not clear, but capacity for performance, central etiologies, biomechanical inefficiencies, and inflammation have all been implicated. There can be a pain-fatigue complex, as described in adults with CP
- Typical aging includes gradual decline in strength, endurance, and motor performance if there is no ongoing exercise or activity program. In general, there is poor participation in exercise and activity by children and adults with disabilities. Inactivity may be the foundation of injury, pain, or change in function and skills
- Musculoskeletal pain has been attributed to underlying weakness, spasticity, malalignment, deformities, poor biomechanics, repetitive activities, arthritis, unwitnessed injuries, and fractures
- Neurogenic pain can be caused by entrapment, radiculopathy, stenosis, and tethering
- Overweight and obesity are common with aging, often because of poor nutrition choices, limited activity, or the balance between them. Increased weight may lead to change in biomechanics, poor endurance, and can result in musculoskeletal pain complaints
- Significant change in motor performance can be associated with:
  - Spinal stenosis
  - Tethering
  - Syrinx
  - Other developmental abnormalities
  - Fractures

- Osteoporosis, called secondary osteoporosis, should be expected in children and adults with a history of limited weight bearing and weakness; it is unclear if osteoporosis increases or changes with age or menopause
- Mental health issues may have been present in childhood. Depression may increase with increasing isolation and lack of organized activities for adults
- Conditions with multiple organ system involvement require monitoring of those systems:
  - Spina bifida and/or spinal cord injury: GU, GI, Chiari/hydrocephalus, pressure ulcers, autonomic dysreflexia, lymphedema, latex allergy
- Cerebral palsy: GU, GI, pulmonary, seizures, oral health
- Down syndrome: Endocrine, cognition, GI, hearing, cardiovascular
- Intellectual disability: Cardiovascular, pulmonary, seizures, oral health

Risk Factors for Pathologic Aging

- Severity of disability and existing associated or additional medical conditions
- Type of cerebral palsy
- ASIA score, including motor/sensory level (see Rating Scales chapter)
- Presence of Chiari malformation, other spinal deformity, or instability

Clinical Features of Pathologic Aging

- Progressive loss of skills, weakness, or deconditioning
- Progressive pain complaints
- Refusal to participate in prior typical activities
- Significant increase in or new onset of spasticity
- Decline in bladder or bowel control
- Increased need for assistance and change in living arrangement
- Tetraplegia, which is a decline from previous exams and functional status

Natural History

- Typical aging for adults with early onset disabilities includes gradual decline in strength, flexibility, and endurance without routine exercise and activity. This often results in a modest decline in function into middle age
- Pain complaints can begin as early as late teens and early 20s
- For CP, GMFCS levels III–V are at risk for decline after age 8 years and within adolescence and early

adulthood, while GMFCS levels I and II are fairly stable. The GMFCS level at around age 12 is highly predictive of motor function in adulthood. On average, functional abilities at age 25 years should be maintained for at least another 15 years
- Many adults with motor impairments choose to use a wheelchair or power mobility for energy conservation
- In general, most adults with childhood onset disabilities are healthy. Those with more severe impairments or additional health conditions usually have more difficulties and ill health

Diagnosis

Differential diagnosis for significant loss of function
- Stenosis
- Tethering
- Syrinx
- Chiari compression
- Unknown anatomic developmental abnormality

History
- Decline in function or performance: though progressive weakness, sensory changes, or spasticity are often difficult to elicit
- Pain complaints, limiting activities
- Change in bladder/bowel habits
- May note change in swallowing or eating

Exam
- Comparison to previous exams is most helpful
- May note new or unexpected upper or lower motor neuron signs
- Evaluation involving activity usually best identifies areas of weakness or pain
- Examine using typical challenge tests for musculoskeletal pathologies, although manual muscle test is usually not as helpful with underlying spasticity

Testing
- Plain x-rays can identify areas of degenerative joint disease
- MRI is required when spinal compression is considered, and anesthesia or sedation may be needed. CT myelogram may be desirable if there has been instrumentation near the area of question
- Electrodiagnosis can often help identify lower motor neuron pathology or peripheral entrapments. Be aware of existing underlying neuropathies, based on peripheral vascular status

Section III: Special Issues

Pitfalls

- The expectation that all changes in function are because of the existing disability and aging, and not due to pathology, therefore not proceeding with further evaluation

Red Flags

- Progressive loss of function
- Change in neurologic exam
- Change in urinary function

Treatment

Medical

- Spinal compression pathologies usually are not amenable to medical management
- Typical nonsteroidal anti-inflammatory medications, analgesics, or anti-seizure medications may be helpful for pain control
- Spasticity management with medications, botulinum toxin or phenol injections, or intrathecal baclofen can be considered
- Adjustment to orthoses, wheelchairs, assistive devices, or the environment can improve function and pain management

Exercises

- Strengthening
- Flexibility
- Aerobics
- Aquatics
- Routine exercise programs: monitor function, maintain performance, and manage pain

Modalities

- Heat
- Ice
- Ultrasound
- Transcutaneous electrical nerve stimulation
- Neuromuscular electrical stimulation
- Kiniseotaping
- Body weight support

Injection

- Botulinum toxin or phenol injections for spasticity management
- Trigger point injections
- Joint or bursal injections
- Epidural injections for symptoms related to radiculitis or stenosis

Surgical

- Decompression
- Fusion for multilevel involvement or listhesis
- Intrathecal balcofen pump for spasticity
- Consider an inpatient rehabilitation admission post-procedure to assure mobilization and return to a higher level of performance

Consults

- Neurosurgery or orthopedic-spine surgery

Complications of treatment

- Progressive loss of function

Prognosis

- Highly variable

Suggested Readings

Kemp BJ, Mosqueda L, eds. *Aging with a Disability: What the Clinician Needs to Know.* Baltimore: The Johns Hopkins University Press; 2004.

O'Brien G, Rosenbloom L, eds. *Developmental Disability and Ageing.* London: MacKeith Press; 2009.

Turk MA, Logan LR, Kanter D. Aging with pediatric onset disability and diseases. In: Alexander MA, Matthews DJ, eds. *Pediatric Rehabilitation: Principles and Practice.* New York: Demos Medical Publishing; 2009.

Benign Mechanical Back Pain of Childhood

Kevin P. Murphy MD

Description

Back pain which is focal, activity related, improved with conservative care (CC), rest, activity limits, ice, massage, core strengthening, NSAIDs.

Etiology/Pathogenesis

- Macro- and microtrauma to the immature musculoskeletal system

Epidemiology

- Up to 20% of youth (younger than age 15) have experienced back pain at some point in their young life
- Up to 74% of school backpackers. More common with heavy backpack (>10%–20% body weight), female gender, large BMI, single shoulder strap

Risk Factors

- Obesity
- Positive family history
- Deconditioning or inactivity
- Poorly supervised and equipped recreational activity

Clinical Features

- Focal segmental pain on palpation, postural adjustments or with mechanical stress or strain. Associated with a particular time and event. Neurologically intact

Natural History

- Improvement over 2 to 4 weeks with CC

Diagnosis

Differential diagnosis

- *Fibromyalgia*: Myofascial pain, diffuse. Sleep disturbance, headaches, fatigue, problematic relationships, obesity, deconditioning associated. Polysomnography often positive. Cultural and familial traits often present (female > male). Treat with CC, low-impact aerobics, education, counseling, weight management

- *Spondylolysis*: From repetitive spinal hyperextension. Only one newborn reported with condition. Incidence in general population ≈5% by age 7. L5/S1 midline pain, worse with hyperextension/axial loading; beltline radiation. Treat with CC; bracing and segmental fusion in more severe cases (unrelenting symptoms often with spondylolisthesis)
- Radiculopathy, discogenic pain/slipped vertebral epiphysis, iliac apophysitis, "kissing" spinous processes, spinal dysraphism/stenosis, transitional vertebrae, other discogenic
- *Typical Scheurermann's disease*. Repetitive microtrauma to immature fatigued adolescent thoracic vertebral bodies. Familial traits noted. Incidence in general population (0.5%–8%). Adolescent mid-thoracic pain/kyphosis; subacute to chronic onset; worse with axial loading/heavy activity. Treat with CC; bracing; surgery in more severe cases (thoracic kyphosis > 75°)
- *Atypical Scheurermann's disease*. Thoracolumbar apophysitis not meeting usual criteria
- *Congenital decompensating kyphosis*
- *Discitis*: Aseptic (viral/disc degeneration) versus septic (*Staphylococcus aureus*); rare; high fever, leukocytosis, cultures may be positive. Refusal to sit/stand; constipation; ileus. Biopsy may be necessary. Treat with hospitalization, IV hydration, anti-inflammatories/antimicrobials (vancomycin)
- *Vertebral osteomyelitis* (anterior spinal elements with/without paravertebral collections); Pott's disease(tuberculosis)
- *Child abuse*: Soft tissue injuries more common than fractures; posterior rib/spinous process fractures in up to 30%. Skeletal survey helpful; multiple injuries/multiple healing stages
- *Referred pain*: Pyelonephritis, pneumonia, endocarditis, choleocystitis, nephrolithiasis, pancreatitis, mega colon, constipation/ileus, hiatal hernia/reflux
- Other: Psychogenic, juvenile arthritis, renal osteodystrophy, pelvic inflammatory disease,

pregnancy, trauma, osteoporsis with compression fractures, ankylosing spondylitis, sickle cell crisis

History
- Activity related

Exam
- Focal segmental pain
- Neurologically intact

Testing
- A clinical diagnosis. If not improving with 2 to 3 weeks of CC then all other causes need to be ruled out. Further evaluation includes plain radiographs (e.g., thoracic, Scheurermann's disease with three or more anterior wedge vertebral bodies greater than 5°, irregular vertebral end plates/Schmorl nodes), lumbar with obliques (e.g., spondylolysis with fracture of pars interarticularis and classic "scotty dog" sign, unilateral or bilateral), CBC/chemistry panels, inflammatory markers (ESR, CRP, Lyme, RF, ANA, etc.), bone scan and MRI (e.g., discitis with inflammation of the disc space involving vertebral bodies, one level above and below). CT (bone tumors/fractures)

Pitfalls

Benign spinal tumors
- *Osteoid osteoma*: Intense focal nighttime pain; not activity related. Almost "always" relieved by aspirin/NSAIA. Painful scoliosis associated. Bone scan shows early lesion before CT/radiographs. Spinal nidus usually in posterior elements. Treat with surgical excision versus CT-guided radiofrequency ablation
- *Osteoblastoma*: Bone scan identifies; CT with intralesional stipple ossifications; surgical excision. Common in pelvis
- *Eosinophylic granuloma*: Associated Hand-Schuller-Christian (bone lesion, exophthalmus, diabetes insipidus) and Letter-Siwe disease (malignant histiocytosis x). Self-healing with no treatment possible
- *Aneurysmal bone cyst*: Posterior spinal elements; may extend to vertebral body/rib; common in pelvis. Often not found until nerve root/cord compression; Treat

with surgical resection; possible segmental fusion; CT with cystic fluid level
- *Fibrous dysplasia*: Endocrinopathies associated; café au lait spots; diabetes, hyperthyroidism, precocious puberty; McCuene-Albright syndrome. Common in pelvis

Red Flags

Malignant spinal tumors
- *Ewing's sarcoma*: Codman triangle (triangular area of subperiosteal bone created when a lesion raises the periosteum from bone; generally caused by a tumor or subperiosteal abscess), "onion skin appearance"; MRI diagnostic; surgery, chemotherapy, radiation
- *Osteogenic sarcoma*: Codman triangle, "sunburst" pattern; MRI diagnostic; wide surgical excision, chemotherapy
- *Metastatic*: 90% of malignant spinal tumors are secondary not primary sites. Neuroblastoma. Wilm's tumor (hemihypertrophy associated). Spinal cord tumors. Leukemia/lymphoma

Treatment
- CC; better equipment, facilities, training/coaching, low-impact aerobics, postural adjustments, attitudinal encouragement

Modalities
- Superficial heat/cold
- Avoid ultrasound over open physes

Injections
- Generally not utilized < age 12

Prognosis
- Excellent

Helpful Hints
- Mom is usually correct and not to be taken lightly

Suggested Readings
Abel MF. *Orthopedic Knowledge Update*. Rosemont, IL: American Academy of Orthopedic Surgeons; 2006.
Staheli LT. *Fundamentals of Pediatric Orthopedics*, 4th ed. Philadelphia: Lippincott, Williams and Wilkins; 2008.

Bladder Management

Ed Wright MD

Definition and Etiology of Neurogenic Bladder

Bladder or sphincter, motor or sensory dysfunction caused by a lesion in the brain, spinal cord, or the peripheral nervous system.

Spinal cord pathology results in the majority of bladder sphincter dysfunction. Spinal dysraphism, most often mylelomeningocele, is by far the most common and well-studied cause of pediatric neurogenic bladder. Sacral agenesis and causes of tethered cord such as lipomeningocele and spinal bifida occulta are other congenital causes. Acquired spinal cord conditions, including trauma as well as vascular insults, tumor, and transverse myelitis, make up the remainder of spinal cord-related bladder sphincter dysfunction. Brain origins of a less destructive and compromising form of neurogenic bladder include cerebral palsy, stroke, and tumors. Brainstem lesions, below the pontine micturition center, have findings more consistent with spinal cord rather than brain pathology.

Normal Bladder Function and Measurement in Children

A healthy bladder stores and empties in a synergistic pattern and grows over time. Storage requires a compliant, relaxed detrusor and a competent bladder outlet. The bladder outlet is composed of the smooth muscle extension of the bladder neck, known as the internal sphincter and a continuously firing striated external sphincter. Normal emptying results from a completely contractile detrusor coordinated with a quiescent urethral sphincter.

Expected bladder capacity is predicted by the equations:

$$2 \times \text{age (years)} + 2 = \text{capacity (ounces) for children less than 2}$$
$$\text{Age (years)}/2 + 6 = \text{capacity (ounces) for children 2 and older}$$

Urodynamics Normal Parameters

Leak point pressure (LPP): the pressure at which urine leaks around a urethral catheter: <40 cm H_2O

Detrusor filling pressure: <40 cm H_2O

Bladder pressure change with filling: < 10–15cm H_2O

Normal voiding pressure: boys: 50–80 cm H_2O, girls: 40–65 cm H_2O

Briefly, urodynamics (UDS) are performed with a triple lumen catheter in the bladder. One opening remains at the highest point of urethral resistance as the site of LPP measurement. A second is within the vesicle to measure filling and emptying pressures. The third is used for filling the bladder. A second catheter is inserted in the rectum to measure abdominal pressure artifact. Simultaneous, needle electromyography recordings of the sphincter detects denervation, overactivity, and the synergy pattern with the detrusor. Optional video cystography provides details of bladder configuration and ureteral competence.

Uropathology of Bladder Sphincter Dysfunction

Studies of children with myelomeningocele have provided us our greatest understanding of developmental bladder pathology and its sequelae. Disordered innervation of the bladder and sphincter (usually striated sphincter) results in one of four functional bladder types. The presence of simultaneous contraction of the detrusor and sphincter, called detrusor/sphincter dyssynergia (DSD), is the least safe bladder type, creating risks of bladder hypertrophy, ureter dilatation, and eventually, kidney infection and scarring.

Evaluation of Bladder Sphincter Dysfunction

Myelomeningocele

Goals of evaluation and treatment are (1) early detection and treatment of a high-pressure system, (2) continence by school age, and (3) independence. Upper tract deterioration begins early when there is untreated DSD, an elevated leak point, or an elevated filling pressure. Therefore, to achieve the first goal newborn investigation, beginning after spinal closure, includes urinalysis, ultrasound (US) of the urinary tract, post void/leak residual catheterization measurement, and, in most centers UDS. Voiding cystography is obtained if there is evidence of high detrusor pressures or reflux. If there is evidence of

239

Types of Bladder Sphincter Dysfunction

Detrusor/sphincter activity	Impact on storage	Impact on emptying	Clinical sequelae if untreated
Detrusor ++/Sphincter ++ (DSD)	Low capacity, high pressure	Incomplete, high pressure	Frequency, small volumes, incontinent voids, UTI's, detrussor hypertrophy, reflux, and upper tract damage
Detrusor ++/Sphincter −−	Low capacity	Complete	Frequent, incontinent voids. Eventual detrusor hypertrophy leads to reflux and upper tract damage.
Detrusor −−/Sphincter ++	Excessive compliance	Retention with overflow leakage	Overflow incontinence, further detrusor decompensation, UTI's, and reflux
Detrusor −−/Sphincter −−	Low capacity	Constant leak	Incontinent voids and UTI's

a high-pressure system, treatment is initiated. The extent and frequency of follow up evaluation is dependent upon age, bladder type, and interval infections but generally is 3 to 4 times per year in the first year of life. Frequency of follow-up can decline with age and stability. There are continuous risks for deterioration of the voiding pattern with the development of a tethered cord. This can occur with growth, spine surgery for kyphoscoliosis, and with weight gain. UDS data provides an objective measure of changes in spinal cord function and should be continued regularly into adulthood.

Acquired spinal cord lesions

Children with spinal cord injury require a different path to evaluation and treatment. Typically they have experienced normal bladder function and growth prior to their injury. There urologic investigation should begin only after they emerge from spinal shock. As a result they will have begun symptomatic treatment prior to formal urologic assessment. A baseline US should be obtained at or around discharge from rehabilitation and UDS should occur no earlier than 6 weeks. Changes in detrusor sphincter dynamics can occur for up to 2 years following injury so physiatric assessment should include ongoing voiding histories with a focus on infections, changes in continence, frequency, and post void residuals. Ultrasound and UDS should occur at least annually until bladder sphincter function is clearly stable and safe. Annual US should continue to adulthood with UDS every 2 years. Similar to tethering in spinal dysraphism, posttraumatic syringomyelia and spine surgery for scoliosis present the possibility of late changes in bladder function for children with acquired spinal cord lesions.

Cerebral origin detrusor dysfunction

This is best characterized as detrusor overactivity and results in urgency with or without incontinence. Continence can be delayed or unobtainable and is multifactorial. It is influenced by overall development, degree of cognitive, communicative, and mobility impairments, previous treatments, including limb botulinum toxin injections, or rhizotomy, and inattention. There is less often true DSD.

Medical management of detrusor sphincter dysfunction

For all spinal cord related uropathology clean intermittent catheterization (CIC) at appropriate intervals allows for low pressure, complete bladder emptying. This reduces both reflux and UTI risks. Anticholinergics, most often oral oxybutinin 0.3 to 0.6 mg/kg/day (max 15 mg), reduce detrusor tone during filling and emptying. This facilitates continence, reduces DSD, reflux risks and detrusor hypertrophy. Intravesical instillation of oxybutinin 0.3 to 0.9 mg/kg/day during CIC is used when oral dosing is inadequate or produces side effects. Combining CIC with oxybutinin allows the vast majority of children with spinal cord related detrusor sphincter dysfunction to achieve safe detrusor pressures and eventual continence. Fluid intake, bladder capacity and pressures influence CIC frequency which, in practice, varies from 6/day in infants to 5/day in school age children with myelomeningocele. Depending on bladder capacity and pressures children with acquired injuries may perform CIC less frequently. Botulinum toxin injection with up to 300 Units can be injected into the bladder every 6 to 9 months as an alternative method of detrusor relaxation.

Proper training in technique for complete bladder emptying and compliance are important to infection prevention. Reused supplies are not related to more UTI's. Other efforts at UTI prophylaxis include urine acidification, saline bladder rinses, and oral (Septra 2 mg/kg/day) chemoprophylaxis.

Independent intermittent catheterization can be considered at 6 to 9 years for a child with good dexterity and a supportive environment. If continence is a challenge between CIC, children with low sphincter tone deserve a trial of an alpha agonist, such as ephedrine, to enhance internal sphincter resistance. Crede voiding (a method of pushing the hand over the bladder to attempt to empty it) is not efficacious even in those with absent sphincter tone as it does not provide reliable emptying. Regular bowel evacuation is an important element of bladder function since impaction can alter bladder filling and emptying. Soiling can increase the risk of UTI.

Detrusor dysfunction in cerebral injury is primarily an issue of urgency and incontinence with little risk of UTI or pressure related uropathology. Judicious use of anticholinergics to avoid urinary retention is appropriate.

Surgical Management of Detrusor Sphincter Dysfunction

For spinal cord-related uropathology surgical procedures exist to: (1) increase bladder outlet resistance, (2) improve ease of catheterization, and (3) enhance bladder capacity and reduce pressures.

For bladder neck incompetence, outlet resistance can be achieved temporarily by injection of various bulking agents, or addressed more permanently through various sling suspension techniques or implantation of an artificial urinary sphincter. The bladder neck can also be obliterated in favor of creating a continent catheterizable stoma. Continent stomas for CIC can be used for children with normal bladder capacity who need easier catheterization access. Cutaneous appendicovesicostomy (Mitrofanoff) or ileal tube (Monti) procedures are commonly used stomas. They can be positioned either in the midline (umbilical) or the right lower quadrant. As these stomas are typically competent, CIC compliance is required to prevent excessive detrusor pressures. When bladder capacity is inadequate, augmentation procedures include ileum or colon cystoplasty; in which the bowel segment is detubulated, left attached to its mesenteric vascular supply, and reshaped to form a cup to cover an opened detrusor.

Suggested Readings

Bauer SB. Neurogenic bladder: etiology and assessment. *Pediatr Nephrol.* 2008;23:541–551.

deJong TPVM, Chrzan R, Klijn AJ, Dik P. Treatment of the neurogenic bladder in spina bifida. *Pediatr Nephrol.* 2008;23:889–896.

Kaefer M, Zurakowski D, Bauer SB, et al. Estimating normal bladder capacity in children. *J Urol.* 1997;158:2261–2264.

McGuire EJ, Woodside JR, Bordin TA, Weiss RM. Prognostic value of urodynamic testing in myelodysplastic patients. *J Urol.* 1981;136:205–209.

Stephenson TP, Wein AJ. The interpretation of urodynamics. In: Mundy AR, Stephenson TP, Wein A, eds. *Urodynamics: Principles, Practice and Application.* Edinburgh: Churchill Livingstone; 1986.

Verpoorten C, Buyse GM. The neurogenic bladder: medical treatment. *Pediatr Nephrol.* 2008;23:717–725.

Bowel Management

Maureen R. Nelson MD

Bowel continence is important for physical and social health. When children begin school 91% to 94% will be continent. Those who are not continent of bowel might have a problem due to neurogenic bowel or other anatomical etiologies, but do not usually. About 95% of the children who have incontinence have no physiologic, neurologic, or other bowel problem. Fecal incontinence is commonly related to delayed toilet training. Children with neurodevelopmental disorders are more likely than other children to have constipation and delayed bowel training. The most common cause for incontinence in childhood is retention or constipation.

Anatomy and Physiology

The autonomic nerves control the colon, rectum, and internal anal sphincter. The parasympathetic innervation is from S2-4, the sympathetic innervation is from lower thoracic and lumbar levels, and the voluntary motor and sensory fibers to the external anal sphincter are from S2-4 via the pudendal plexus. The gastrocolic reflex increases peristalsis for about 30 minutes after eating. When the rectum becomes full it initiates relaxation of the internal anal sphincter. The external anal sphincter contracts and other nearby voluntary muscles may assist. When it is socially convenient, the external sphincter may relax and defecation occurs.

Bowel Management

The goal of bowel management is a daily bowel movement in a manner that is socially continent. The approach to good bowel management includes drinking plenty of fluids, and eating fruits, vegetables, and other sources of fiber. An osmotic laxative may be helpful. Timing of 30 minutes after the evening meal to sit on the commode is frequently helpful. If there is significant constipation, it should be cleaned out before beginning the regular bowel program.

In neurogenic bowel, osmotic laxative and high-fiber diets are used, along with digital rectal stimulation and/or suppository. A stool softener and stimulant are generally used. An enema may be needed initially to clean out the bowels. It is important to get to the commode since sitting upright allows gravity to assist with emptying and also shortens the length of the colon. In an upper motor neuron injury, there is a spared anal and bulbocavernosus

reflex and digital stimulation may work well alone. This is frequently found in someone with tetraplegia due to SCI. Many lesions are mixed upper and lower neuron. There is also delayed colonic transit time after SCI, and early on there may be an ileus. Some say that suppositories and digital stimulation are ineffective in a person with a lower motor neuron (LMN) lesion with a flaccid sphincter and recommend a manual evacuation in this case. Most children with spina bifida are reported to have LMN bladders, as do children with lower level SCI, and many can have a successful bowel program as suggested above. If it is not effective, some choose to have a surgical intervention.

A malone anterograde continence enema (MACE) is a catheterizable appendicocecostomy, which can be used to flush an enema once or more a week to empty the bowels.

If there is partial or intact bowel sensation present biofeedback may be useful. Anorectal manometry is performed, with sensation determined to be good if a balloon inflated with less than 10 mL of water is felt. The external sphincter can be trained with biofeedback by repeatedly inflating and deflating the balloon. This can improve the voluntary control of the external anal sphincter, and thereby improve bowel continence.

Early after SCI, TBI, or other trauma constipation is extremely common. The injury itself, anesthesia, immobility, and use of large amounts of narcotics have a significant impact. Thickening agents used for liquids can exacerbate the problem. There is commonly a lack of privacy in the hospital so some individuals may suppress having a bowel movement due to inability to comfortably get to a commode.

X-rays of the abdomen are variable for the evaluation of constipation. Transabdominal ultrasound of the rectum is shown to differentiate as it shows enlarged rectal diameter of >3.5 cm in children with constipation compared to 2.1 to 2.4 cm in children without constipation.

The most common cause for incontinence in childhood is retention or constipation. Reducing constipation also improves urinary symptoms. Constipation is defined to be present if, during an 8-week time frame there are at least two of the following: two stools or less per week, incontinence at least once a week, painful or

Bowel Medications

Medication	Effect	Side effects
Bulk-forming		
Psyllium	Absorbs water to promote peristalsis and reduce transit time	Cramps, obstruction, bloating, flatulence
Stool softeners		
Docusate	Allows water and fat to enter stool	Diarrhea, rash, throat irritation
Stimulants		
Senna	Local irritant to colon to increase peristalsis	Nausea, diarrhea, emesis, cramps
Saline laxatives		
Magnesium citrate	Distends colon & increases peristalsis	Diarrhea, hyper Mg, cramping; electrolyte imbalance
Saline enema	Flush distal colon	
Hyperosmolar		
Polyethylene glycol	Catharsis by electrolyte and osmotic effect	Nausea, malaise, dizzy, diarrhea, headache
Glycerin suppository	Local irritant; osmotic dehydrating colon	
Theravac minienema	Locally triggers peristalsis of colon	Diarrhea

hard stools, prolonged postponement, presence of large mass of impaction, or giant stools obstructing the toilet.

Of the children who have incontinence, 95% have no physiologic neurologic or other bowel problem but have functional constipation, the cause of which is likely multifactorial. It is important to do a thorough history and physical to rule out any physiologic etiology. Some children have incontinence simply due to lack of readiness for toilet training. This is more common in children with autism, ADHD, and developmental disorders, as they commonly have more difficulty with attention, fine motor skills, and motivation. The key is to do a bowel clean out, with enemas or medications via mouth, or sometimes medications via nasogastric tube, in an attempt to avoid enemas. Then a behavioral toilet-training program is critical with regular toileting, liquids and fiber in the diet, and sometimes medications.

Secondary or voluntary soiling commonly has a psychologic cause and may be related to a specific event or trigger. Twenty-five percent of children who are abused or neglected have incontinence.

Bowel patterns change with age from an average of three bowel movements daily for neonates to about 1.7 daily at 1 year. Preschoolers vary from three times daily to every other day. There are cultural differences in age at potty training, with age for achieving bowel control worldwide ranging from age 1 to 4 years.

Suggested Readings

Nelson VS, Hornyak JE. Spinal cord injuries. In: Alexander ME, Matthews DJ, eds. *Pediatric Rehabilitation: Principles and Practice*, 4th Ed. New York: Demos; 2010:261-276.

Nijman RJM. Diagnosis and management of urinary incontinence and functional fecal incontinence (encopresis) in children. *Gastroenterol Clin N Am.* 2008;37:731-748.

Palliative Care in Pediatric Rehabilitation Medicine

Rita Ayyangar MBBS

Description

Pediatric Palliative Care(PC) originated from the hospice movement and has evolved into its own specialty. The WHO (1998) defines it as

- Active total care of the child's body, mind and spirit, and also involves giving support to the family.
- Begins when a life-limiting illness is diagnosed, and continues regardless of whether or not a child receives treatment directed at the disease and even when cure remains a distinct possibility.
- Health providers must evaluate and alleviate a child's physical, psychological, and social distress.
- Effective palliative care requires a broad inter-disciplinary approach that includes the family and makes use of available community resources; it can be successfully implemented even if resources are limited.
- It can be provided in tertiary care facilities, in community health centers and schools and even in children's homes.

Categories of Conditions Appropriate for Pediatric Palliative Care (also called ACT/RCPCH categories)

- Helps with communication with parent about expected course and other care providers re: when to consult PC
- Helps with planning for individual patients and families and for resources
- Helps with Research- when to introduce PC, how to alter services based on category, allocation of resources based on your programs category distribution
- Four Categories
1. Conditions for which curative treatment is possible but may fail
   - Advanced or progressive cancer with a poor prognosis
   - Complex and severe congenital or acquired heart disease
2. Conditions where premature death is inevitable; requiring intensive long term treatment to maintain quality of life
   - HIV infection
   - Cystic Fibrosis
3. Progressive conditions in which treatment is exclusively palliative

Metabolic Disorders

- Certain chromosomal abnormalities
- Muscular Dystrophy
4 Conditions involving severe, non-progressive disability, causing extreme vulnerability to health complications

- Severe Cerebral Palsy
- Hypoxic or anoxic brain injury
- Holoprosencephaly or other brain malformations
- Neurologic sequelae of meningitis and other infectious disease

Elements in Approach to Pediatric Palliative Care

Physical concerns
- Identify pain or other symptoms
  - Develop a pharmacologic and non-pharmacologic plan

Psychological concerns
- Identify child and family fears and concerns
- Identify child and family coping and communication styles
- Assess child's prior experiences with dying and traumatic life events, gauge child's understanding of death concept and assess family resources for bereavement support
- Refer to mental health professional as appropriate

Spiritual concerns

■ Review child's hopes, dreams, values, meaning of life, role of religion and prayer
■ Allow time for child and family to reflect on life's meaning and purpose
■ Refer to culturally appropriate spiritual care provider

Advance care planning

■ Identify decision makers
■ Discuss illness trajectory, assess child and family's understanding of prognosis and help determine probable time of death (hours, days, weeks or months) as best as able.
■ Identify goals of care with family and patient and communicate to treatment team
  – Curative, uncertain or primarily comfort care
  – Advanced directives- valid for those over 18 years of age
    ○ Instructive directive e.g. living will
    ○ Proxy directive e.g. durable power of attorney
■ Anticipatory guidance regarding physical changes at time of or near death, treatment plan including who to call, who will manage symptoms, and how.

Practical concerns

■ Establish communication and coordination with health care team
■ Establish child's and family's preference of location of care
■ Address changes in functional abilities, assessing need for equipment
■ Assess financial burden of illness on family and offer assistance through social services or community supports

Barriers to Care

■ Child dying before parent is not natural order, therefore remains emotionally difficult
■ Prognostication for children with very complex problems is extremely challenging
■ Discordance between parent/patient and physician perception of what constitutes good quality of life
■ Ethical, legal and health policy issues pertaining to medical decision making
  ○ Adolescent rights to medical decision making
  ○ Primary health care team may need to advocate for wishes of child and family in context of local and state law

■ Eligibility for hospice care
  ○ Many hospice facilities lack pediatric expertise
  ○ Children with complex medical conditions may require care such as assisted ventilation that is not reimbursable under existing systems of hospice insurance and may need 'bridging' care

Pediatric Habilitation and Rehabilitation is defined as the process of enhancing the acquisition or restoration of skills by a child who was born with or has had an illness or injury causing disability, with the goal of maximizing the physical, functional, emotional and spiritual development of the child.

Goals include:

■ Maximize self sufficiency and function
■ Minimize burden of care and discomfort

Comparing Philosophies

Rehabilitation	Palliative care
Acute and chronic disorders	Life threatening and chronic disorders
Enhance physical, functional, emotional and spiritual development of child	Total care of body, mind and spirit
Minimize burden of care and enhance comfort	Relieve physical and psychological discomfort, and social distress
Directed at child, environment and family, resources	Child, family environment and resources
Interdisciplinary team approach	Interdisciplinary team approach
Prognosis guides focus	Prognosis guides focus

Contrasting the Two

Rehabilitation	Palliative care
Emphasis on function, reducing burden of care	Emphasis on symptom relief, increasing comfort and relieving distress
Geared toward restoration and functional recovery	Geared toward acceptance of poor prognosis
Expertise in disability related issues	Expertise in end of life issues

Section III: Special Issues

Dietz's Four Phases of Cancer Rehabilitation

1. Preventive- Interventions and measures to reduce the impact of anticipated disabilities and maximize physical and psychological functioning and health through exercise, nutrition, counseling and education.
2. Restorative- Interventions and measures aimed at restoring function to premorbid state and is the goal of acute rehabilitation programs. These may include curative or reconstructive surgical and medical treatments, and physical, occupational and speech therapy.
3. Supportive- Includes interventions to reduce secondary disabilities and handicap e.g. use of adaptive devices such as a walker or cane, use of a prosthesis, hand splint etc.
4. Palliative- As the disease progresses focus shifts to symptom relief, pain control, prevention of complications such as bed sores, deterioration due to inactivity and immobility, provision of comfort and psychological support

Deconditioning, fatigue and weakness are common problems in the patient with chronic disease particularly if it is progressive or at end stage as may be seen with various cancers. Rehabilitation goals may need to be adjusted for the different categories of care (ACT/RCPCH). As an example for ACT III category of Progressive conditions in which treatment is exclusively palliative, the rehabilitation strategy would hinge on flexibility. Initially, one would focus on maintaining optimal function thru exercise and energy conservation techniques; then the focus would shift to adaptive equipment and load modification. Secondary impairments e.g. contractures would need to be addressed as the disease progresses and focus on socialization and leisure activities maintained throughout.

As can be seen Palliative Care and Rehabilitation Medicine have many similarities in approaches. The best care for children with chronic conditions then may be one that integrates both palliative care and rehabilitative principles.

These may be applied throughout the continuum of care of an individual beginning at initial presentation, proceeding through diagnosis and disease modification to death; changing emphasis in concordance with the disease state. Rehabilitation may be the primary focus through the preventive and curative phase, with an overlap during the life prolonging phase and a shift in focus to palliative care during the life closure, dying and bereavement periods.

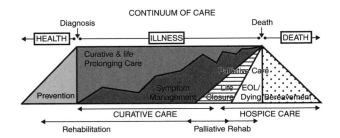

Health to death: Integrating rehabilitative and palliative care.

Suggested Readings

Himelstein, BP, Hilden JM et al: Pediatric Palliative Care. In NEJM 350 (17), April 2004, pp. 1752–1762.

Olson E, Cristian A: The role of rehabilitation medicine and palliative care in the treatment of patients with end-stage disease. In Physical Medicine and Rehabilitation Clinics of North America Volume 16, Issue 1, February 2005, pp. 285–305.

Santago-Palma J, Payne R: Palliative Care and rehabilitation. In Cancer Aug 2001, 92 (4 supplement): 1049–52.

Polytrauma in Pediatric Rehabilitation

Adrienne G. Tilbor DO

Description

Polytrauma is defined as injury to more than one body system, or at least two serious injuries to one body system.

Types

- Traumatic brain injury (TBI)
- Spinal cord injury (SCI)
- Burns
- Orthopedic injuries
- Organ injuries
- Ocular trauma
- Thoracic injuries
- Vascular trauma

Etiology

- Motor vehicle crashes
- Falls
- Violence (penetrating and blunt)
- Nonaccidental trauma
- Sports incidents
- Bicycle crashes
- Recreational vehicle trauma
- Pedestrian trauma
- Child abuse

Epidemiology

- Trauma is the major cause of morbidity and mortality in children and the predominant cause of death in children older than 1 year of age
- Death from unintentional injury accounts for 65% of all injury deaths in those <19 years
- The incidence of multiple trauma among all pediatric trauma admissions is 10%
- Each year, 20,000 children and teenagers die as a result of injury
- The highest incidence of pediatric trauma is in the spring and summer
- A male predilection: 3 to 1
- The average age of children with multiple injuries is <10 years

Pathogenesis

Varies with combination of injuries

Risk Factors

- Lack of helmet use
- Lack of seatbelt and child safety restraints
- Intoxicated motor vehicle drivers
- Unsafe home environment
- Increased handgun use
- Increased proclivity for violence

Clinical Features

- Alteration in mental status, including loss of consciousness
- Fractures
- Paraplegia or tetraplegia
- Burns
- Hemorrhage
- Respiratory distress
- Retinal hemorrhages
- Fever
- Seatbelt sign

Natural History

- Burns more common in ages 1 to 4 years
- Upper limb fractures more common in ages 5 to 9 years
- Lower limb fractures and TBI more common in teens
- SCI is relatively uncommon although cervical spine injury must be considered in small children with severe trauma, especially TBI, due to their relatively large head size which provides a fulcrum that increases risk
- Spinal Cord Injury Without Radiographic Abnormality (SCIWORA) in 10% to 20% of children with SCI
- Thoracic injury occurs in approximately 5% of children hospitalized with trauma
- Blunt abdominal trauma involves renal injury in 10% to 20% of trauma cases
- Most child abuse occurs in children younger than 3 years of age, with one third being younger than 6 months

Diagnosis

Differential diagnosis
- Child abuse
- Unexplained shock
- Acute abdomen

History
- Lethargy, confusion, light headedness
- Weakness or lateralizing neurological findings
- Incontinence or seizures
- Loss of consciousness >1 minute
- Abdominal/thoracic/skeletal pain
- Multiple episodes of emesis
- Headache
- Memory loss
- Behavior disturbance

Exam
- Glasgow Coma Scale
- Unilateral dilated pupil
- ASIA Impairment scale
- Depressed or basilar skull fracture
- Bulging fontanel
- Stridor, pulsatile bleeding, expanding hematoma, cold limb, absent pulse
- Diplopia, corneal abrasions, abnormal red reflex, and ruptured globe in ocular trauma
- Abdominal wall bruising, abrasion, and friction burns

Testing
- CT scan: brain/chest/abdomen/spine/pelvis/face
- EEG
- EKG, chest radiograph
- Blood work to assess organ function and nutritional status
- Magnetic resonance imaging of brain or spine
- Audiologic testing
- Ophthalmologic/neuro-ophthalmologic evaluation
- Videofluoroscopic swallow function study
- Electrodiagnosis: NCS and EMG
- Urodynamic studies
- Neuropsychologic testing

Pitfalls
- Inability to preserve cerebral oxygenation and perfusion is the leading cause of death and the principle determinant of outcome in CNS injury
- Secondary problems such as uncontrolled hypotension and hypoxia cause substantial morbidity

Red Flags
- Cerebral edema
- Low cerebral perfusion pressure and high intracranial pressure
- Poor pupillary response
- Decerebrate or decorticate posturing
- Ventilatory failure

Treatment

Medical
- Pain control
- Early use (first week) of antiepileptic medication for posttraumatic seizure prevention
- Acute treatment for hyperpyrrexia (cooling)
- Manage autonomic dysfunction (tachycardia, diaphoresis, dystonia, fever, hypertension)
- Low air loss beds to prevent pressure ulcers
- DVT prophylaxis or treatment
- Appropriate nutritional supplementation
- Selected medications for treatment of sleep disorder, attention/cognition, pain, anxiety/depression, spasticity/dystonia

Exercises
- Range of motion and strengthening
- Wheelchair mobility
- ADLs, oromotor exercises
- Visuoperceptual activities, exercises balance/coordination

Modalities
- Heat
- Intraoral/orofacial/limb vibration
- Functional electrical stimulation
- Kinesiotaping

Injection
- Botulinum toxin injection
- Motor point blocks with phenol

Surgical
- Neurosurgery for intracranial injury
- General pediatric surgery for gastrostomy tube
- Orthopedic surgery for fractures

Consults
- Neurosurgery
- Orthopedic surgery
- Ophthalmology

- Neurology
- Endocrinology

Complications
- Posthemorrhagic hydrocephalus
- Thyroid dysfunction

Prognosis
- Depends on injuries and effective trauma care from pre-hospital through rehabilitation

Helpful Hints
- May uncover injuries (especially fractures) as child becomes more alert and aware of discomfort

Suggested Readings
Jaffe KM. Pediatric trauma rehabilitation: a value-added safety net. *J Trauma*. 2008;64(3):819-823.

Niedzwecki CM. Traumatic brain injury: a comparison of inpatient functional outcomes between children and adults. *J Head Trauma Rehabil*. 2008;23(4):209-219.

Section III: Special Issues

Sexuality in Children with Disabilities

Nancy A. Murphy MD FAAP FAAPMR

Description of Sexuality

Intimately linked to basic human needs of being accepted, displaying and receiving affection, feeling valued and attractive, and sharing feelings.

- Relates to anatomic and physiologic function, as well as sexual knowledge, beliefs, attitudes, and values
- Extends beyond genital sex to gender-role socialization, physical maturation and body image, social relationships, and future social aspirations

Background

- Teens with disabilities express desires and hopes for marriage, children, and normal adult sex lives
- Teens with disabilities are as sexually experienced as other teens
- Youth with disabilities are often erroneously regarded as child-like and asexual, or inappropriately sexual and with uncontrollable urges
- Society may hinder sexual development more than the disability itself

Sexual Development and Disability

- Ages 0 to 3: Masturbation is normal; teach public versus private behavior
- Toddlers: Teach body parts and "good touch-bad touch"
- Ages 5 to 8: Teach basics of good relationships and social responsibility
- Ages 8 to 11: Emphasize healthy diet, hygiene, good communication, and knowledge of puberty to promote healthy body image
- Adolescence: Address sexual function, contraception, sexually transmitted diseases (STDs), values, intimacy, and love
- Barriers include the lack of age-appropriate peers, lack of privacy, and overprotection

Health Maintenance and Puberty

- Children with disabilities are 20 times more likely to experience early puberty
- Idiopathic precocious puberty affects 1 in 1000 girls overall, but 20% of girls with spina bifida
- Abnormal uterine bleeding during the first 2 years after menarche is usually related to anovulatory bleeding, but may be due to thyroid disease or antiepileptic and neuroleptic medications
- The CDC (Centers for Disease Control and Prevention) recommend the 3-dose series of human papilloma virus (HPV) vaccine for all females aged 11 to 12 years (can be administered after 9 years of age; catch-up vaccination is recommended for females aged 13-26 years who have not been previously vaccinated)
- Menstrual history should include: date of menarche; frequency, duration and quality of menstrual periods; dysmenorrhea
- Pap smears are recommended by 3 years from onset of sexual intercourse or by age 21 years
- Pelvic exams should be modified with frog-leg position, V position, or elevation of the legs without hip abduction to increase comfort and decrease anxiety

Sexual Function and Fertility

- Sympathetic nervous system (T11-L2) regulates psychogenic arousal
- When rectal sensation, anal wink, and bulbocavernosus reflexes are absent, sexual stimulation should target arousal rather than orgasm
- Fertility is generally preserved in females but reduced in males with spina bifida and spinal cord injury
- Women with spina bifida have a 5 in 100 risk of bearing children with neural tube defects; recurrence reduced by 50% to 75% with 4 mg folic acid for ≥3 months before and 1 month after conception
- Genetic counseling is essential to reduce disability recurrence

Contraception

- Antiepileptic drugs can induce hepatic enzymes and decrease effectiveness of estrogen containing contraceptives
- Increased risk of thrombosis with estrogen-progestin containing contraceptives
- Barrier devices contain latex; contraindicated in latex-sensitive persons
- Polyurethane condoms provide less protection against pregnancy and STDs and tend to break during intercourse

- Medroxyprogesterone acetate (depo-provera) injections can minimize or eliminate menstrual flow, but accelerate bone mineral density losses

Sexual Abuse

- Children with disabilities are sexually abused at a rate that is 2.2 times of that for typical children
- Increased vulnerability due to dependence on caregivers, limited social skills, poor judgment, inability to report abuse, and lack of knowledge and strategies to defend themselves
- Recognize subtle changes (bowel or bladder function, appetite, mood, sleep, behavior, participation) that may suggest abuse

Sexuality Education

- Youth with disabilities are entitled to the same sexuality education as their peers, with modifications to promote understanding
- Individualized education plans (IEPs) should include sexuality education: body parts, puberty, personal care and hygiene, medical examinations, social skills, sexual expression, contraception, rights and responsibilities of sexual behavior
- Appropriate education may reduce risk for sexual abuse, pregnancy, and STDs

Helpful Hints

- Children and adolescents with disabilities are sexual persons
- Introduce issues of psychosexual development early and continue regularly
- Promote self-care and social independence
- Advocate for developmentally appropriate sexuality education in home, community, and school settings

Suggested Readings

Alexander MS, Alexander CJ. Recommendations for discussing sexuality after spinal cord injury/dysfunction in children, adolescents, and adults. *J Spinal Cord Med.* 2007;30:S65-S70.

Greydanus DE, Omar HA. Sexuality issues and gynecologic care of adolescents with developmental disabilities. *Pediatr Clin North Am.* 2008;55(6):1315-1335.

Murphy NA, Elias ER. Sexuality of children and adolescents with developmental disabilities. *Pediatrics.* 2006;118(1):398-403.

Index